CLASSICAL
HOMEOPATHY

MEDICAL GUIDES TO
Complementary & Alternative Medicine

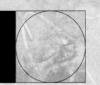

CLASSICAL HOMEOPATHY

MICHAEL CARLSTON, MD, DHt
Assistant Clinical Professor
Department of Family and Community Medicine
University of California—San Francisco
San Francisco, California

Series Editor MARC S. MICOZZI, MD, PhD
Executive Director
The College of Physicians of Philadelphia
Adjunct Professor of Medicine and Rehabilitation Medicine
University of Pennsylvania
Philadelphia, Pennsylvania

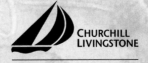

CHURCHILL
LIVINGSTONE

An Imprint of Elsevier Science
New York   Edinburgh   London   Philadelphia

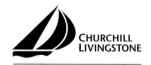

CHURCHILL LIVINGSTONE

An Imprint of Elsevier Science

The Curtis Center
Independence Square West
Philadelphia, Pennsylvania 19106

CLASSICAL HOMEOPATHY   ISBN 0-443-06565-9

NOTICE

Complementary and alternative medicine is an ever-changing field. Standard safety precautions must be followed, but as new research and clinical experience broaden our knowledge, changes in treatment and drug therapy may become necessary or appropriate. Readers are advised to check the most current product information provided by the manufacturer of each drug to be administered to verify the recommended dose, the method and duration of administration, and contraindications. It is the responsibility of the licensed prescriber, relying on experience and knowledge of the patient, to determine dosages and the best treatment for each individual patient. Neither the publisher nor the editors assume any liability for any injury and/or damage to persons or property arising from this publication.

Library of Congress Cataloging in Publication Data
Classical homeopathy / [edited by] Michael Carlston
        p.; cm. – (Medical guides to complementary & alternative medicine)
    Includes bibliographical references and index.
    ISBN 0-443-06565-9
    1. Homeopathy. I. Carlston, Michael. II. Medical guides to complementary and alternative medicine.
    [DNLM: 1. Homeopathy. WB 930 C614 2003]
    RX71 .C534 2003
    615.5'32—dc21

                                                        2002073670

Publishing Director: Linda Duncan
Publishing Manager: Inta Ozols
Associate Developmental Editor: Melissa Kuster Deutsch
Project Manager: Linda McKinley
Designer: Julia Dummitt

KI-MVY

Printed in the United States

Last digit is the print number: 9 8 7 6 5 4 3 2 1

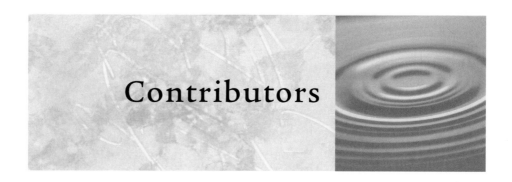

Contributors

DEBORAH GORDON, MD
Associate Faculty
Hahnemann College of Homeopathy
Point Richmond, California

STEVEN KAYNE, PhD, MBA, LLM, FRPharmS, FCPP, FFHom (Hon)
Hon Consultant Pharmacist
Glasgow Homeopathic Hospital
Visiting Lecturer in Complementary Medicine
University of Strathclyde
Glasgow, Scotland

RICHARD PITT, RSHom (NA), CCH
Director
Pacific Academy of Homeopathy
San Francisco, California

MICHAEL QUINN, RPh
Founder and Chief Pharmacist
Hahnemann Pharmacy
President
Hahnemann Laboratories, Inc.

JULIAN WINSTON, B.ID
Director Emeritus
National Center for Homeopathy
Alexandria, Virginia

This book is dedicated to those who are unafraid
to ask questions in their desire to learn

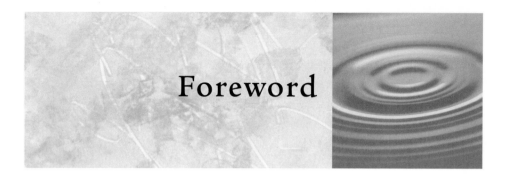

Foreword

As complementary and alternative medicine (CAM) becomes an increasingly prominent part of our health care system, more knowledge about these practices is needed. Homeopathy is a CAM system that few professionals know about and fewer still understand. Often it is confused with herbalism, thought to be simply the use of small amounts of drugs, and approached as if it were simply an alternative to disease treatment by conventional medicine. It is none of these. Controversy and bias around homeopathy is often heated and rarely based on factual data. Thus there are gaps between public and professional interest, skeptic and advocate opinion, and conventional and complementary practitioner knowledge. This book can fill those gaps.

Homeopathy was extensively practiced in the United States and Europe at the turn of the last century and is still widely used in many places of the world today. Many American medical schools were begun as homeopathic but closed after the Flexner report in 1916 and the advent of laboratory-based medicine. Homeopathy was vigorously suppressed in the United States and almost died out. Ironically, as its popularity waned in the United States, homeopathy spread widely in South America and India, where it is extensively used today for serious conditions. Interest in and use of homeopathy in the United States and Europe is now on the rise again as the public seeks nontoxic and holistic approaches to health care. This book is the first comprehensive introduction for nonhomeopathic professionals about homeopathy—and its history, regulation, practice, and research—to originate from America since the rise in interest in CAM.

The book begins with a rationale for why health care practitioners should study and learn this system of medicine. It gives a succinct overview of the principles and history of homeopathy and its development. It addresses why patients seek it, how it is practiced, what it does and does not work for, and summarizes the current state of the science in a balanced and evidence-based manner. It gives the reader information about training, licensure and liability, drug production and regulation, self-case use, and costs. In short, this book has everything the practitioner needs to know to understand issues of homeopathic practice and where to get more information or training.

Homeopathy will, like other areas of CAM, eventually find its proper place in medicine. This book will go a long way in helping that process along. Dr. Carlston is to be commended for taking a clinical approach, balanced with evidence, to homeopathy. Although research is important, and more is needed, medicine ultimately begins and ends in the clinic. The strength of homeopathy comes from its gentle nature and holistic view, its foundation in the dynamics of clinical practice, and its vision of the healing capacity of the person. It has a lot to teach us about the process of healing, and this book is one of our best guides.

WAYNE B. JONAS, MD
Director
Samueli Institute for Information Biology
Director (1995-1999)
Office of Alternative Medicine, National Institutes
of Health

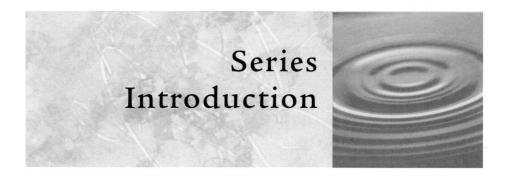

Series Introduction

The aim of this series is to provide clear and rational guides for health care professionals and students so they have current knowledge about the following:

- Therapeutic medical systems currently labeled as *complementary medicine*
- Complementary approaches to specific medical conditions
- Integration of complementary therapy into mainstream medical practice

Each text is written specifically with the needs and questions of a health care audience in mind. Where possible, basic applications in clinical practice are explored.

Complementary medicine is being rapidly integrated into mainstream health care, largely in response to consumer demand and in recognition of new scientific findings that are expanding our view of health and healing—pushing against the limits of the current biomedical paradigm.

Health care professionals need to know what their patients are doing and what they believe about complementary and alternative medicine. In addition, a basic working knowledge of complementary medical therapies is increasingly important for practitioners in primary care, some biomedical specialties, and the allied health professions. Complementary therapies expand our view of the art and science of medicine and make important contributions to the intellectual formation of students in health professions.

This series provides a survey of the fundamentals and foundations of complementary medical systems practiced in North America and Europe. Each topic is presented in ways that are *understandable* and that provide an important *understanding* of the intellectual foundations of each system—with translation between the complementary and conventional medical systems where possible. These explanations draw appropriately on the social and scientific foundations of each system of care.

Rapidly growing contemporary research results are also included where possible. In addition to providing evidence regarding the conditions for which complementary medicines may be of therapeutic benefit, guidance is also provided about when complementary therapies should not be used.

This field of health is rapidly moving from being considered *alternative* (implying exclusive use of one medical system or another) to *complementary* (used as an adjunct to mainstream medical care) to *integrative medicine* (implying an active, conscious effort by mainstream medicine to incorporate alternatives on the basis of rational clinical and scientific information and judgment).

Likewise, health care professionals and students must move rapidly to learn the fundamentals of complementary medical systems in order to better serve their patients' needs, protect the public health, and expand their scientific horizons and understandings of health and healing.

MARC S. MICOZZI, MD, PhD
Philadelphia, Pennsylvania
1997

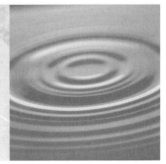

Series Editor's Preface

*E*xtraordinary claims require extraordinary results. The history of homeopathy, its purported mechanism of action, and recent research results all appear extraordinary when seen through the lens of the contemporary biomedical paradigm. As biomedicine increasingly turns its attention to investigation of "alternative" and complementary therapies, encouraged by popular interest and use, research studies are increasingly yielding positive results with alternative modalities that were only recently thought not to work *because they could not work*, as was once famously stated for homeopathy itself. The goal of this book series, *Medical Guides to Complementary and Alternative Medicine*, is to present information on the historical and scientific basis of healing traditions outside biomedicine with the hope of expanding the biomedical paradigm to be more inclusive of all observed healing phenomena.

Many contemporary medical researchers and practitioners assume that once empiric observations prove that alternative modalities work, then a priori their mechanisms of action must lie easily within the realm of explanations offered by the contemporary medical paradigm. Problematically, when research designs are created to test alternative therapies, controls are created for presumed mechanisms of action within the biomedical paradigm without regard to the actual mechanisms proposed by alternative practice traditions themselves.

Empiricism has been well established as the basis of scientific observation and of rational medical practice since the time of Sir Francis Bacon. On the other hand, positing mechanisms to explain empiric observations is always bounded by the prevailing paradigm of the time. The medical paradigm has evolved through time and will not likely remain frozen much longer in its twentieth-century reductionist, materialist version.

In perhaps no area of alternative medicine are these issues as delineated as in homeopathy. If all explanations of health are to be materialist explanations, as in the biomedical paradigm, homeopathy falls far short. If we are to recognize that there is a nonmaterial, "energetic" aspect to healing (as proposed by Ayurveda, Chinese medicine, many manual therapies, and of course, "energy healing," among other modalities), then homeopathy may manifest itself in an entirely nonmaterial mechanism.

In the United States, homeopathy and so-called *allopathic* medicine (a name conferred on regular medicine by homeopaths in mid-nineteenth century) have defined their practices at least partially in distinction and opposition to each other through the years. As stated by the great nineteenth-century physician Oliver Wendell Holmes, "I care little for homeopathy, and even less for so-called alleopathy." In this, he was setting aside debates about mechanism in favor of empiricism. The only rational basis for medical practice is whether treatment alleviates human suffering and prolongs or improves human life.

When the prevailing system of healing is unable to cope with the disease burden of a suffering population, which is increasingly afflicted with stress-related conditions of all types, it is useful to consider alternatives that have "survived" over time (as Dr. Carlston aptly puts in his volume) the standardization of medical practice into one relatively narrow realm. The survival of alternative practice such as homeopathy may ultimately contribute to our own survival as a healthy civilization.

MARC S. MICOZZI, MD, PhD
Bethesda, MD
November 2001

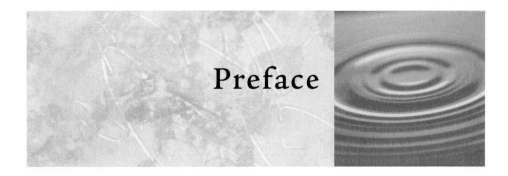

Preface

> "The physician's highest calling, his only calling, is to make sick people healthy—to heal, as it is termed."
>
> SAMUEL HAHNEMANN, *Organon of Medicine*[1]

In the opening sentence of homeopathy's founding document, Samuel Hahnemann declares his conviction that the patient's well-being is the only vital consideration in medicine. Debates about medical theories and the economics of health care have meaning only when considered in light of the patient's health; if it doesn't help the patient in some way, it doesn't matter. Conversely, if it does help the patient, it must not be withheld. Like many of the best ideas, this one is obvious. Unfortunately, sometimes we forget even obvious truths.

In February of 1994, my father-in-law was seriously ill. He spent 1 week in an intensive care unit (ICU) at Stanford Hospital. The families of each of the ICU patients sat together in a room waiting for the brief periods when two families members could go in to hold the hand, stroke the hair or talk to our usually unconscious loved one. Each family supported the other ones with amazing compassion and sensitivity. In many ways we formed an extended family in the ICU waiting room. The emotions of this newer, larger family rose and fell with the condition of each of the patients, our missing family sheltered in the ICU.

While waiting for my turn to visit, I read a brief news item about Columbia University opening an alternative medicine center. At the same time, I overheard a conversation between two women whose husbands had been in the ICU for many weeks. With their waning hope they lagged behind the other families who had just rushed in for their 10-minute visit. One woman said to the other, "You are Chinese, aren't you? The doctors say that my husband's kidneys are failing and there isn't much they can do. A friend of mine had a problem that an acupuncturist cured, so it makes me wonder. Is there anything in Chinese medicine that can help the kidneys?" The Chinese-American woman responded by saying that she had heard of some treatments that might help. Their initial optimism quickly faded after one of the women raised the concern that the doctors were likely to refuse to allow such treatments or would, at the least, be upset by their wish to try. The women decided it was best not to upset the physicians trying so hard to save their husbands' lives.

I wonder how often a tragic scene like this passes without an interested eavesdropper to later recount the tale. There is simply no ethical rationale for denying any safe and potentially effective treatment to any patient. As a physician, I am embarrassed and disappointed by our patients' opinions of us. I am upset that patients are afraid to discuss complementary therapies with their physicians. As it did in this incident, this fear seems to arise from patients' convictions that their physicians are hostile to these therapies.

There has been a barrier between medical orthodoxy and other forms of health care. Somehow, the health care used by 80% of the world's population has come to be labeled *alternative medicine*.[2] As we form an increasingly global society, conventional physicians and other Western health professionals are beginning to accept that human beings have been using these methods because they are effective, although to an unknown degree. With this newfound respect, there is much that can be learned from the "other" forms of medicine in use today. Although few people with whom I discussed this issue several years ago believed a medical détente could occur in our lifetimes, the injustice of the schism made me optimistic it would eventually be bridged. However, I must confess surprise at the speed with which this philosophic healing is taking place. The ill-founded barrier is crumbling rapidly. Writing this book is an attempt to further the process.

OVERVIEW

The goal of this book is to familiarize the reader with homeopathic medicine in its classic form. We will attempt to convey an understanding of homeopathy's unique view of health and disease, its place (current and ideal) within the health care system, and a taste of homeopathic clinical practice. My perspective, and the perspective of this book, is that patient well-being is paramount and homeopathic medicine is an effective means of achieving that aim. In fact, as a doctor practicing both conventional and homeopathic medicine, my experience has been that homeopathy often works better than conventional medicine for many common chronic health problems.

This book should be especially interesting to students of the health professions, practicing health care providers with a limited understanding of homeopathic medicine, and academicians desiring a fundamental understanding of homeopathic medicine. We begin with a discussion of the philosophic principles of homeopathic medicine. This is followed by consideration of where homeopathy has been and where it is currently, in a cultural, historical, and scientific context. Later sections of the book delve into the clinical practice of homeopathy, including discussions of the types of health problems particularly suited to homeopathic treatment. Hahnemann's motto for homeopathy, which is translated as "to taste and understand," seems a good idea. Thus I have incorporated an appendix with specific treatment suggestions for some common medical problems, so that the reader can test homeopathy in a small way. Homeopathic medicine can be a powerful medical tool that demands careful application to achieve success. Therefore, this book is not a substitute for proper homeopathic or conventional medical training. Both require a great deal more information and experience than can be contained in one book.

Another limitation of this book is in the restriction of the homeopathic philosophy discussed.

Recently some clinicians have begun using homeopathic remedies in many new and controversial ways. Because these approaches and controversies are in their infancy and will require many more years to be fairly evaluated, they are not the subjects of this text on the classical application of homeopathy in medicine.

This book is the outgrowth of a homeopathic elective that I have taught since 1993 in the School of Medicine of the University of California, San Francisco (UCSF). The course has been popular, averaging well over 100 health-sciences students per class. My side of that learning experience was critical to the evolution of this text.

I am sympathetic to the point of view that criticizes the common use of what would appear to be placebo dilutions in homeopathy. Despite many years of witnessing the beneficial effects of all levels of homeopathic dilutions in clinical practice, I am still puzzled. How could homeopathy be more than placebo? Placebo should not consistently produce the effects I have seen in patients with all varieties and severity of complaints. Very good clinical, animal, and basic science research has often documented significant differences between placebo and homeopathic dilutions. I know that, using homeopathy, I can routinely help patients with problems for which my regular medical training offered next to nothing. However, how can dilutions past Avogadro's number retain biological activity? In all honesty, I am still amazed that homeopathy works as often as it does.

In the final analysis, this mystery is fascinating. Scientists need mysteries. Without the unknown to explore, there is no need of science. As a scientist, I see homeopathy as the most intriguing form of healing in the world. This book is an exploration of the fascinating science of homeopathy. I hope that reading it will challenge your thinking about homeopathy and about the practice of medicine, regardless of your preconceptions. My greatest hope is that it will, in some way, positively affect your treatment of your patients.

References

1. Hahnemann S: *Organon of Medicine*, ed 6 (original 1842) (trans Kunzli J, Naude A, Pendelton P), Los Angeles, 1982, JP Tarcher.
2. Farnsworth N et al: Medicinal plants in therapy, *Bull World Health Organ* 63:965–981, 1985.

Acknowledgments

I would like to acknowledge the assistance of several people. First, the medical students at UCSF and the family practice residents at Sutter Hospital Santa Rosa for their questions that illuminated the essential components of this text. For the wisdom of their medical perspectives, Wayne Jonas, Marc Micozzi, Paul Erickson, Kristin Dillon, and Marisha Chilcott. For early editorial assistance, Meg Stemper. For all of the work from the publishing staff at Elsevier Science, particularly Inta Ozols, Jennifer Watrous, Kellie White, and Melissa Kuster.

Mike McConnell at Graphic World Publishing Services for ironing out the wirnkles. For immense research assistance over many years, the newly retired medical librarian Joan Chilton. For their hard work and perseverance, Stephen Kayne, Julian Winston, Deborah Gordon, Richard Pitt, and Michael Quinn. For their patience, Morgan, Rachel, and Marissa Carlston. Most importantly, for her support, my "in house" editor and spouse, Melanie Carlston. I hope the result is worthy of the considerable efforts of this remarkable group.

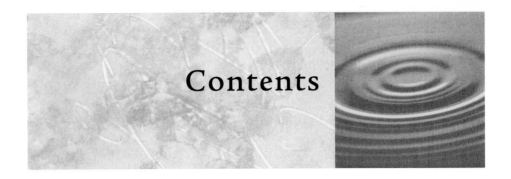

Contents

CLASSICAL
HOMEOPATHY

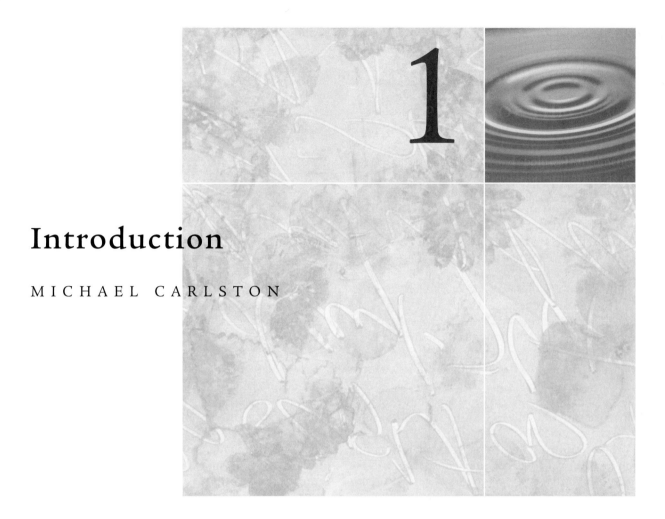

Introduction

MICHAEL CARLSTON

WHY LEARN ABOUT HOMEOPATHY?

There are several reasons why a physician or any other medical professional ought to learn about homeopathic medicine. In addition to the health benefit if homeopathy works, study of homeopathy can impart knowledge and unique homeopathic perspectives that will benefit even a skeptical student and his or her patients.

The most important reason to study any medical therapy is for the benefit the therapy can offer to patients. Although homeopathy has not been studied as extensively as almost anyone would like, homeopaths have accumulated two centuries worth of documented clinical evidence of homeopathy's efficacy in a very broad range of illnesses. Recent research tends to support this experiential evidence. Homeopathy first became famous as a means of successfully treating the horrible epidemics of the nineteenth century. Because we are now threatened by the rise of new microbial diseases and the waning effectiveness of antibiotics, other options are urgently needed. Homeopathy can often provide an effective alternative to antibiotics. Homeopathy's most unique capability is to alleviate chronic illness; because treatment of chronic illness is conventional medicine's greatest weakness, homeopathy may be the ideal form of complementary medicine.

Another reason to study homeopathy is its popularity. Regardless of a physician's own interest in homeopathy, some of his or her patients are very likely to be using it. At a minimum, physicians must learn about the uses and misuses of homeopathic medicine for their patients' safety.

Eisenberg and others conducted a landmark study of "unconventional medicine" that determined that roughly 600,000 American adults saw homeopathic practitioners in 1990, and another 1.2 million used homeopathy for self-care.[1] Over the past decade, figures show that sales of homeopathic medicine have been rising at an annual rate of approximately 20%.[2]

A 1997 survey by Landmark Healthcare found that 5% of the American adult population, approximately 9 million people, reported use of homeopathic products in the prior year; 73% of that use was for self-treatment.[3]

David Eisenberg and colleagues followed up on their 1990 data with another national survey in 1997. They found that the use of homeopathy increased fivefold to 6.7 million adults—3.4% of the adult population. They also found that self-care use increased to more than 82%, meaning that 5.5 million American adults were using homeopathy independent of any professional supervision.[4]

A linear projection of these data suggests that the number of adult Americans using homeopathy by 2002 has risen to 12 to 13 million, with 8 to 10 million using it on their own. Although many of the most popular homeopathic products sold in the United States are specifically intended for use by children, we have no national data regarding the extent of pediatric use.

Self-treatment predominates the homeopathic landscape and its repercussions must highlight any consideration of homeopathy by American health care providers. In their first survey, Eisenberg and colleagues found that more than 60% of those using unconventional therapies did not tell their conventional physicians. This was disturbing proof of patients' mistrust of their conventional physicians' attitudes. Unfortunately, the second survey did not find any improvement in the following years. Patients have simply been unwilling to speak to their conventional physicians about their use of alternative therapies. Assuming this figure is applicable to homeopathy, approximately 6 to 8 million Americans use homeopathic medicines every year without the knowledge of their conventional physician or the supervision of a professional homeopath. Their conventional physicians therefore do not know whether the effects, beneficial or adverse, their patients are experiencing are from the covert use of homeopathy or from conventional treatment.

Assuming this pattern of nondisclosure holds true for homeopathic patients (we have no data to support or confirm this supposition), that minority

who do inform their physicians are likely to be more knowledgeable about the subject than their physicians. Only rarely do patients tell me they discussed their use of homeopathy with their "other" doctors. When a patient reports that a conventional physician has even the most meager knowledge of homeopathy, it is a rare event. This ignorance can be harmful to the patient and embarrassing to the physician.

Homeopathic medicine's philosophy of healing and understanding of illness adds tremendously to the practice of medicine. Hering's Laws of Cure, for example, helps the physician determine whether a patient's response to any therapy is curative or suppressive (Box 1-1). This method of analysis is applicable whether the treatment is homeopathy, acupuncture, conventional medication, or surgery. The family practice residents and medical students in my classes have been excited about the philosophic understanding of health they have gained from studying homeopathy. They have a hunger to make sense of their growing experience of clinical medicine. Homeopathic philosophy can help them achieve an understanding beyond what they learn in their conventional training.

One of the most striking differences between conventional medicine and homeopathic clinical practice is the patient interview. The homeopath needs a tremendous amount of precisely detailed information to select, from the large number of potential

BOX 1-1

Hering's Laws of Cure[5]

Dr. Constantine Hering, the father of American homeopathy, taught that the healing process progresses as follows:

1. Symptoms are resolved in reverse order; that is, healing progresses from the most recent condition to the oldest
2. The recession of the symptoms progresses from the upper body parts downward to the lower body parts
3. The symptoms that are resolved first are those that affect the deeper organs and tissues, whereas those that are resolved later are more superficial
4. Improvement occurs with the more important organs and systems first, then moves on to the less important ones

homeopathic medicines, the appropriate medicine for each patient. The patient interview and physical examination is the sole means of acquiring this information. Laboratory testing and other modern diagnostic methods have yet to be correlated with homeopathic prescribing. The homeopath must develop interviewing skills to a very high degree to obtain the necessary information. On several occasions, nonhomeopathic medical school faculty members have suggested to me that medical students should receive their training in proper interviewing skills from homeopaths because of the care with which homeopaths interview patients.

HOMEOPATHY AND CONTROVERSY

Homeopathy is a soup made from the shadow of a pigeon that starved to death.

ABRAHAM LINCOLN

When Abraham Lincoln was assassinated, William Seward, the Secretary of State, was also wounded by Booth's gunfire. Like many of America's mid-nineteenth century elite, Seward's physician, Dr. Tullio Verdi, was a homeopath. The Surgeon General, Joseph K. Barnes, was first on the scene, and he cared for both men until Dr. Verdi arrived. Barnes then reported to Verdi the care he had provided to Seward.

The Surgeon General's actions provoked controversy within the fledgling American Medical Association (AMA). The controversy involved what officially constituted unethical behavior on the part of Lincoln's physician, and led to his censure by the Washington Medical Society. The Surgeon General had violated the AMA's "Consultation Clause," which banned its members from consulting with homeopaths or even providing treatment to a patient who had seen a homeopath until that patient formally discharged the homeopath.

Fortunately this degree of hostility has been relegated to the history books. Research evidence that this unorthodox therapy might actually be effective has helped open serious consideration of homeopathy. However, homeopathy has often been controversial. Although its history does not lack for colorful and dramatic personalities, the controversial aspect of homeopathy is primarily a result of its fundamen-

tal philosophic opposition to the world-view of conventional medicine.

The name for conventional medicine's therapeutic philosophy is *allopathy,* meaning *against suffering,* whereas homeopathy's philosophy is based on the concept of *similar to suffering.* Although homeopathy is almost purely *homeopathic,* allopathic medicine is far from truly *allopathic.* Allopathic medicine includes a philosophic hodgepodge of methods, including some that could even be called homeopathic. Uncomfortably, it was Samuel Hahnemann, the founder of homeopathy, who named allopathic medicine. In many ways homeopathic medicine has helped allopathic medicine define itself over the past two centuries by providing a clear-cut and consistent model of what allopathic medicine is not.

Homeopathy's "similar to suffering" theory refers to the therapeutic use of substances that, when ingested, create symptoms identical to those the patient is experiencing. This defining principle is diametrically opposed to the therapeutic approach of orthodox medicine, whose aim is to prescribe pharmacologic substances that will oppose the patient's symptoms. Homeopathy and conventional medicine also have opposing interpretations of the nature of those symptoms. The homeopath believes the symptoms result from the organism's effort to heal itself, whereas the allopath tends to view the symptoms as equal to the problem. If you look at the index of the *Physicians' Desk Reference,* you will find that it is largely made up of "anti" medication; antacids, antiarthritics, antibiotics, anticoagulants, anticonvulsants, antidepressants, antiemetics, antihistamines, and antiinflammatories, for example. Whereas the homeopath gives a remedy to act in concert with the patient's symptoms, the allopath prescribes to obstruct those symptoms.

This fundamental principle of homeopathy makes more sense as our scientific understanding of human physiology advances. When my medical school microbiology professor lectured to our class about evidence that the symptoms we experience in acute infectious diseases are the result of the immune system's mobilization to combat the disease and are not the direct effect of the microorganism, I recognized the "homeopathy" in the physiology. It makes sense, then, that a substance that accentuates the symptoms already produced by the body could assist the healing process by augmenting the already operating source of those symptoms—the immune response.

The most fervent, almost rabid, opposition to homeopathy arises from the common use of homeopathically diluted medications that do not contain any scientifically measurable amount of the medicinal substance. Homeopathic medicines are commonly diluted beyond the point where Avogadro's hypothesis suggests that not even one molecule should remain of the original substance. Because Avogadro's number is one of the fundamental constants in chemistry, this is a formidable intellectual barrier. Although there are scientific theories that might explain away the problem, all of them are controversial. Critics therefore believe homeopathic treatment is solely placebo, and forget that this dilution process is secondary to the primary principle of "like cures like." Homeopaths believe that the effectiveness of homeopathic treatment extends well beyond the placebo effect, which inevitably benefits all groups of patients.

The principles of homeopathic medicine can be applied without using dilutions that appear to challenge Avogadro's hypothesis. Since Avogadro's constant was discovered, many homeopaths have refused, on intellectual grounds, to use medicines diluted past this point. Today this attitude is most common in France. What really is most essential to homeopathy is the primary hypothesis of like cures like.

In some quarters, entrenched bias against homeopathy has been so unyielding that positive evidence from clinical trials, even well-conducted, randomized, and controlled ones, has been ignored. An interesting example of perceived bias against homeopathy in academic medicine occurred in 1989. It followed the publication of a clinical trial demonstrating homeopathy's effectiveness. An editorial in *Lancet*, entitled "Quadruple-blind," commented on this double-blind, randomized clinical trial of homeopathic treatment for influenza.[6] The trial demonstrated a very positive result in favor of the homeopathic treatment. Expresssing instinctive reservations, the editorialist mused about the number of levels of blinding that would be required for a favorable homeopathic trial to be accepted as a true result. He humorously commented that antihomeopathic bias was so entrenched that it might be necessary to blind the journal reader to the fact that the tested substance was homeopathic.

Ideally, a large number of clinical trials would have been performed to document the effectiveness of homeopathy for a large range of medical diagnoses. Unfortunately, this is not the case. Those who believe that homeopathy is effective must continue to produce high-quality research.

However, the limited proof available in the published literature does not justify delaying the use of homeopathy until more proof is accumulated. In the past decade, a number of homeopathic clinical trials have been published in many of the best medical journals. Although inconclusive, the balance of this literature is favorable to homeopathy.[7,8] Few alternative therapies are represented as well as homeopathy in the conventional medical literature.

This is the age of evidence-based medicine, based on the concept that rigorous clinical trials can help delineate the ideal way to practice medicine. Although I believe that this careful, objective consideration will undoubtedly improve the quality of health care we provide to our patients, it is impossible, at least for the foreseeable future, to base all treatment on the results of clinical trials.

The biggest impediment to the realization of evidence-based medicine is the paucity of clinical trials. Although it is estimated that more than one million clinical trials have been conducted, additional estimates are that these mountains of data provide evidence of effectiveness for only 5% to 15% of orthodox medical interventions.[9] Medicine, in all its therapeutic diversity, clearly needs more clinical research. Unfortunately, patients are unable to delay their illnesses until the ideal treatment has been determined. Usually, treatment recommendations must be made in relative ignorance.

Most of the remaining problems of applying research findings to clinical practice involve issues that were summarized by the famous nineteenth century social scientist and homeopathic advocate, Mark Twain, who (borrowing from Benjamin Disraeli) wrote, "There are three kinds of lies—lies, damned lies and statistics." The goal of medical research is to use lessons learned to improve the clinical practice of medicine. However, the precise conditions of a clinical trial are seldom encountered amidst the complexities of "real world" medicine. Generalizing from even the best clinical trials and then implementing the findings into patient care is a difficult and sometimes treacherously misleading process. In the final analysis, clinicians, and our patients, must unavoidably rely largely on our clinical judgments.

More than a decade ago Prince Charles called for members of the British Medical Association to seriously consider the potential of complementary medicine. Faced with a royal admonition, the Association issued a report on the nature and potential efficacy of various forms of complementary medicine. The rather insubstantial and brief statement on homeopathy could be summarized as, "Homeopathy doesn't work because it couldn't work." Although many British physicians now refer patients to homeopaths, and 20% of all Scottish general practitioners have been trained in homeopathy, other physicians maintain a stubbornly unscientific attitude and refuse to objectively consider research evidence.[10-12] They base their arguments upon the absence of a proven mechanism for the action of the most highly diluted homeopathic medicines.

Homeopaths believe that this posture is akin to disavowing the existence of gravity because of an inability to prove how it works. Similarly, most scientists believe that unexpected results need to be looked at critically; however, when results are confirmed, theories must be revised to encompass the new information. The apparent contradiction becomes a valuable means of enlarging our understanding of the world.

The homeopathic sentiment is best expressed by the quotation from Hahnemann at the beginning of the preface. *The physician's highest calling, his only calling, is to make sick people healthy—to heal, as it is termed.* The homeopath's mission is to heal the sick. It is important to try to understand the tools we use for the patient's benefit. However, as an empiricist, the homeopath is quite happy to use a tool that is not fully understood, provided it helps the patient. Patients benefit by receiving care from a physician who is knowledgeable about homeopathic medicine. Many medical problems, for which no effective conventional treatments are available, respond well to homeopathic treatment. Some of these homeopathic treatments are quite simple and can be learned by studying this book. Others are more complicated and require consultation with a homeopathic specialist.

Fortunately, medical students are beginning to learn about homeopathic medicine in medical schools. A 1995 survey found that 11% of American medical schools taught something about homeopathic medicine.[13] By 1998 this figure had risen to 57%, and more than 15% of medical schools required some instruction in homeopathy.[14]

There remains a great deal of ignorance about homeopathy within the conventional medical community. Misconceptions are the norm. Homeopathic practitioners readily admit our own ignorance of the mechanism of its action as well as uncertainty about its limitations and ideal clinical methodology. As more students are educated about homeopathy, some of them will conduct clinical trials and basic sciences research that will give us the answers we seek and, perhaps, settle some or all of the controversy surrounding homeopathic medicine.

References

1. Eisenberg D et al: Unconventional medicine in the United States, *N Engl J Med* 328:246-252, 1993.
2. Herbal and homeopathic remedies: finally starting to reach middle America? *OTC News and Market Report* 223-238, July 1991.
3. Landmark Healthcare, Inc.: *The Landmark report on public perceptions of alternative health care*, Sacramento, 1998, Landmark Healthcare.
4. Eisenberg D et al: Trends in alternative medicine use in the United States, 1990-1997: results of a follow-up national survey, *JAMA* 280:1569-1575, 1998.
5. Swayne, J: *Homeopathic method*, London, 1998, Churchill Livingstone.
6. Quadruple-blind, *Lancet* 1(8643):914, 1989.
7. Kleijnen J, Knipschild P, ter Riet G: Clinical trials of homoeopathy [published erratum appears in *BMJ* Apr 6;302(6780):818, 1991] [see comments]. *BMJ* 302(6772):316-323, 1991.
8. Linde K, Clausius N, Ramirez G et al: Are the clinical effects of homeopathy placebo effects? A meta-analysis of placebo-controlled trials [see comments] [published erratum appears in *Lancet* Jan 17;351(9097):220, 1998]. *Lancet* 350(9081):834-843, 1997.
9. Bero L, Drummond R: The Cochrane collaboration, *JAMA* 274:1935-1938, 1995.
10. Reilly D: A certificate of primary care homeopathy, *Br Homeopath J* 83:57-58, 1994.
11. Swayne, J: Survey of the use of homeopathic medicine in the UK health system, *J R Coll Gen Prac* 39:503-506, 1989.
12. Fisher P, Ward A: Complementary medicine in Europe, *BMJ* 309:107-111, 1994.
13. Carlston M et al: Alternative medicine education in US medical schools and family practice residency programs, *Fam Med* 29:559-662, 1997.
14. Barzansky B et al: Educational programs in US medical schools, 1998-1999, *JAMA* 282:840-846, 1999.

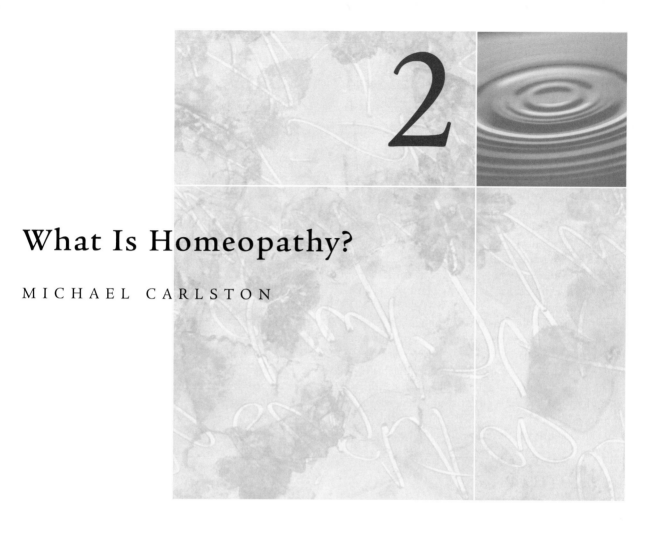

What Is Homeopathy?

MICHAEL CARLSTON

Aude sapere ("Dare to taste and understand")

HAHNEMANN'S *motto for homeopathy*

Many physicians and lay people are very confused about what homeopathy really is. Although many tenets of homeopathic philosophy are open to debate, antagonism toward homeopathy is surprisingly ill informed. Ironically, conventional medicine's summary judgment against homeopathy derives from a misunderstanding of homeopathic principles. Thoughtful consideration of a system of healing requires a sound understanding of the method, including its principles and clinical practice. The system of homeopathy is so complex and different from conventional medicine that it requires careful thought to intelligently accept or reject its principles.

The most common misconception has been that *homeopathic medicine* is synonymous with *natural medicine.* Although this sounds nice, it is inaccurate. Even if true, this definition would not shed much light, because what exactly is natural medicine? Naturopaths, the most established group of health professionals specializing in natural medicine, usually learn about homeopathy as only one of many therapies during their training. Although homeopathic medicines, or *remedies,* as they are often called, are often manufactured from naturally occurring materials, this is not a requirement of the homeopathic pharmacopoeia. Homeopathic theory advocates using remedies to heal the patient by stimulating his own

7

healing powers. Although this theory, if proven true, would effect what might be called a *natural healing*, it is unclear what such healing would mean compared with other forms of natural medicine. Such imprecision seems to make the identification of homeopathy as "natural" more misleading than helpful.

An American medical student's first exposure to homeopathy traditionally occurs when the phrase "homeopathic dosage" is used to castigate a physician who prescribed a subtherapeutic dosage of a conventional medicine. The assumption is that homeopathy has something to do with using insufficient quantities of medicine. Without investigating further, the student would not learn that homeopathic manufacturing involves a process of serial dilution of the medicinal agent, sometimes to an improbable extreme. Further investigation is unlikely given the perceived certainty that this pharmacologic nihilism must be a therapeutic blind alley.

In truth, the controversial process of dilution does not define homeopathy. Herein lies the irony: conventional medicine's rejection of homeopathy has been based upon the issue of ephemeral dosages, although such dilutions are not essential to homeopathy. If homeopathy cannot be defined simply as the use of fantastical dilutions, how then should it be defined?

DEFINITIONS

The National Institutes of Health opened the Office of Alternative Medicine (OAM) in 1992 (since upgraded to center status as the National Center for Complementary and Alternative Medicine [NCCAM]). One of the OAM's early efforts to bring some order to the amazingly diverse realm of complementary and alternative medicine was a classification schema.[1] Among the alternative fields of practice identified by NIH–OAM (Box 2-1), homeopathy was listed under "Alternative Systems of Medical Practice," along with Traditional Oriental Medicine, African Traditional Medicine, Naturopathic Medicine, and Native American Health Care Practice, among others (Box 2-2). Although this framework is useful, its ability to define homeopathy and other forms of alternative medicine is clearly limited by the tremendous differences within its broad categories. Practitioners of these traditions usually find little that is familiar in the methods of the other traditions.

BOX 2-1

Alternative Medicine Classification by NIH–OAM

Mind-body interventions
Bioelectomagnetic applications in medicine
Alternative systems of medical practice
Manual healing methods
Pharmacological and biological treatments
Herbal medicine
Diet and nutritional therapy

NIH–OAM, National Institutes of Health-Office of Alternative Medicine.

BOX 2-2

Alternative Systems of Medical Practice by NIH–OAM

- African traditional medicine
- Alcoholics Anonymous
- Anthroposophically extended medicine
- Ayurvedic medicine
- Curanderismo
- Environmental medicine
- Herbal medicine
- Homeopathic medicine
- Native American Indian health care practices
- Naturopathic medicine
- Santeria
- Shamanism
- Traditional Oriental medicine

NIH–OAM, National Institutes of Health-Office of Alternative Medicine.

The attempt to define homeopathy correctly begins simply with its name. *Homeopathy* means "similar to disease" or "similar to suffering." The clinical application of this principle defines homeopathic medicine.

Use of this essential homeopathic principle stretches far beyond the confines of the two centuries-old homeopathic medical tradition. The aspect of homeopathy defined by the homeopathic medical tradition and the broader usage of the similarity principle will be discussed in greater detail in Chapter 3. Homeopathy as a system of medicine originated in Germany with the experiments of Samuel Hahnemann. Reviewing Hahnemann's life story is a good place to begin our investigation.

HAHNEMANN'S STORY

As a conventionally trained physician, Hahnemann used the methods of his time, the late eighteenth century. These methods included a variety of practices that had changed very little in centuries. Patients were bled to reduce lung congestion, whether caused by pneumonia or heart failure. Various agents were applied to the skin to create blisters, in the belief that they would purify the body by causing it to excrete toxins. Chemicals such as mercury and arsenic were given to patients in poisonous doses. History records the deaths of many people, including heads of state, hastened, if not directly caused, by the medical care they received during this time in the history of conventional medicine.

When Hahnemann observed the clinical response of his patients to these treatments, he was understandably disturbed. Often, the only apparent effects of these treatments were adverse ones. Pressed by the economic necessity of providing for his young and growing family, he was caught in a moral dilemma. His practice of medicine was no different from that of the rest of his medical community, but he perceived that this standard care was harmful to his patients. If he acted in accordance with his beliefs and the Hippocratic dictum—First do no harm—he would have to eliminate much of his medical practice. On the other hand, he needed to support his family. Why should he suffer economically when his colleagues harmed their patients, made a living, and won praise for their injurious methods?

Hahnemann wrote the following of his decision:

To become in this way a murderer, or aggravator of the sufferings of my brethren of mankind, was to me a fearful thought, — so fearful and distressing was it, that shortly after my marriage I completely abandoned practice and scarcely treated anyone for fear of doing him harm, and—as you know—occupied myself solely with chemistry and literary labors.[2]

Hahnemann possessed an easy facility with languages. He put this gift to use when he decided to abandon his clinical practice and earn his livelihood translating medical texts into German from French, Latin, Italian, and English. His work as a translator provided his family with adequate means for their survival, and simultaneously allowed him to remain true to his convictions.

Hahnemann gained more than economic subsistence from this work. The translations brought him into close contact with the ideas of the most prominent physicians of his time and the masters of antiquity. These ideas influenced his subsequent medical practice. His clinical practice changed, and Hahnemann acquired a reputation for unorthodoxy.

Hahnemann vigorously espoused unpopular opinions criticizing conventional medicine. These forceful declarations alienated the medical community. When he lectured in the University of Leipzig he was described as a "raging hurricane." Hahnemann's fury and his apparently foolish ideas made him a lightning rod for ridicule. Ironically, much of the ridicule was for ideas we now accept as conventional medical wisdom.

One of his unorthodox opinions was the belief that the life circumstances of his patients could severely affect their health. Consequently, he insisted that his patients change harmful circumstances whenever possible.

For example, the prevailing medical opinion was that exercise was unhealthful. Hahnemann argued otherwise. To his detractors, one of the proofs of Hahnemann's ignorance was his family's practice of going on long walks for health. Hahnemann emphasized the important contribution of lifestyle to health.

Disease engendered by prolonged exposure to *avoidable* noxious influences should not be called chronic. They include diseases brought about by:

the habitual indulgence in harmful food or drink;
all kinds of excesses that undermine health;
prolonged deprivation of things necessary to life;
unhealthy places, especially swampy regions;
dwelling only in cellars, damp workplaces, or other closed quarters;
lack of exercise or fresh air;
physical or mental overexertion;
continuing emotional stress;
etc.

These self-inflicted disturbances go away on their own with improved living conditions if no chronic miasm is present, and they cannot be called chronic diseases.[3]

Hahnemann's belief in the prime importance of a healthful lifestyle persisted throughout his lengthy medical career. In his seminal work, *Organon of Medicine,* he wrote:

If someone complains of one or more trifling symptoms that he has noticed only recently, the physician should not consider this a full-fledged disease requiring serious medical attention. A slight adjustment in the mode of living usually suffices to remove this indisposition.[3]

Today's homeopathic practitioners are truly Hahnemann's descendants in their staunch advocacy of lifestyle modification over the use of prescription medication. As demonstrated by Goldstein,[4] not only do homeopaths advocate lifestyle change, but they are extraordinarily successful at helping their patients implement these health habits.

In 1792, Hahnemann was placed in charge of an asylum for the insane. Perhaps as a consequence of this experience, Hahnemann was among the first European or American physicians to speak out against the violent treatment directed against patients with mental illness.[5,6]

It is impossible not to marvel at the hard-heartedness and indiscretion of the medical men in many establishments for [the insane], who . . . content themselves with torturing these most pitiable of all human beings with the most violent blows and other painful torments. By this unconscientious and revolting procedure they debase themselves beneath the level of the turnkeys in a house of correction, for the latter inflict such chastisements as the duty devolving on their office, and on criminals only.[2]

Many of Hahnemann's controversial opinions are now widely accepted by physicians. Nearly any modern physician who awoke to find his or her colleagues poisoning their patients with arsenic, using bloodletting, inducing vomiting and diarrhea, torturing the mentally ill, and urging their patients to avoid exercise at all cost would be as outraged as Hahnemann was 200 years ago.

Hahnemann's Experiments with Quinine

Perhaps Hahnemann would have faded entirely from medical history were it not for an incidental discovery he made regarding the clinical effects of quinine. Malaria was a widespread health problem in Europe during Hahnemann's lifetime, and quinine was the mainstay of conventional treatment. In 1790, while translating one of the most highly regarded medical texts of the time, Cullen's *Materia Medica*, Hahnemann was upset by Cullen's claim that quinine was

an effective treatment for malaria because it was bitter and astringent. Cullen's belief was coherent with the precepts of Galenic Greek medicine, which, although nearly two millennia old, were still generally accepted as correct. Hahnemann rejected Cullen's claim on the basis of his experience that many other substances that were even more bitter and astringent had no effect at all on malaria.

Ever the inquisitive scientist, Hahnemann, apparently in a fit of pique, ingested a dose of quinine to determine its actions. He was surprised to discover that he developed a headache, fever, diarrhea, and chills. The surprise arose from his recognition of a paradox—that the symptoms created by quinine were the characteristic symptoms of malaria, the very disease quinine treated so effectively.

Hahnemann reflected upon this experience and searched the classical medical literature for similar information about parallels between toxic and beneficial effects of medicines. He also recognized the clinical application of this *like cures like* principle in the conventional treatment of tertiary syphilis by his contemporaries. Although syphilis was well known for causing bone destruction, gingivitis, and copious salivation, standard conventional treatment was mercury, which induced the same physiologic response. Physicians used the patient's copious salivation as an indication that an adequate dose of mercury had been administered. Not only was this another example of the effectiveness of the like-cures-like approach, this treatment appeared to deliberately utilize the approach.

The implications of this principle gradually became apparent to Hahnemann. Over the next several years Hahnemann slowly transformed his clinical practice, refocused his writings on his newly developing theories (most notably his "Essay on a New Principle for Ascertaining the Curative Power of Drugs, with a Few Glances at Those Hitherto Employed") and founded the medical system called *homeopathy.*

HOMEOPATHIC PRINCIPLES

Homeopathic medicine is so different from conventional medicine that the two could seldom be confused. However, arguments over which features are essential to a homeopathic definition have raged for nearly 200 years. This text is focused on the classic foundations, the core of homeopathy as espoused and practiced by Hahnemann. That perspective will guide this discussion.

Hahnemann knew nothing of injecting diluted substance into acupuncture points, using electronic devices to guide remedy selection, or mixing a collection of homeopathic remedies together and labeling them for one specific illness. All of these are common practices today. Hahnemann, like many modern classical homeopaths, would likely wonder what these methods have to do with homeopathy. This speculation is not based upon a judgment of merit or efficacy. Simply, these approaches, good or ill, are at best very distant relations or offshoots of homeopathic medicine.

Homeopathy in its classical form is founded on the following four principles: (1) like cures like, (2) provings, (3) single medicine, and (4) minimal dose. Each of these tenets warrants detailed consideration.

posophists use diluted medicinal agents and prescribe them to patients based upon general characteristics of each patient's personality. Nearly 500 years ago, Paracelsus wrote that a plant that was growing in the moist darkness hidden among other plants was a source of medicine for a person who was shy and withdrawn. Although classical homeopaths do not view any of these approaches as purely homeopathic, Paracelsus' intuitive perception of similarity is one with which they feel a great deal of sympathy.

Hahnemann made a pivotal recognition of the similia principle in the action of quinine, and two centuries later his homeopathic explanation of quinine's antimalarial effects is as good as any other we have.[7,8] Quinine's direct actions on the malarial organism are controversial. It is also intriguing that overdoses of quinine led to a disease called black water fever, which is characterized by hemorrhagic fever, often fatal and very similar to malaria.[9]

LIKE CURES LIKE

Considering the paradoxic therapeutic action of quinine and mercury, Hahnemann recalled the admonition to let like cure like from writings attributed to Hippocrates, as well as Paracelsus' correlate, the "Doctrine of Signatures." Hahnemann's experience, coupled with the words of these great masters, encouraged him to develop this approach for use in clinical practice. This method of using a substance that creates certain symptoms to treat a patient suffering the same symptoms is the defining principle of homeopathic medicine. It is the cornerstone of homeopathy. This importance is reflected in the system's name: *homeo-pathy* is literally "similar to suffering."

Hahnemann did not invent the use of like cures like, and this approach is not unique to homeopathy (see Chapter 3). On the other hand, homeopathic medicine is unique in the unwavering application of the homeopathic principle to every patient in every clinical encounter.

A certain measure of debate centers on the question of what exactly does *like* mean? What elements of the patient's makeup are open to selection as homeopathic characteristics and how alike must *like* be?

Some health care practitioners connect their patients to various electrical devices to determine which homeopathic medicine they need. Anthro-

PROVINGS

Hahnemann's intention to use a homeopathic approach was initially stymied by medicine's relative ignorance of the effects of medicinal substances on the human organism. He needed considerably more information; specifically, he needed to identify detailed indications as to when to give a certain medicine to a certain patient. Obviously, it is impossible to recognize similarity between patient and treatment without being familiar with both sides of the like-cures-like equation. Carefully taking the patient's history is crucially important, but at best can provide only half of the needed information. What does the drug do to the human organism? What are the symptoms created by the drug? The practitioner needs fully developed information on the drug side of the equation as well.

To develop this requisite knowledge base, Hahnemann began testing the commonly used medicines of the time and other promising substances in hopes of using their homeopathic characteristics to treat patients. Hahnemann recruited his family, friends, and colleagues to ingest the test substances and record the symptoms they experienced. These symptoms were compiled and became the initial pool of homeopathic pharmacologic knowledge.

In German, these experiments were called *Pruefung* (literally, "test").[10] Now the term used is *proving.* This testing process is quite similar to Phase I drug trials in today's conventional medicine. The intention of a Phase I trial is to discover the damaging adverse effects of a medication. In a way, homeopaths are seeking those adverse effects, hoping to use them to heal their patients. Although Galen, one of Western medicine's great progenitors, had suggested testing medicines on healthy people, Hahnemann appears to have been the first to systematically employ this method. As a result, some recognize this testing process as the beginning of clinical pharmacologic research.[11]

This systematic, experimental approach to medicine was extremely important to Hahnemann and the establishment of homeopathy in patient care. Homeopaths claimed the superiority of their methods in part because of this carefully analytic approach to clinical medicine that was lacking in the conventional medical practices of their time. In the preface to his *Materia Medica Pura,* Hahnemann wrote:

I am not going to write a criticism of the ordinary Materia Medica, else I would lay before the reader a detailed account of the futile endeavors hitherto made to determine the powers of medicines from their color, taste and smell.[12]

Hahnemann believed that careful scientific experimentation was most important, and that theoretic speculations (such as the conventional practice of divining the action of a drug by its color, taste, and smell) were second-rate in comparison.

The day of the true knowledge of medicines and of the true healing art will dawn when men cease to act so unnaturally as to give drugs to which some purely imaginary virtues have been ascribed, or which have been vaguely recommended, and of whose real qualities they are *utterly* ignorant; and which they give mixed up together in all sorts of combinations. . . . By this method no experience whatever can be gained of the helpful or hurtful qualities of each medicinal ingredient of the mixture, nor can any knowledge be obtained of the curative properties of each individual drug.[12]

Hahnemann's guidelines for homeopathic provings were quite specific and carefully considered.

As regards my own experiments and those of my disciples every possible care was taken to insure their purity, in order that the true powers of each medicinal substance might be clearly expressed in the observed effects. They were performed on persons as healthy as possible and under regulated external conditions as nearly as possible alike.[12]

If the subjects intentionally or accidentally stepped out of these disciplined experimental conditions (e.g., through injury, overindulgence, vexation, fright), no further symptoms were recorded to avoid contaminating the data. If some lesser insult suggested the possibility of interference, the subsequent symptoms were marked as being of potentially questionable origination.

Hahnemann and his students discovered that each medicine or remedy created a large number of reactions, many of which are familiar to conventional physicians as commonly recognized disease characteristics such as cough, headache, or back pain. Because each person proving a remedy would respond somewhat differently from the others, precise information was important. Equally important was comparing the responses of the provers to ascertain the most fundamental and characteristic healing qualities of each substance.

Hahnemann soon learned that, just as there are precise symptomatic distinctions between remedies, people respond in their own unique manners to every disease. Although the general pathologic changes were the same (a pneumonia is a pneumonia), careful observation revealed distinct differences among patients. Some patients with pneumonia had painful coughs, some had coughs that paradoxically improved when they lay down, and some were chilly while others felt hot during the illness. Many patients experienced a tremendous variety of associated symptoms, irrelevant to conventional diagnosis but important to the homeopath precisely because they were unusual.

These individual peculiarities lead the homeopath to use different remedies for different patients with the same conventional diagnosis. The individual variability among patients and remedies has far-reaching consequences in the clinical practice of homeopathy and for researchers investigating its effectiveness. Fortunately for patients, but unfortunately for homeopaths, each patient produces only a fraction of the fully developed complex of the homeopathic symptoms engendered by the remedy that will help. Some of the symptoms developed by the proving subjects are rarely, if ever, seen in clinical practice. The art of homeopathic clinical practice lies in eliciting the symptoms from the patient and then recognizing the same pattern amongst the palette of more than 1500 homeopathic remedies.

In addition to provings, there are other sources of indications for homeopathic remedies. For example, the recorded symptoms of poisonings can suggest clinical applications of diluted poisons to the homeopath. Undoubtedly, the most important source of additional information about homeopathic remedies comes from records of symptoms cured in the clinical use of the remedy. Some argue that this information is even more reliable and more important than symptoms learned from provings.

SINGLE MEDICINE

Today it is difficult to find a health food store in the United States that does not sell homeopathic medicines, and almost all of them sell homeopathic combination remedies. The number that sell individual remedies is much smaller. These combinations are mixtures of several different homeopathic medicines. Because these combinations are rarely tested by traditional provings, they are the focus of controversy within the professional homeopathic community.

Hahnemann reviled the customary practice of mixing several medicinal agents because of the uncertain effects and potential danger to the patient. It is ironic that so much of homeopathic medicine is now this type of polypharmacy. Modern homeopaths practicing in the classical homeopathic tradition criticize this mixed approach for essentially the same reasons given by Hahnemann. Although it is difficult or impossible to assess self-care practices that were used two centuries ago, too many lay people using homeopathy today seem to operate by the antihomeopathic belief, "If a little bit is good, more must be better," and so run the risk of overmedicating themselves with homeopathic remedies. Although in my own clinical experience adverse effects of this approach are uncommon, they do seem to occur, so a more cautious approach appears warranted.

MINIMAL DOSE

Homeopathic use of microdoses is not only controversial; its historical development is shrouded in mystery. Homeopathic remedies are made from an incredible variety of substances. Plants, minerals, and animal poisons make up the largest groups of remedies. Because these substances are then diluted and shaken (succussed) serially, many homeopathic remedies are *postavogadran* dilutions (Box 2-3). This means that it is unlikely that there is even one molecule of the original substance remaining in many of the tubes of homeopathic remedies sold in the United States.

Hahnemann initially administered his medicines in the dosages used by conventional physicians. There were problems with this approach. Clinical experience taught Hahnemann that conventional dosages of homeopathic remedies often temporarily intensified patients' symptoms. In addition, patients would transiently develop symptoms of the remedy from which they did not previously suffer. To circumvent this undesirable tendency toward adverse effects, Hahnemann began diluting the medicines he used.

In the preamble to *Materia Medica Pura,* Hahnemann recounts a case of a cleaning woman disabled by a collection of symptoms, including abdominal pain, irritability, and insomnia:

I gave her one of the strongest homeopathic doses, a full drop of the undiluted juice of bryonia root,* to be taken immediately, and bade her come to me again in 48 hours.[12]

His footnote (*) refers to a more recent change in dosing of homeopathic remedies:

According to the most recent development of our new system the ingestion of a single, minutest globule, moistened with the decillionth (x) development of power

---

BOX 2-3

Commonly Sold Homeopathic Dilutions Relative to Avogadro's Number

1X = 1 part in 10
3X = 1 part in 1,000
6X = 1 part in 1,000,000
12X (or 6C) = 1 part in 1,000,000,000,000
Avogadran limit here
12C = 1 part in 1,000,000,000,000,000,000,000,000,000
30X = 1,000,000,000,000,000,000,000,000,000,000
30C = 1,000,000,000,000,000,000,000,000,000,000,000,000,000,000,000,000,000,000,000,000

Professional homeopaths often use 200C (i.e., 1 followed by 400 zeros), 1M (i.e., 1 followed by 2,000 zeros), or "higher" potencies.

would have been quite adequate to effect an equally rapid and complete recovery; indeed, equally certain would have been the mere olfaction of a globule the size of a mustard seed moistened with the same dynamization, so that the drop of crude juice given by me in the above case to a robust person, should not be imitated.[12]

To allay the reader's concern, it should be known that the patient recovered and, like many a modern patient, did not return for the follow-up appointment. When a skeptical colleague tracked the patient to her village, she reportedly told him this:

What was the use of my going back? The very next day I was quite well, and could again go to my washing, and the day following I was as well as I am still. I am extremely obliged to the doctor, but the like of us have no time to leave off our work; and for three weeks previously my illness prevented me from earning anything.[12]

The homeopathic process of dilution and succussion is carried to such a remarkable degree that many cannot think clearly about the system of homeopathy beyond this issue. They ignore the other principles, most notably the *similia* doctrine, and erroneously view the entire system as a simple matter of diluting medicinal substances beyond the possibility of pharmacologic action. Nor is this misconception held only by detractors. Some health care practitioners now inject acupuncture points with diluted substances of all sorts and call it homeopathy, even though they ignore the fundamental doctrine of like cures like in this process.

Although Hahnemann routinely recorded his experiments and clinical treatments in the same detail as the case of the washerwoman above (recall my abbreviated retelling of one of his cases), no one has found any record explaining the rationale behind the mechanics of Hahnemann's very specific process of dilution and succussion. Many have theorized that Hahnemann's Masonic affiliation led him to knowledge of alchemic principles and then to this alchemy-like process. However, there is no direct evidence to support this claim. We do know that Hahnemann's motivation for dilution was to minimize adverse effects by administering the minimal dose. The process of succussion is more mysterious, as is the rationale for the specific proportions he chose for his dilutions. Late in his life Hahnemann altered his dilution procedure and thereby generated controversy about the relative merits of this later protocol, a controversy that lasts to this day. In view of the great deal of information we possess regarding Hahnemann's

thinking and his patient records, our ignorance on this seemingly important matter is notable. This uncharacteristic vacuum suggests that Hahnemann might have intended secrecy, perhaps lending credence to the theory of Masonic influence. Some think that Hahnemann simply did not believe his reasoning was important enough to write down. He was merely attempting to create a uniform dilution.

HOMEOPATHIC VIEW OF HEALTH AND DISEASE

Homeopaths since Hahnemann have always viewed symptoms of illness a bit differently from conventional physicians. Homeopaths emphasize the importance of the precise characteristics of each patient's symptoms, because they are the means the homeopath uses to ascertain the pattern of each individual's unique response to his illness. The specific distinguishing features help the homeopath sort out the patient in front of him from all others with the same disease condition.

Homeopaths also view symptoms as signposts indicating the manner in which the organism is working to restore itself to health. In other words, symptoms are not bad in themselves, nor are they the disease. Symptoms are a consequence of the body's work to regain health. Treatment should thus be directed at improving healthy response and correcting underlying imbalance, which then, secondarily, will relieve the symptoms.

Furthermore, there is a hierarchy of symptoms. Some symptoms are more important than others. Generally speaking, mental and emotional disturbances are more important than dermatologic complaints and even rarely some serious physical conditions. For example, a patient who is emotionally disturbed is sicker than a patient with a disfiguring skin rash. Likewise, a lively, energetic, and socially involved paraplegic is healthier than an able-bodied person who is crippled by anxiety or depression. A positive response to treatment is reflected in the movement of the disorder from deeper (more important) to more superficial symptoms. Interpreting the pattern of symptoms following treatment tells the homeopath whether the treatment was beneficial or harmful. The homeopath must use the analysis framework provided by homeopathic theory to correctly evaluate clinical information and determine the subsequent course of treatment. The answer to the question "Was my treatment effective?" must meet very specific criteria recognized throughout the world's homeopathic community. As a result, two homeopaths will rarely disagree in their assessment of the changes in a patient's health. In many ways homeopathic principles create a formalized process leading to a determination very much in harmony with the common sense perspective of laymen.

Disturbances in the deepest aspects of a patient's being are reflected in the patient's mind and body. This is the nature of disease. Pursuing this line of thought to its logical conclusion, some homeopaths (including Hahnemann) have identified spiritual dysfunction as the primal origin of disease. Few have gone so far as to claim it as the exclusive disease-generating force, generally allowing that external forces (e.g., lifestyle and exposure to health-damaging influences) also play a part. Clearly, philosophical considerations are more central in the clinical practice of homeopathy than they are in conventional medicine. Because homeopathy is a highly structured approach to healing, compared with the empirical bent of conventional medicine, this difference is not surprising.

SURVIVAL OF HOMEOPATHY

One way to answer the question "What is homeopathy?" is to borrow from modern pop psychology by answering, "Homeopathy is a survivor." Given the controversy surrounding and even encouraged by Hahnemann and his therapy, the fact that this medical system survived and even came to flourish in the early nineteenth century is intriguing. The principal reason for the rise of homeopathy is a familiar and important one—effectiveness. Homeopathic treatment was at least as successful as conventional medical treatment. There is evidence that strongly suggests that homeopathy was superior to conventional therapies in the treatment of epidemic diseases. The first big advances in the popularity of homeopathy came through the relative success homeopaths achieved treating the typhoid and cholera epidemics that swept through early nineteenth-century Europe.

Although the ability to alleviate suffering is the most attractive feature to the largest constituency, philosophy is important as well. The current homeo-

pathic resurgence is fueled in part by interest in its philosophy and identity as a "natural" form of healing. The homeopathic view of disease and health differs from that of most orthodox physicians. Whereas some find the philosophic perspectives of homeopathy controversial, they are quite appealing to others. Many people live their lives aspiring to certain ideals. People who highly value emotional well-being or spiritual principles often find appealingly familiar echoes of those values and principles in homeopathic medicine. Choosing homeopathy gives them a way to incorporate their broadest ideals into their health care.

Homeopathy has always been the medical perspective of a minority. As a dissenting minority, homeopathy and the homeopathic community have forged a contrarian identity. This alternative perspective attracts individuals who, for a variety of reasons, reject orthodox opinions, medical and otherwise. In this sense, the homeopathic community sometimes provides a comfortable home for people who find themselves at odds with the larger society. This group represented a larger portion of the homeopathic community in the past than it does today. However, despite this rapprochement, homeopathic principles simply do not allow this system of medicine to be entirely compatible with conventional medicine.

Homeopathy survives because it provides certain elements missing in conventional medicine. It is another option, sometimes complementary to conventional medicine, sometimes an alternative, and sometimes even hidden within the practice of conventional medicine.

SUMMARY

Writing a century ago in his essay "What Is Homeopathy?" James Tyler Kent wrote:

Then to the question, what is homeopathy? I must answer, *no man knows! God* only knows the length and breadth of the intricate, unfathomable mystery. The knowable part of this science, if I may use the word, consists in observing the sick-making phenomenon of drugs and the phenomena of sickness, gathering and grouping the similars, selecting with the likeness in view and waiting for results.[13]

Although Kent might have believed the attempt futile, my fullest answer to "What is homeopathy?" is the entirety of this book. Many of the ideas presented in this chapter are discussed in greater detail later in the chapters that follow. Hopefully you now know enough to have more (and better) questions than you did before. Continued reading should answer many of those questions, but it will inevitably lead you to others that are currently unanswerable. Although "currently unanswerable" may disappoint some readers, the truth is there is a very great deal we do not know about homeopathy, and, in Kent's view at least, "currently unanswerable" might be an overly optimistic assessment.

References

1. Alternative Medicine: Expanding horizons: A report to the National Institutes of Health on alternative medical systems and practices in the United States, NIH Publication No. 94-066, December 1994. US Government Printing Office, Washington, D.C. Prepared under the auspices of the Workshop on Alternative Medicine, Chantilly, VA, Sept 14-16, 1992.
2. Dudgeon RE, editor: *The lesser writings of Samuel Hahnemann.* New Delhi, 1999, B. Jain, p 512 (original 1851).
3. Hahnemann S: *Organon of medicine,* ed 6, Los Angeles, 1982, JP Tarcher (original 1842).
4. Goldstein MS, Glik D: Use of and satisfaction with homeopathy in a patient population, *Altern Ther Health Med* 4(2):60-65, 1998.
5. Gamwell L, Tomes N: *Madness in America: cultural and medical perceptions on mental illness before 1914,* Binghampton, New York, 1995, Cornell University Press.
6. Dudgeon RE: *Lectures on the theory and practice of homeopathy,* London, 1854, Leath and Ross.
7. Foley M, Tilley L: Quinoline antimalarials: mechanisms of action and resistance and prospects for new agents, *Pharmacol Ther* 79(1):55-87, 1998.
8. Slater AF: Chloroquine: mechanism of drug action and resistance in *Plasmodium falciparum. Pharmacol Ther* 57 (2-3):203-235, 1993.
9. Garrett L: *The coming plague: newly emerging diseases in a world out of balance,* New York, 1994, Penguin Books, pp 447-448.
10. Coulter H: *The origins of modern western medicine, J.B. Van Helmont to Claude Bernard.* Washington, DC, 1988, Wehawken Book Company, p 311.
11. Kaptchuk TJ: Intentional ignorance: a history of blind assessment and placebo controls in medicine, *Bull Hist Med* 72(3):389-433, 1998.
12. Hahnemann S: *Materia medica pura,* New Delhi, 1995, B. Jain (originally published in 1811).
13. Gypser KH, editor: *Kent's minor writings on homeopathy,* Heidelberg, 1987, Karl F. Haug Publishers, p 147.

Suggested Readings

Bradford TL: *The life and letters of Dr. Samuel Hahnemann,* Philadelphia, 1895, Boericke and Tafel.

Coulter H: *The origins of modern western medicine: J.B. Van Helmont to Claude Bernard,* vol 2, Washington, DC, 1988, Wehawken Book Company.

Dudgeon RE: *Lectures on the theory and practice of homeopathy,* London, 1854, Leath and Ross.

Haehl R: *Samuel Hahnemann, his life and work,* 2 vols, Homeopathic Publishing, New Delhi, B. Jain, 1983 (translated by M Wheeler, WHR Grundy; edited by FE Wheeler, JH Clarke; originally published in 1922).

Hahnemann, S. *Organon of medicine,* ed 6, Los Angeles, 1982, J. P. Tarcher (original 1842).

Hobhouse RW: *Life of Christian Samuel Hahnemann, founder of homeopathy,* Rosa CW Daniel, New Delhi, B. Jain, 2001 (originally published in 1933).

Jutte R et al: *Culture, knowledge and healing: historical perspectives of homeopathic medicine in Europe and North America,* Sheffield, England, 1998, European Association for the History of Medicine and Health Publications.

Vithoulkas G: *Science of homeopathy,* New York, 1980, Grove Press.

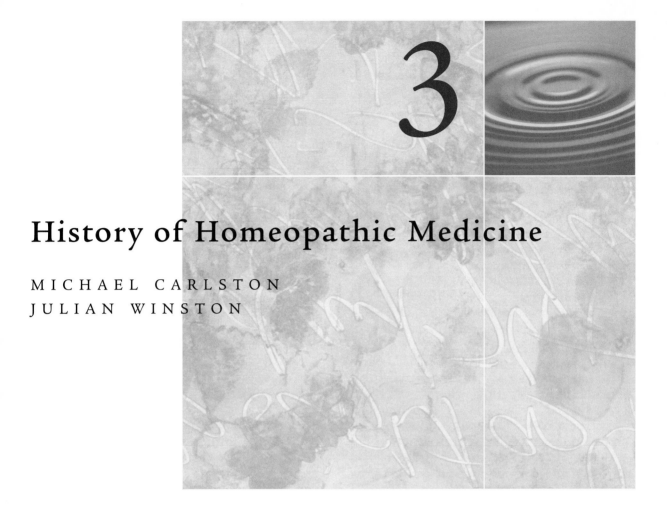

History of Homeopathic Medicine

MICHAEL CARLSTON
JULIAN WINSTON

HOMEOPATHY BEFORE HAHNEMANN

"The same substances that cause strangury, cough, vomiting and diarrhea will cure those diseases."[1]

HIPPOCRATES

Homeopathy has always been controversial. Hahnemann was compelled to move to another country to escape the political and social pressure brought to bear on him and his students. In fairness to his detractors, Hahnemann probably contributed substantially to the conflict, because he was not at all gentle in his public criticisms of the methods and ethics of his opponents. After Austria's emperor died, he placed an advertisement in a major newspaper blaming the emperor's orthodox physicians for the death.

Although homeopathic history is rich with colorful and dramatic personalities, the controversy surrounding homeopathy has always had more to do with its fundamental philosophic opposition to the world-view of conventional medicine than with personalities. This polarity is so deeply ingrained that orthodox medicine's most widely used philosophic name, *allopathy,* was devised by homeopaths. In many ways, homeopathic medicine has helped allopathic medicine define itself over the past two centuries.

But how does homeopathy define itself? The idea of using like to cure like did not spring unique and fully born from Hahnemann's brain. Hahnemann recognized this principle, familiar from the writings of Hippocrates, manifesting in his experience with patients. He resurrected the phrase *similia similibus curantur* ("let likes cure likes") from Hippocratic literature and did not claim that the fundamental principle of his method was new. Hahnemann's special contribution along this line was to promote a highly systematic approach to healing founded on this principle. His system encompassed a rigorous process of testing potential therapeutic agents, specific methods of processing the raw material, and detailed protocols for applying the principles to patient care. He named this system *homeopathy,* from the Greek words *homoios* ("similar") and *pathos* ("suffering").

Hahnemann's contribution was significant, but to fully understand homeopathy we must consider principles that have not necessarily been labeled homeopathic. A work by Boyd[2] from 1936 includes an interesting discussion of Hahnemann's philosophic forebears. Dudgeon's[3] 1852–1853 lectures given at London's Hahnemann Hospital and Harris Coulter's[4] series on the history of Western medical thought are other excellent sources of information. Often unwittingly, like has been used to treat like worldwide throughout medical history, under differing names, to varying degrees, and with differing details of application. Other homeopathic principles have appeared in varying guises over the millennia.

Hippocrates

Many writings have been passed down from the school of thought identified as *Hippocratic.* Although we know that Hippocrates was not the author of many of these writings, they do represent a relatively consistent viewpoint compared to the hodgepodge of theories expounded six centuries later by Galen, another founding father of Western medicine. This ancient Hippocratic corpus in many instances advocates the use of like to treat like. For example, "So that which produces urinary tenesmus in the healthy, cures it in disease."[1] Another passage, translated by Jones, makes the point even clearer:

The pains (complaints) will be removed through the opposite of them, each according to its own characteris-

tics. So warm corresponds to the warm constitution which has been made ill by cold; so correspond the others. Another type is the following: through the similar the disease develops and through the employment of the similar the disease is healed.[1]

One of the Hippocratic writings records the following as the recommended treatment for a patient with suicidal mania (quoted in Dudgeon): "Give him a draught made from the root of mandrake, in a smaller dose than will induce mania."[3]

Compare that clinical recommendation with this excerpt from a modern reference discussing the ill effects of mandrake (*Mandragora officianarum*):

Because of the high content of scopolamine in the drug, poisonings lead at first to somnolence, but then also, after the intake of very high dosages, to central excitation (restlessness, hallucinations, delirium and manic episodes), followed by exhaustion and sleep.[5]

The modern description of the mania-inducing effects of this plant makes its selection as a Hippocratic prescription for a mental disorder clearly harmonious with Hahnemann's later teaching.

The therapeutic recommendations in the Hippocratic corpus were not purely or even predominantly homeopathic. Both allopathic and homeopathic approaches were advocated, sometimes in the same sentence: "If this held in all cases it would be easy, now according to the nature and cause of the disease to treat according to the contrarium and now according to the nature and origin of the disease through the similar."[1]

Even before Hippocrates, the role for *similia* in the practice of medicine was recognized by many traditions. Ayurvedic medicine encompassed the use of similars, enumerating it as one of the possible therapeutic approaches to the patient. The Egyptian Ebers papyrus from 1,500 BCE advocated using the eyes of pigs to treat blindness. Also suggesting similars, this document gave instructions on the use of fish heads to treat headaches in human sufferers.

Similar concepts influenced Galen, a Greek physician living in Rome in the second century. His independent thinking was reflected at times in his contentious self-confidence. Galen's synthesis of the competing trends of empiric and philosophic medical traditions made his writings the foundation of Western medicine for 1400 years. Although Galen actively opposed the Doctrine of Signatures, various medical historians point out that he "carried on" or "paid lip service" to the use of similars. Because they are so at odds with the mass of the Galenic literature, it appears that his writings advocating the use of similars are either theoretic anomalies or untidy remnants in his synthesis of earlier medical thought.[6,7]

Paracelsus

Another of the recognized fathers of Western medicine was Philippus Aureolus Theophrastus Bombastus van Hohenheim, more commonly known as Paracelsus (b. 1494?, d. 1541). Some observers view Hahnemann's homeopathy as the child of the Doctrine of Signatures so vigorously advocated by Paracelsus. Hahnemann and Paracelsus shared many more beliefs than just the *similia* principle. It is tempting to view Paracelsus as Hahnemann's intellectual forefather. Closer investigation suggests that the lineage is contestable, particularly when we consider other antecedent medical philosophies that in some way defended the *similia*. Although the philosophy and writings of Paracelsus were very likely to have some influence on Hahnemann, the same can be said of Hippocrates and other advocates of the *similia* principle.

Similia and the Doctrine of Signatures
Because through the art of chiromancy, physiognomy and magic it is possible to recognize in the external appearance, the peculiarities and virtue of every root and herb by its signature, shape, form and color, and it requires no further testing or long experience. Does not the leaf of the thistle stick like needles? Because this sign has been found by magic, there is no better herb for internal sticking than the thistle.

PARACELSUS, Quoted in Boyd[2]

Because Paracelsus sometimes mentioned the use of a certain plant that was shaped like the diseased organ he was treating, some claim that his version of the Doctrine of Signatures was based simply upon shape. However, Paracelsus' use of *similia* was more complex. For example, he valued the herb *Hypericum perforatum* (St. John's Wort) even more than present-day American consumers, advocating it for all manner of disease: "The *Hypericum* is almost a universal medicine."[2] Although he did look at the plant's visible characteristics, he made a broad intuitive jump, linking *Hypericum*'s perforated leaves to an ability to drive away spirits, toxins, and parasites that had invaded the patient. Similarly, he wrote that the shy,

cowering nature of a plant growing in the underbrush indicated its usefulness for a shy, cowering patient. Similarity as perceived by Paracelsus was a match between his perceptions of the patient's inner nature and the healing qualities of the substance.

Boyd argued that these similarities are magical, not physiologic; that they are more intuitive or perhaps capricious than similarities discovered by the process of homeopathic testing (proving). He wrote, "In contrast the fundamental implication of the modern simile is: the similarity of a 'drug' to a disease is determined by a complete study of the real physiologic actions ascertained by actual experimentation upon a reasonable number of subjects."[2] Boyd tried to distance the modern simile of homeopathy from the magic simile of Paracelsus and others. However, throughout homeopathic history there have been homeopaths who emphasized the primacy of spirit over physical reality to an extreme degree.

A current example is supplied by Rajan Sankaran, a widely respected Indian homeopathic physician. Dr. Sankaran emphasizes the importance of proving symptoms developed by people who do not even ingest the homeopathic preparation being tested.

The most characteristic symptoms of the drug were produced in a woman (seminar participant) who had not taken the proving dose! She developed symptoms that she had never experienced before in her life, and they coincided with those who had taken the dose. A similar phenomenon was observed again at the Spierkeroog (N. Germany) seminar, where bacillinum was proved. The best provings were from those who had not taken the dose. This is enough to set the mind thinking for a long time.[8]

Boyd would have great difficulty characterizing information gathered from Sankaran's provings as physiologic.

In other examples of *similia*, Paracelsus has been quoted as stating the following: "Contraria contraries curantur, that is heat dispels cold; that is false and has never been so with drugs,"[9] "The simile, according to which you should treat, gives understanding to healing,"[2] and "Never a hot illness has been cured by something cold, nor a cold one by something hot. But it has happened that like has cured like."[7]

Both Paracelsus and Hahnemann applied the *similia* principle with great subtlety. Such subtle application demands that the physician comprehend the qualities that distinguish one patient or medicine from every other because of the precise concordance between patient and remedy. Individual inconsistencies or quirks are not trifles to ignore; rather, they are the key to unlocking the most difficult cases. Uniquely individual characteristics must be respected and understood to successfully treat the patient.

The obverse of this philosophic coin is that disease categories are imprecise. One patient's disease is unlike every other. Although two patients can suffer asthma, the specific qualities of their asthma and many other characteristics of each patient differ from the other. Much of the time, the imprecision of disease categories makes them practically useless. Just as each patient is unique, so is each patient's treatment different.

Paracelsus and Hahnemann held vitalistic medical viewpoints, in keeping with the spiritual values of their worlds. Paracelsus explained this viewpoint as follows:

The visible body has its natural forces, and the invisible body has its natural forces, and the remedy of all diseases or injuries that may affect the visible form are contained in the visible body, because the latter is the seat of power that infuses life into the former, and without which the former would be dead and decaying. If we separate the vital force from the physical form, the latter dies and putrefies.[9]

Hahnemann's take on the subject was that "without the vital force the material organism is unable to feel, or act, or maintain itself . . . without the vital force the body dies; and then, delivered exclusively to the forces of the outer material world, it decomposes, reverting to its chemical constituents."[10]

Accompanying the belief that healing comes from the inner, or more spiritual, essence of man was the belief that illness was a trial, and overcoming it purified the patient. Successfully navigating a disease purged and strengthened the patient. This is another philosophic canon of homeopathy that had been espoused by Hippocrates. Whereas homeopaths call it a *healing crisis*, others call this principle *"coction"*— essentially cooking out the impurity. Although ancient, the idea had fallen out of favor until Paracelsus revived it.

Other Philosophic Similarities

Paracelsus insisted upon consideration of the entirety (anatomie) of the patient and of the drug. On the patient side of the equation, homeopaths call this the totality of symptoms. A clear image of each must be developed in the mind's eye of the physician.

Now the anatomie of this external man should be completely developed by the physician and indeed so completely that he cannot find a little hair on the head, nor a pore which he has not found ten times before. Because from this out of the anatomie, the physician goes to the prescription, that limb to limb, arcanum to arcanum, disease will be placed to disease.

PARACELSUS, From *Paragranum*, 8, 87
(Sudhoff edition)

Because out of the entire man comes health, not out of crumbling fragments, and that is never considered in colleges and has at all times merely patched, not warm to cold, constrictive to laxative, that is not a basis for a physician and never has been.

PARACELSUS, From *De caduco matrices* 1, 606
(Huser edition)

So now you know what arsenic is, so heal accordingly to the content of the anatomie, the arsenic with arsenic, as anatomie teaches you.

PARACELSUS, From *Labyrinth. Med.*, 9, 120
(Sudhoff edition)

Pharmaceutical matters were very important in the case of Hahnemann and Paracelsus. Not only were their thoughts about the materials of medicine defining and similar to each other, their parallel relationships with the apothecaries were at best strained. These shared attitudes and beliefs generated much of the controversy surrounding their professional lives.

Both men believed that medications should be administered in a manner beyond considerations of material dosage. Long before the controversy arising from homeopathy's conflict with Avogadro's theorem, Paracelsus wrote the following:

Because drugs should be administered not with the weight but beyond the weight. Because who can weigh the beams of the sun, who can weigh the air or the spiritum arcanum? No one. But now in what way should drugs be administered? The drug should work in the body as a fire. . . . Can one find the weight of fire? No, one cannot weigh fire. Now a spark is without weight. Also the same is to be understood of the administration of drugs.

PARACELSUS, From *Vom Ursprung un Herkommen der Franzosen*, 7, 300–302 (Sudhoff edition)

Hahnemann and Paracelsus each extolled the virtues of the inner essence (Paracelsus called it the *arcanum*) of the medicine. Paracelsus wrote the following:

[one must] understand that the power all lies in a simple and the same simplicia needs nothing else than alchemy . . . it lies in the extraction and not in the composition.

PARACELSUS, From *Paragranum,* 8, 84
(Sudhoff edition)

Hahnemann wrote the following in his *Organon of Medicine:*

If this mechanical process is properly carried out according to these instructions, the medicinal substance that seems to us in its crude state only matter, sometimes even nonmedicinal matter, is at last completely transformed and refined by these progressive dynamizations to become a spirit-like medicinal force. This spirit-like medicinal force by itself is no longer perceptible to the senses, but the medicated globule acts as its carrier.[10]

Although Paracelsus claimed that iron miners could be cured by the toxin that poisoned them, he also maintained that the elemental poison had to be purified by the healer to become curative. He believed that processing a material could change its medicinal character, just as Hahnemann wrote centuries later: "And thus it is to be understood with regard to others, that what may be harmful to us through our hands, the same is also again fashioned by our hands into a remedy" (quoted in Coulter, p. 384).[7]

Controversy

Like Hahnemann, Paracelsus fought with the apothecaries. As a group, the apothecaries were powerful and formidable adversaries. This social reality does not appear to have tempered the attacks mounted by Paracelsus or Hahnemann. Paracelsus demeaned the pharmacists' practice of mixing medicinal substances and vociferously proclaimed their lack of integrity, as would Hahnemann centuries later.

The battle against the medical establishment was boundless. Again like Hahnemann, Paracelsus was not at all interested in excusing the failings of his professional brethren. He energetically and venomously ridiculed other physicians:

Not one of you will survive, even in the most distant corner, where even the dogs will not piss. I shall be monarch and mine will be the monarchy. . . . And I do not take my medicines from the apothecaries, their shops are just foul sculleries which produce nothing but foul broths. But you defend yourselves with belly-crawling and flattery. How long do you think it will last? . . . Let me tell you this,

the stubble on my chin knows more than you and all your scribes, my shoebuckles are more learned than your Galen and Avicenna, and my beard has more experience than all your high colleagues.[11]

All disease, except such as come from mechanical causes, have an invisible origin, and of such sources popular medicine knows very little. Men who are devoid of the power of spiritual perception are unable to recognize the existence of anything that cannot be seen. Popular medicine knows therefore next to nothing about any diseases that are not caused by mechanical means, and the science of curing internal disease. . . . The best of our physicians are the ones that do the least harm. But unfortunately, some poison their patients with mercury, others purge them or bleed them to death. There are some who have learned so much that their learning has driven out all their common sense, and there are others who care a great deal more for their own profit than for the health of their patients.[9]

Paracelsus died at age 47 or 48. Supposedly his death was the result of a push off a cliff; the rumor was that thugs hired by the local medical school supplied the push.

Paracelsus recognized the *similia* and other approaches to healing, and although there are parallels with and undoubted influences on Hahnemann and homeopathic thinking, Paracelsus was not a homeopath.

Swedenborg

Over many centuries physicians, philosophers, and mystics have discussed varying shades of *similia.* Certain plants or minerals are thought to be "like" certain patients. That similarity could be morphologic, physiologic, or perceived as some sort of mystical congruence. One of the great champions of this doctrine was the Swedish scientist and mystic Emanuel Swedenborg. The core of Swedenborg's mystical belief was in some ways *similia* writ large over the entirety of creation, and it held strong appeal to homeopaths.

Like many members of the Western intelligentsia and arts community (e.g., Goethe, Linneaus, Coleridge, William Blake, Balzac, Baudelaire, Ralph Waldo Emerson, Elizabeth Barrett Browning, Dostoevsky, Thomas Cole, Frederick Church, Yeats), many of the greatest homeopaths of the nineteenth century studied the spiritual philosophy of

Swedenborg.[12] John James Garth Wilkinson, an English homeopathic physician, was particularly important because he introduced homeopathic medicine to the English upper class and the royal family. Wilkinson was introduced to homeopathy by his Swedenborgian friend, Henry James, Sr., who had overcome a personal crisis through reading Swedenborg's writings.

Swedenborg believed there was a precise correlation between the physical world and higher spiritual realms. Entities in the higher realms would manifest in a cruder manner on lower realms down to the physical realm where we live. For example, Swedenborg considered the sun the manifestation of God's loving energy on the physical plane:

The first step down is the celestial heaven, which in its celestial love corresponds most closely to the One itself. The spiritual heaven is the next step down, a lesser representation, corresponding to celestial love, the love of one person for another. . . . The natural heaven is the lowest level of heaven. The world of spirits is the next level. Here men are opened to and discover their inner nature. And the world of spirits interacts with the inner processes of mind. Man's mind itself is a series of levels corresponding to all levels of the spiritual world, ranging from almost pure feelings to thoughts and ideas, to speech and gestures, to the body itself. Beyond man, animals, plants, and the physical world are further lower-order correspondents to the One. This whole series of existences corresponds to the One God who is thereby everywhere manifest. Not only man is made in the image, but creation itself is a series of images.[13]

As described by Van Dusen, this view of reality makes everyday experiences deeply symbolic and richly meaningful. Some homeopaths believed that accessing these higher realms through the medium of homeopathically potentized remedies brought healing down to the human realm. One of the most famous homeopathic physicians was Swedenborgian James Tyler Kent.[14] Kent wrote that a man who did not believe in God could not become a homeopath. However, another Swedenborgian, Constantine Hering, who was an equally important homeopathic physician and Hahnemann's most important pupil, wrote, "While there is good reason why Swedenborgians might prefer homeopathic treatment, there is none at all that homeopaths be Swedenborgians."[15]

Swedenborg lived a century before Hahnemann. His thought influenced many of Hahnemann's greatest contemporaries, including Goethe, who corresponded with Hahnemann and may have been treated by him. Despite the tantalizingly close connections, we have no evidence of a direct influence from Swedenborg to Hahnemann.

Hahnemann's Teachers

As noted previously, Hahnemann did not claim that he invented homeopathy out of nothingness. He credited his teacher with his achievements as a physician—"All that I am as a physician I owe to Quarin."[2] We also know that Quarin's teacher, Stoereck, advocated testing drugs for their opposite effects:

If stramonium makes the healthy mentally sick through a confusion of the mind, why should one not determine whether it gives mental health in that it disturbs and alters the thoughts and sense in mental disease, and that if it gives health to those with spasms, to try and see if, on the other hand, they get spasms.[2]

These influences are inadequate to account for all that Hahnemann created. The practices of Hippocrates and others contained only portions of the system Hahnemann developed. However, the quasi-homeopathic ideas expressed by Hahnemann's immediate forebears are evidence that the system of homeopathy represented an evolutionary development rather than a revolution in medical thought.

Summary

It can be reasonably argued that *similia* is still a part of modern conventional medicine. Consider the list in Table 3-1 of conventional treatments used for their homeopathic or *similia* effects.

Importantly, the applications of *similia* listed in Table 3-1 are unintentional and are easily recognizable only to homeopaths. Conventional physicians are not using "like to cure like" if they do not know they are doing so. When a conventional physician mirrors the practices of a homeopath in this way, it is entirely accidental.

Hahnemann's system of medicine looks much less radical when viewed in context. Homeopathy as a system of medicine grew out of a long-standing, albeit minority, tradition. The most prominent feature of that tradition was the *similia* doctrine. Modern homeopathy is an expression of several

TABLE 3-1

Conventional Treatments Used for Their Homeopathic or Similia Effects

Treatment	Causes and Cures
Methylphenidate hydrochloride (Ritalin)	Hyperactivity
Digitalis	Rapid heart beats
Aspirin	Fever and GI bleeding (cancer)
Radiation	Cancer
Chemotherapy	Cancer
Red pepper (capsicum)	Pain
Quinine	Symptoms of malaria
GABA	Narcolepsy

GABA, γ-Aminobutyric acid; *GI*, gastrointestinal.

ancient principles of medical thought, including the doctrine of similars.

HOMEOPATHY IN THE UNITED STATES

Nineteenth Century American Prominence

Homeopathy arrived in the United States in 1825, brought by Hans Burch Gram, a doctor of American birth who was trained in Denmark by a pupil of Hahnemann's. Within a few years of his return to New York, Dr. Gram converted several "regular" practitioners in the New York City area, and these physicians became the leaders of homeopathy in the state. This group was responsible for teaching homeopathy to several other physicians who, in turn, spread it to other states—New Jersey, Rhode Island, Massachusetts, Connecticut, Indiana, and Illinois.

At the time, almost all states had abandoned the practice of licensing physicians. There were many practitioners of botanic medicine, some of whom learned from Native American herbalists. At a time when regular medical training consisted of 4 months of lectures and 2 years of preceptorship, the care offered by herbalists was often better than the bleeding, purging, and administration of mercury compounds prescribed by the "regulars." Homeopathists stood apart from herbal practitioners in that most

homeopaths were converts from conventional medicine.

At about the time that Gram settled in New York, William Wesselhoeft and Henry Detwiller, two German physician immigrants living near Bethlehem, Pennsylvania, began studying Hahnemann's books, *Organon of Medicine* and *Materia Medica Pura*, sent to them by Dr. Stapf, a pupil of Hahnemann. When Detwiller cured a patient with a homeopathic dose in 1828, the two became homeopaths and introduced the system to others in their community.[15]

Constantine Hering, trained in medicine in Germany, had been working as a botanist in Surinam, South America. Introduced to homeopathy while a medical student, he practiced in South America before moving to the United States in 1833. He found the practice of homeopathy well underway in the German communities around Philadelphia, and he became the guiding force that brought the homeopathic movement together. In 1835 he founded, together with several other physicians, the first medical school in the world to teach homeopathy. Although the Allentown Academy, as it was called, lasted for only a few years, it became the training ground for some of the finest homeopathic doctors—the teachers of the next generation.

In 1844 Hering, with a group of doctors from New York and Boston, founded the American Institute of Homeopathy (AIH)—the first national medical organization, antedating the AMA by three years. The AIH has actively promoted homeopathic medicine and the dissemination of related medical knowledge ever since.

In 1847, conventional physicians formed their own national association—the American Medical Association (AMA). The question almost immediately arose as to what position the AMA would take in relation to homeopathic physicians. After considerable discussion, the AMA adopted the position that those "adhering to an exclusive dogma" (i.e., homeopaths) could not be members of the association and, furthermore, no member of the association was allowed discourse with such practitioners. Nearly two decades later, the White House physician was almost removed from the Washington Medical Society because, in the aftermath of the Lincoln assassination, he had talked to the physician of Secretary of State Seward, a homeopath. The hostility of the AMA toward homeopathy continued into the twentieth century.

In 1848, in Philadelphia, Hering, joined by Dr. Williamson and Dr. Jeanes, founded the Homeopathic Medical College of Pennsylvania, later to become the Hahnemann Medical College. Dr. Hering, often referred to as the father of American homeopathy, was a prover of many remedies, and the author of *The Guiding Symptoms,* a 10-volume *Materia Medica* that is in use to this day.

The practice of homeopathy continued to spread. Its growth was twofold. On one hand, many practitioners were graduates from the increasing number of homeopathic medical colleges that were founded between 1850 and 1880. Colleges were begun in New York, Boston, Chicago, St. Louis, Cincinnati, Detroit, Louisville, Detroit, and Des Moines, and by 1880 these colleges had placed about 5000 homeopathic physicians into practice.

The other impetus for growth came from the lay users of homeopathy. In 1835, Constantine Hering wrote *The Homeopathic Domestic Physician,* a book that gave instructions for using homeopathic medicines in domestic situations. Over the next 45 years, other domestic manuals were printed, and these books and their accompanying kits often became the only medical advice available to the far-flung pioneer communities. A doctor at the 1869 meeting of the AIH observed that "many a woman, armed with her little stack of remedies, had converted an entire community to homeopathy."[16]

At the Centennial Exposition in Philadelphia in 1876, the AIH held its first International Congress, and more than 700 homeopaths from around the world were in attendance. But the movement was beginning to split apart from within. The split had started in 1870 when Carroll Dunham, MD, the AIH president, proposed that the organization open itself to all medical practitioners—even if those joining were not committed homeopaths. His hope was that the "pure" homeopaths within the organization would teach the method to those who had but a smattering of knowledge. This "opening" was decried by the "pure" homeopaths.

At the same time, homeopathic schools were teaching less of the method taught by Hahnemann and more of an eclectic blend of therapeutics that combined simplified homeopathic therapeutics with conventional allopathic medicine. By the 1876 meeting, factions began to form. Dunham, try as he might, could not pull them together. The AIH gradually fell into the hands of the "half-homeopaths," and

the "pure" homeopaths established the International Hahnemannian Association (IHA) in 1880. Hering, who had been the glue in homeopathy, died in 1880, and the movement began to founder. Although "half-homeopaths" continued to run the AIH and the schools, a new leader arose among the "pure" homeopaths.

James Tyler Kent, an eclectic trained physician in St. Louis, was introduced to homeopathy when he consulted a local homeopath to treat his wife. Kent emerged as one of the prominent homeopathic practitioners and educators for the next 30 years. In 1890, Kent moved to Philadelphia and established the Post Graduate School of Homoeopathics. Kent's *Lectures on Homeopathic Philosophy* and *Lectures on Materia Medica,* still in print, were derived from his lectures at this school. With the help of his pupils, Kent assembled the *Repertory of the Homeopathic Materia Medica*—the classic reference work still used worldwide. Before Kent moved to Chicago in 1900, the free clinic at the school had treated more than 40,000 patients and the school had trained 30 physician who became the leaders in the homeopathic movement in the next century.[17]

Twentieth Century Decline and Resurgence

While new innovations were being made in the fields of transportation, communications, and architecture, medicine, too, was experiencing changes. Pasteur's germ theory had become well established. The German chemical industry developed a number of synthetic drugs, among them aspirin, and an eager public was beginning to use them. The French physiologist Claude Bernard had described the body as a machine that responded to the laws of chemistry and physics, and medicine began to be driven by "science" and moved into areas of increasing specialization.

Organized homeopathy, already experiencing a split within its ranks, did not cope well with the rise of "modern medicine." Beginning in 1900, homeopathy in the United States experienced a sudden and seemingly final decline. Although there were 12,000 "homeopathic graduates" in the United States at the turn of the century, most were homeopaths in name only. Few of them were really educated in the philosophy of homeopathy, and most were using both allopathic and homeopathic medicine according to their whim. Only about 2000 were members of the AIH, and fewer than 150 were members of the IHA, the professional association for the few that practiced "pure" homeopathy.

To understand how homeopathy stayed alive we must first look at the factors that led to its demise. One factor in homeopathy's decline was the rise of allopathic pharmaceutic companies, which earned significant profits during the Civil War and were investing the money in the medical establishment.

These companies slowly moved from traditional botanic medical products into the production and sale of "patent" medicines—compounds whose formulation was proprietary to the company. As historian Harris Coulter says:

The flooding of medical practice with these "proprietaries" represented the final conquest of the medical profession by the patent-medicine industry. . . . it was the newest avatar of the profession's unrelenting desire to simplify medical practice. The compounding of medicines were centralized, and the physician was spared the intellectual effort required to obtain knowledge of his principal means of cure. Instead of learning the powers and properties of medicinal drugs, he had only to memorize the names of series of specific compounds and prescribe them for the disease names of his patients.[18]

At about the turn of the twentieth century, the AMA decided to accept advertising for pharmaceutic products in its journal. Advertisements could list a product's ingredients—although the actual formula need not be printed—and its therapeutic indications. Advertisers flocked to the journal and drug companies became the largest source of income for the AMA.

A second factor in homeopathy's decline was the opening of the AMA to homeopaths. In 1901, the AMA changed its code of ethics to allow membership to "every reputable and legally qualified physician who is practicing or who will agree to practice nonsectarian medicine."[18,21] In 1903, the AMA rescinded its "consultation clause," which prohibited AMA members from consulting with homeopaths, and invited homeopaths back into the organization. Saying that it was time to forget sectarian differences, the AMA espoused the development of "modern medicine" and "scientific medicine." Local AMA societies began to recruit physicians. It was allowable to practice homeopathy—as long as you did not state publicly that you were doing so. Wrote one homeo-

path to a homeopathic journal: "I thought there would be an opportunity to discuss homeopathic principles and homeopathic remedies if I joined the county and national societies of the old school, and so put some leavening into the lump. I found, however, that I was counting without my host. Such discussions were not permitted, so I am coming back."[19] Dr. J. N. McCormack, the brains behind the drive to bring homeopaths into the AMA, noted in 1911, "We must admit that we have never fought the homeopath on matters of principle; we fought him because he came into our community and got the business."[19] "The homeopaths," says Coulter, "were caught off guard by this onslaught and it produced a crisis in the new school's affairs through the whole of the decade."[19]

A third factor in homeopathy's decline was the poor quality of instruction in homeopathic schools. Most of the graduates, never having been taught homeopathic principles, saw little difference between homeopathy and conventional medicine. They were taught a mish-mash of therapeutics that, when tried, more often than not failed them, and they "slipped" into a regular practice. The AMA, seeing this trend for homeopaths to resort to everything but homeopathy, saw it not as a lack in their homeopathic training but as a proof that education in "scientific medicine" was worthwhile.

There was a sharp drop in the number of graduates of homeopathic schools between 1895 and 1905. By 1910 the schools were already floundering.[20]

In 1909, the Carnegie Foundation, wishing to give money to medical schools but not having any standard by which to judge them, commissioned educator Abraham Flexner to conduct a survey of American medical schools. Flexner visited all medical schools in the United States and wrote an 846-page report that was issued by the Carnegie Foundation. Flexner noted the drop in the number of homeopathic school graduates: "In the year 1900 there were twenty-two homeopathic colleges in the United States; to-day there are fifteen; the graduating classes have fallen from 418 to 246. As the country is still poorly supplied with homeopathic physicians, these figures are ominous."[21] Although Flexner commented on the need for continued homeopathic education, his report was extremely critical of the facilities of the 15 homeopathic colleges still in operation. Many of them had inadequate facilities in general, and those that had adequate facilities had little clinical training for the students. Said Flexner:

Logically, no other outcome is possible. The ebbing vitality of homeopathic schools is a striking demonstration of the incompatibility of science and dogma. One may begin with science and work through the entire medical curriculum consistently, espousing everything to the same sort of test; or one may begin with a dogmatic assertion and resolutely refuse to entertain anything at variance with it. But one cannot do both. One cannot simultaneously assert science and dogma; one cannot travel half the road under the former banner, in the hope of taking up the latter, too, at the middle of the march.[21]

The result of the Flexner report was the closing of many medical schools, including most of the homeopathic schools. Between 1911 and 1926 there was a precipitous drop in the number of homeopathic colleges in operation. By 1922 all but three—Hahnemann in Philadelphia, New York Homeopathic Medical College, and Hahnemann San Francisco—had closed.[22]

A fourth factor in homeopathy's decline was the lack of commitment and the poor quality of homeopathic medicine practiced by many of those who called themselves homeopaths. This lack of commitment is personified by Dr. Royal Copeland, president of the AIH in 1908. Copeland was an 1889 graduate of the Homeopathic department of the University of Michigan at Ann Arbor. He was professor of Materia Medica at Ann Arbor, and was elected mayor of Ann Arbor in 1901. He was Dean of New York Homeopathic Medical College from 1908 to 1923. He served as Health Commissioner for the city of New York from 1918 to 1923 and was elected Senator from New York in 1923, serving until his death in 1938.

As Senator, Copeland introduced the legislation that would become the Food, Drug, and Cosmetic Act of 1938. This Act created the Food and Drug Administration. The problem for homeopaths was that Copeland (and many others) were trained in the "name" homeopathy but not at all in the "practice" of it. Judging by his 1934 "domestic manual," which has not a mention of homeopathy in it, Copeland had ceased practicing homeopathy by that time.[23]

In 1919, Dr. Edwin Lightner Nesbit commented on the decline of homeopathy in the *Journal of the American Institute of Homeopathy (JAIH):*

When Copeland says, "If homeopathy had strength enough, and vigor enough and old-time stamina enough to fight its battles now as it did in the pioneer days, it could accomplish enough in this generation," etc. I say,

"Yep, attaboy, and me too," meaning "amen." Only from this practitioner's viewpoint I would say, if our homeopathic leaders—like Copeland—had their vision enough ten years ago to see the inevitable trend of their truckling to non-homeopathic "standards" and to stand for "standards" of their own devising alone, the homeopathic branch of the medical profession would have had more and better colleges of its own today than our pioneers ever dreamed.[24]

Kent died in 1916. His pupils, in large part, helped to keep homeopathy in the United States alive during a time when it was seen as "grandma's medicine" and not scientific and modern.

With the 1920s approaching, homeopathy's facade was barely standing. Even the homeopathic successes in The Flu Epidemic of 1918 were of little consequence. Although the mortality rate for patients receiving homeopathic treatment was between 1% and 3% (considerably lower than the mortality rate of between 25% and 30% for those receiving allopathic treatment), the differences caused not a stir from the conventional medical establishment.[25-28]

A myth lays the demise of homeopathy at the feet of the "fanatical" high-potency prescribers, thereby blaming the very people who were responsible for preserving homeopathy in the United States. Although pseudohomeopathy failed to work for its practitioners and their patients, those who were using real homeopathic care knew its value. Like a persecuted sect that survives through the centuries by passing information from generation to generation, those who understood homeopathy as the methodology outlined by Hahnemann managed to keep it alive.

One of the leaders of the next generation was Julia M. Green. Green was born in 1871 and died in 1963. Her life spans the time from the beginning of the decline of homeopathy almost through its resurgence. Trained in medicine at Boston University (a homeopathic school) she began her medical practice in Washington, DC, in 1900. In 1921, spurred by her vision, 12 homeopathic physicians assembled to start a new organization. One of the first orders of business was to establish a postgraduate training program for physicians. The first course, 6 weeks long, ran in 1922. In 1924, the organization was officially incorporated as the American Foundation for Homeopathy (AFH). The AFH postgraduate school began to train a number of physicians who would keep homeopathy alive in the coming years.

The collapse of the homeopathic edifice was clearly seen by Rudolph Rabe, MD, an 1896 graduate of New York Homeopathic Medical College. In an essay in 1926, Rabe clearly saw the demise of homeopathy and placed the blame squarely on the shoulders of the profession itself and those who curry favor with the dominant school to the detriment of their own. Said Rabe:

We invite to our national medical conclaves and banquets, men prominent in the professional and office life of the old school and then pat ourselves vigorously on the back, for the glory of our achievement. But do we really achieve anything worthwhile by these press-agent methods? Does all this diplomatic tomfoolery bring us anywhere? We doubt it and look in vain for evidence. Has any Old School college seriously taken up the study and investigation of homeopathy? If so, we have not heard of it. On the contrary, the juggernaut of established medicine continues to roll relentlessly on and to flatten out all doctrinal differences. In keeping with every other department of American national life, we are undergoing a process of standardization, which is killing all individuality. We have become 'good fellows,' who applaud vociferously every compliment thrown at us, but in our eager running after the glittering chariots of the old school, are divesting ourselves more and more of such shreds of principle as are left to us. The end is easy to foretell.[29]

Rabe was 44 when he penned this piece, and he lived to see his fears play out. Four years after he wrote this, his position as instructor of Materia Medica at New York Homeopathic Medical College was abolished.

In 1935, the AMA's Council on Medical Education and Hospitals said it would no longer carry schools of sectarian medicine on its approved list. New York Homeopathic Medical College became New York Medical College, and other hospitals removed the word *homeopathic* from their names. Although these hospitals assured their homeopathic staff that they would not be dropping homeopathy, it was gradually phased out as the hospitals came under the control of conventional physicians.[29]

The Social Security Act, passed by the Roosevelt administration in 1935, was perceived by the AMA as an imminent threat. The fear of socialized medicine was very real to conservative medical professionals who were wary of any incursion into traditional American freedoms. For all of their differences, homeopathic physicians were as conservative a lot as their AMA colleagues. Lucy Stone Herzog, MD, an 1891 graduate of Cleveland Homeopathic Medical College, took the lead in attempting to form a united front with the AMA. A national committee was formed to act as a liaison with the AMA to protect the interests of the medical profession. In retrospect, the fears were unfounded. Although nothing much came of the joint committee in regard to the Social Security Act, the perceived acceptance of the AMA was important to homeopaths, and desire to forge stronger links between the two schools grew.

Royal E. S. Hayes was a graduate of the New York Eclectic Medical College in 1898. He was an early member of the IHA and served as the organization's president in 1926. He practiced in Waterbury, Connecticut. In a talk to the Connecticut Homeopathic Medical Society in 1951, Hayes recalled what it was like when he joined the Society in 1904:

Only one member was able to cope with chronic disease, improve constitutions or deal homeopathically with severe crises. . . . When a homeopathic remedy was used it was almost certain to be 1X to 6X. The 12th was high and the 30th had no medicine at all. . . . But at that time, not only was straight prescribing and the single remedy not adhered to, such supposed lunacy was tabooed and even booed. . . . While this was going on, perhaps to the lasting benefit of our art, our institutions were gradually "fading away." I mean really fading away. As you know, the external cause of this was pharmacal and medical monopoly in collusion with bureaucratic prerogatives. But ten times more ominous were the internal causes, that is, lack of understanding, fear of disapprobation, appeasement on the part of some, and the serenity and content of the purists. It was almost fatal. Many went over to the conventional caste and the ones tied to hospitals, asylums, clinics and colleges were too few to cope with the external pressure and infiltration. But the loss shocked the remnant into renewed efforts to improve their own therapy and homeopathic standing, so that now we have proportionately more real homeopathic practice with a minimal contingent than we had fifty years ago with a large one.[30]

By the late 1940s, Hahnemann Medical College, the only school ostensibly teaching homeopathy after 1940, was in disarray. The trustees, seeing an inadequate funding base, mandated more students be admitted. With more students, it became harder to teach at the levels required and scholastic standards fell. Some graduates were unable to pass their licensing exams. In 1945, as soon as the pressure to supply physicians for the war eased, the American Association of Medical Colleges and the AMA

Council on Medical Education and Hospitals notified Hahnemann that it was being put on probation. The teaching of homeopathy did not help its probationary standing. In 1947, the faculty and trustees voted to make homeopathy an elective. It became a single course, taught by a single teacher, Garth Boericke. In 1949, the probation was lifted, and Hahnemann Medical College divested itself of homeopathy. Said one student, "Antibiotics came in and homeopathy went out."[22, 23]

All along there were those who thought, somehow, it might be possible to retain whatever vestige of homeopathy there was at Hahnemann, and by doing so retain some amount of legitimacy for the practice. By 1950, it was becoming clear that such a vision was indeed a chimera. When Garth Boericke retired in 1961, homeopathy went with him. An editorial in the *JAIH* in February of 1957 speaks of the time:

Hahnemann was "put on probation." The resultant upheaval brought about a complete reorganization of its teaching program which eventually got Hahnemann "off the hook," but resulted disastrously for homeopathy. . . . but homeopathy cannot exist without practitioners. In essence, homeopathy in this country received its death blow when Hahnemann "got off the hook."[31]

By the late 1940s, homeopathy was in its final decline. Many young doctors had served in the armed forces during World War II and had learned the use of antibiotics and pain killers in the emergency work they did. When they returned, many of them were ready to apply this newfound knowledge to the non-emergency practices of the general practitioner. In the view of a 1948 graduate of Hahnemann, the most significant factor driving physicians into the use of antibiotics and injections was this—they already knew how to do it. And the public was willing and ready to accept the new and modern medicine. Said Rudolph Rabe in 1948:

Families which years ago employed loyal homeopathic doctors are now in the hands of the Old School. They have gone over to the Old School because they understand that school to be "scientific and modern." They want "streamlined" medicine, even though many of them ultimately pay a high price for their folly. Unfortunately, they do not always associate the disasters with their abandonment of homeopathy.[29]

Meanwhile, AFH postgraduate instruction continued under the leadership of a group of doctors who would teach the 6-week course even if only one person enrolled.

Anthony Shupis was a graduate of Hahnemann Medical College in 1938, and was one of the first to take the AFH postgraduate course after World War II. He was president of the Connecticut Homeopathic Medical Society, and spoke these words at the 1948 meeting:

The precipitous drop in the popularity of homeopathy in contrast to its meteoric rise to the present are a frightful phenomenon to behold. What has happened since the turn of this century to cause its undoing? Has time finally erased its utility? Has homeopathy finally proven to be just another passing fad to be regarded as just an "historical curiosity" or will Hahnemann still refuse to lie quiet in some dusty corner of medical history like other "centenarians"?

Everywhere about us we see our numbers diminishing. Our undergraduate schools are no longer ours, old school physicians have been substituted on the teaching staffs and the control of our hospitals usurped by the surgical and mass drug clique of the dominant school.

Although this is all too true, we are prone to accuse the old school of political skullduggery while whitewashing ourselves. Perhaps it would be better for us to turn about and view our collective selves as we are. In short, perhaps we have been too easily raped.

Let us question ourselves. Are we homeopaths, or better still, are we "fightin" homeopaths? Do we follow the teachings of Hahnemann or are we just graduates from where once homeopathy was only apologetically mentioned? How convincing were our teaching fathers? Have we pursued the study of homeopathy beyond our school borders? If so, how many have done so a whole week? These are but a few of the many questions we must ask ourselves.

How many of us have ever studied *The Organon*, to say nothing of Hahnemann's *Chronic Diseases, Lesser Writings, Materia Medica Pura*, etc., etc.? Have we followed the study of these original teachings with the writings of subsequent workers? Can we honestly say we are really homeopaths? Have we in the treatment of our cases exhausted the possibilities in our search for curative remedies? Have we satisfied Hahnemann's definition of the highest and only calling of a physician? Is it not high time we stopped blaming our "regular" school colleagues? Are not we, ourselves, to blame? Is not our blame the triple chronic state of ignorance, indolence and fear upon which breed the secondary factors to the detriment of our society and cause? It is time we followed Hahnemann's recognition of the outward manifestations alleviating internal ills and ceased suppressing our homeopathic feelings. If we can no longer recruit in our ranks the almost extinct home-opathically-minded graduates, then it falls upon us, as necessary, to attempt to educate our less fortunate regular school graduates. I am certain that there are among them many enlightened open-minded individuals who, given the opportunity, would avail themselves of it if it were offered. If we should attract only one, our purpose would be rewarded and our obligation fulfilled.[30]

The decline of homeopathy through the 1940s was gradual. The 1941 Directory of Homeopathic Physicians in the United States listed more than 6600 names. A number of the people listed had been in practice for more than 50 years—some graduating as far back as 1878. But few new graduates were coming into the marketplace while the old guard was rapidly dying off.

Yet the literature of the IHA at the time is full of vitality. It was as if the essence of homeopathy—the real heart of it—drew in tighter to protect itself from the outside assault. And those who were holding it together should certainly not be forgotten. They held it together by example; they did real homeopathy with their patients, and their patients, in turn, recognized the special nature of the treatment and worked to keep the flame of homeopathy alive.

When homeopaths pulled together with the AMA over the issue of socialized medicine, several homeopaths came to the conclusion that the "regulars" were ready to accept homeopathy—at least as a specialty in therapeutics rather than as an independent medical practice. In 1950, a committee was established by the AIH to investigate the possibility of a specialty board. There was considerable debate. Lewis P. Crutcher, MD, wrote a scathing article in the January 1951 *JAIH*[32] in which he called the attempt to gain recognition by the AMA "cowardly" and said that there are but two schools of medicine: "homeopathic and hypodermic." The drive, he said, was like "asking Protestantism to become a 'specialty' under the control of the Roman Catholic Church." But others within the AIH were urging that links be forged with conventional medicine. In January 1960, AIH President Elizabeth Wright Hubbard announced that the American Board of Homeotherapeutics (ABHT) had been legally incorporated, and they were accepting applications for the specialty designation *DHt*—Diplomate of Homeotherapeutics. It was understood that the AMA would accept homeopathy as a specialty if 100 people registered with the ABHT. When

100 members were finally granted Diplomate status, the AMA questioned the education of a few of those applying, and would not accept them. When others were granted the diplomate—raising the number to 100 again—there were more questions. The AMA never granted the ABHT the status it requested. Although the ABHT is still with us, the AMA has still not recognized homeopathy as a specialty.

In the early 1950s, the leadership of the AIH began to talk about bringing the IHA under its direction. In an editorial in the October 1955 issue of the *JAIH*,[33] Donald Gladish, MD, said it clearly: "As the numbers of the Institute members have fallen, their degree of homeopathicity is increased, partly because nearly all the members of the IHA are also members of the Institute."

Ever since the late 1940s, the annual meetings of both the AIH and the IHA had been held at the same place and time. With membership falling, it was only natural for the two organizations to merge. In December 1959, the *Homeopathic Recorder* ceased publication and was absorbed into the *JAIH*. At the joint meeting in 1960, the IHA disbanded. The AIH, for the first time since 1870, was in the hands of Hahnemannian homeopaths.

The 1950s were dark times. The United States experienced a regressive turn under the influence of Senator Joseph McCarthy. Political and social suppression was rampant. All unconventional ideas were looked upon with suspicion, and many alternative healers were prosecuted.

The stalwarts who kept homeopathy alive during these dark times were few and far between. In 1971, in his book, *Homeopathy: The Rise and Fall of a Medical Heresy*, Martin Kaufman wrote a grim summary: "By 1960, with few notable exceptions, the average homeopath was well over sixty years old. Every year, death further depletes the ranks. With only a few converts, the future looks grim, indeed. Unless this trend can be reversed, homeopathy will not survive for more than two or three decades."[34]

What Kaufman could not foresee was the rise of consciousness that happened in the 1960s and 1970s. While the Vietnam war raged, young people on our home shores flocked to a never-ending stream of Indian gurus and to Timothy Leary's call to "turn on, tune in, and drop out." Some of those heeding this call were medical students who were looking for better ways, and some of them found homeopathy.

One of these young doctors, Richard Moskowitz, summed it up beautifully when he described coming to the postgraduate course at Millersville in 1974 (quoted in Winston):

At first glance, neither the sleepy state college campus where the course was given nor the rumpled clothes and advanced age of the homeopaths who taught it augured well for the future of the profession. Most of the faculty were quite old and semi-retired, and very few were actively earning their living from practicing the method they were teaching us. It was as if a whole generation of the most active, successful experienced practitioners who should have carried the main teaching load were missing.[35] (p 340)

In 1969, Dr. Maesimund B. Panos, who had taken over Julia M. Green's practice in Washington, DC, attended the meeting of the International Homeopathic Medical League (LHMI) in Athens, Greece. One evening, while walking with a group of other attendees to view the sunset over the sea, she fell in beside a young homeopath and struck up a conversation. It was a chance meeting that would change the face of homeopathy in the United States and throughout the world. The young man "with the engaging personality" was George Vithoulkas, a self-taught homeopath who seemed to "understand" homeopathy in greater depth than many of the teachers at the time. In 1974, Dr. Panos brought Vithoulkas to the United States for the joint AFH and LHMI meeting in Washington, DC, introducing him to a whole new generation of homeopaths. The rest is the Rest of the history—this introduction helped fuel homeopathy's resurgence under a group of young physicians like Bill Gray, Dave Wember, Nick Nossaman, Richard Moskowitz, Karl Robinson, Roger Morrison, and Sandra M. Chase—all who went to study with Vithoulkas in Greece, and brought his ideas back to their practices in the United States. It was this group that became the "core" of the teachers for the next generation. Concurrent with these events was the rise of two colleges of naturopathic medicine in the Northwest. John Bastyr, a naturopathic physician who was deeply into homeopathy, helped to found the National College of Naturopathic Medicine in Portland, Oregon. Within a few years, another group of naturopaths founded the John Bastyr College of Naturopathic Medicine (now Bastyr University) in Seattle. These two schools graduated a number of practitioners who became leaders in the homeopathic community through the 1980s and 1990s.

The 1980s and 1990s saw a number of homeopaths from around the world (where homeopathy had continued to flourish), come to the United States to teach seminars and share their knowledge. Through the "dark ages," it was a few homeopaths and their patients who kept homeopathy alive. The AFH set up "layman's leagues," usually under the leadership of a doctor, to educate lay people about homeopathy (but *not* in the practice of it). The way lay people kept homeopathy alive in the United States was very different from the way they contributed to the effort in Great Britain. There, because of the legal system, the lay person was allowed to practice openly. And because so few physicians were interested in learning homeopathy, physicians like John Henry Clarke, frustrated with his efforts to interest doctors, began teaching lay people the principles of homeopathy. This was not the direction in the United States. Although there were lay persons' leagues in the United States, their purpose was to create an interest in homeopathy and generate patients for homeopathic physicians.

In 1946, when Julia M. Green wrote the 40-page "Qualifying Course for Laymen," the thrust was simply to educate people in enough philosophy that they might become good patients.[36] The official role of the lay person was to demand good homeopathy from their physicians. What they would do when homeopathic physicians no long practiced was never discussed.

The first lay course was held by the AFH in 1966. Dean William Boyson assured the Board of Trustees that "the laymen were not being taught remedies nor therapeutics—just philosophy." With the resurgence of homeopathy in the 1970s came an interest in learning more by the lay public. Looking across the sea, they saw the rise of the professional, nonmedical homeopath in the United Kingdom and tried to emulate it at home. The 1980s and 1990s saw the rise of several part-time educational programs (similar to those in the United Kingdom) that were training nonmedical practitioners. The question of the legality of such practice is an issue that concerns the homeopathic community today.

In 1833, when Dr. Quin, the first homeopath in England, came before the Royal College of Physicians, one of the censors advised to leave him alone because (so went the reasoning) homeopathy could not last very long. Two years later, when Hahnemann arrived in Paris, he applied for permission to practice. Several members of the Academy wrote to the Minister of Education and Public Health, protesting Hahnemann's practice and method. Guizot, the Minister, replied, "Hahnemann is a scholar of considerable merit. Science must be free for all. If homeopathy is a chimera or a system without inward application, it will fall of itself."[37] In 1989, when Martin Kaufman, the author of *Homeopathy: The Rise and Fall of a Medical Heresy,* was asked to write a chapter on homeopathy for the book *Other Healers,* he titled it "The Rise and Fall and Persistence of a Medical Heresy."

Early in the first decade of the twenty-first century, homeopathy has shown itself to be not a chimera, and it has certainly persisted. As we pass the two-hundredth anniversary of Hahnemann's first essay about a "new principle for ascertaining the curative power of drugs," we find that homeopathy is alive and well in the United States and worldwide.

References

1. Jones WHS (translator): *Hippocrates,* Cambridge, Mass., 1923, Harvard University Press.
2. Boyd LJ: *A study of the simile in medicine,* Philadelphia, 1936, Boericke and Tafel.
3. Dudgeon RE: *Lectures on the theory and practice of homeopathy,* London, 1854, Leath and Ross.
4. Coulter H: *Divided legacy: a history of the schism in medical thought,* Washington, DC, 1973, McGrath.
5. *PDR for Herbal Medicines,* ed 2, Montvale, NJ, 2000, Medical Economics Company, Inc., 2000.
6. Richardson-Boedler C: The doctrine of signatures: a historical, philosophical and scientific view (I), *Br Homeopath J* 88(4):172-177, 1999.
7. Coulter H: *Divided legacy: the patterns emerge: Hippocrates to Paracelsus,* Washington, DC, 1975, Wehawken Book Company.
8. Sankaran R: *The substance of homeopathy,* Bombay, 1994, Homeopathic Medical.
9. Hartmann F: *The life and doctrines of Phillippus Theophrastus, bombast of Hohenheim known by the name of Paracelsus,* ed 4, New York, 1932, Macoy Publishing and Masonic Supply.
10. Hahnemann S: *Organon of medicine,* ed 6, Los Angeles, 1982, JP Tarcher.
11. Goodrick-Clarke N: *Paracelsus: essential readings,* Berkeley, Calif., 1999, North Atlantic Books.
12. Larsen R editor: *Emanuel Swedenborg: a continuing vision,* New York, 1988, Swedenborg Foundation.
13. Van Dusen W: *The presence of other worlds,* New York, 1974, Swedenborg Foundation.
14. Carlston M: Swedenborgian influences in Kent's homeopathy, *American Homeopath* 2:24-26, 1995.
15. Bradford TL: *Homeopathic bibliography,* Philadelphia, 1892, Boericke and Tafel.
16. Bradford TL: *The pioneers of homeopathy,* Philadelphia, 1897, Boericke and Tafel.
17. Bradford TL: *Biographies of homeopathic physicians,* Philadelphia, 1916, Hahnemann Collection, Allegheny University of Health Sciences. [Bradford's Scrapbooks (35 vols)].
18. Coulter HL: *Divided legacy, science and ethics in American medicine 1800–1914,* vol 3, Washington, DC, 1973, McGrath Publishing.
19. Coulter HL: *Divided legacy, the bacteriological era: a history of the schism in medical thought,* vol 4, Berkeley, Calif., 1994, North Atlantic Books.
20. Kaufman M: *Homeopathy: the rise and fall of a medical heresy,* Baltimore, 1971, Johns Hopkins.
21. Flexner A: *Medical education in the United States and Canada,* New York, 1910, The Carnegie Foundation.
22. Rogers N: *Hahnemann closing: an alternative path: the making and remaking of Hahnemann Medical College and Hospital,* New Brunswick, 1998, Rutgers University.
23. King WH: *The history of homeopathy and its institutions in America,* 4 vols, New York, 1905, Lewis.
24. Nesbit, EL: A Research Institute (letter to the editor), *JAIH* XII(2):149-152, 1919.
25. Dewey WA: Homeopathy in influenza: a chorus of fifty in harmony, *JAIH* XIII(11):1038-1043, 1921.
26. Pearson WA: Epidemic influenza treated by homeopathic physicians, *Homeopathic Recorder* 34:345-348, 1919.
27. *Transactions of the International Hahnemannian Association, 1880–1946.* (Division under Dunham of AIH) Transactions of the American Institute of Homeopathy, 1870, pp 570–589; 1879, p 1180; 1880, pp 144–163.
28. Cook D, Naude A: Myth and fact, *JAIH* 89(3):125-141, 1996.
29. Rabe R: Can the school of homeopathy survive? *JAIH* 42(1):1-4, 1949.
30. Shupis A: Presidential address: the AIH during the 1940-60 period, *Homeopathic Recorder* LXIV(5):123, 1948.
31. Sutherland AD: Homeopathic examining boards (editorial), *JAIH* 50(2):55–58, 1957.
32. Crutcher L: Retrospect and prospect, *JAIH* 44(1):11-15, 1951.
33. Gladish D: A time for decisions, *JAIH* 48(10):314, 1955.
34. Kaufman M: *Homeopathy: The rise and fall of a medical heresy,* Baltimore, 1971, Johns Hopkins University Press.
35. Winston J: *The faces of homeopathy: an illustrated history of the first 200 years,* Tawa, New Zealand, 1999, Great Auk.
36. *The qualifying course for layman,* Washington, DC, 1946, American Foundation for Homeopathy.

37. Haehl R: *Samuel Hahnemann, his life and work,* 2 vols (translated by ML Wheeler, WHR Grundy), London, 1922, Homeopathic Publishing.

Suggested Readings

Boyd LJ: *A study of the simile in medicine,* Philadelphia, 1936, Boericke and Tafel.

Coulter H: *Science and ethics in American medicine: 1800-1914,* Volume III, Washington, DC, 1973, McGrath.

Dudgeon RE: *Lectures on the theory and practice of homeopathy,* London, 1854, Leath and Ross.

Goodrick-Clarke N: *Paracelsus: Essential readings,* Berkeley, Calif, 1999, North Atlantic Books.

Hartmann F: *The life and doctrines of Phillipus Theophrastus, bombast of Hohenheim known by the name of Paracelsus* (ed 4), New York, 1932, Macoy Publishing and Masonic Supply.

Hippocrates: *Hippocrates,* Volume I, Cambridge, Mass, 1972, Harvard University Press.

Kaufman M: *Homeopathy in America: The rise and fall of a medical heresy,* Baltimore, 1971, Johns Hopkins University Press.

Larsen R, editor: *Emanuel Swedenborg: A continuing vision,* New York, 1988, Swedenborg Foundation, Inc.

Van Dusen W: *The presence of other worlds,* New York, 1974, Swedenborg Foundation, Inc.

Winston J: *The faces of homeopathy: An illustrated history of the first 200 years,* Tawa, New Zealand, 1999, Great Auk.

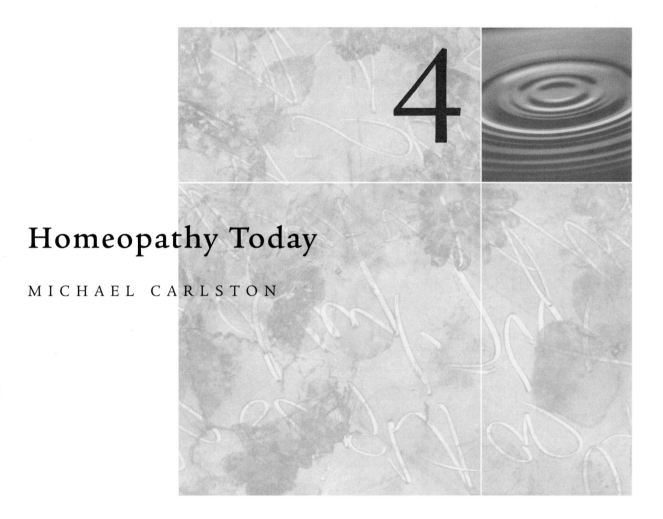

Homeopathy Today

MICHAEL CARLSTON

INTRODUCTION

The world has changed profoundly since Hahnemann's day. His followers have spread homeopathy over much of the world. Simultaneously, they have carried homeopathy, begrudgingly at times, into the modern world. Today the production of homeopathic medicines takes place in gleaming industrial facilities, and even classical homeopaths often use computers to help them select the correct homeopathic remedy.

Although many observers note the historical importance of its early nineteenth-century American golden age, much of homeopathy's worldwide popularity can be attributed to the influence of the British Empire. In the same way that homeopathy came to America in the medical bags of immigrating German homeopathic physicians, it experienced a second wave of expansion via emigration when it was spread throughout the British Empire by British physicians in the mid-to-late nineteenth century. The practice of homeopathy has very deep roots in many of the most far-flung corners of the globe. International gatherings of homeopathic physicians have been the norm for generations.

Although there are considerable differences in homeopathic practice from country to country, they are outweighed by the commonalties among homeopathic patients and practitioners. Worldwide, homeopathic practitioners and patients are tied together by the twin beliefs that healing should be as closely allied to natural processes as possible and that homeopathy works in precisely this manner. Because homeopathic thinking differs qualitatively from conventional medicine, a homeopathic understanding of a patient is available to anyone who studies a few readily available texts. A consequence of this accessibility is that patients are empowered to treat themselves, their families, and their friends. Lay practice and self-care are prominent features of the homeopathic landscape, essential facts for all health care practitioners.

HOMEOPATHY IN THE UNITED STATES

Who uses homeopathy? Who chooses a medical system notorious for its controversial principles, and why do they do so? Despite homeopathy's worldwide popularity, we have relatively little information about homeopathic patients as a group to help us answer these questions. A disproportionate amount of the available data are from studies of what we have come to call *complementary and alternative medicine* (CAM) in the United States. Homeopathy is but a small portion of CAM, and Americans represent a relatively small fraction of worldwide users of homeopathy. It is therefore difficult to answer broad questions about homeopathic patients worldwide. Despite the relative mystery, however, the data are sufficient to conclude that modern homeopathic patients, at least in the Western world, are different from patients who choose only conventional treatment.

Who Uses Homeopathy?

Homeopathy Is Growing Rapidly

One of the signal events in the rising awareness of complementary medicine in the United States was a 1993 article by David Eisenberg and associates in *New England Journal of Medicine*.[1] This study represented the first national measuring stick for "unconventional medicine," as Eisenberg then labeled CAM. The popularity of CAM surprised many and led to a swelling tide of investigation and even greater popularity.

Eisenberg's survey found only modest use of homeopathic medicine in his study population. In 1990, approximately 600,000 American adults saw homeopathic practitioners, a very small fragment of users of CAM at the time. However, the survey made a particularly interesting finding about homeopathy. In addition to the 600,000 adult homeopathic patients, another 1.2 million American adults used homeopathy for self-care.[1] In other words, approximately two thirds of patients using homeopathy did so without professional supervision.

Although the 1990 popularity of homeopathy was small, it had already been growing rapidly. In the 1980s, sales of homeopathic medicine rose at an annual rate of approximately 20%.[2] Evidence is accumulating that this rising interest has not abated, but that the pace of homeopathic expansion has actually accelerated.

In 1997, a survey by Landmark Healthcare[3] found that 5% of the American adult population (approximately 9 million people) reported use of homeopathic products in the prior year. Self-treatment accounted for 73% of that use. In addition, 61% of those who had heard of homeopathy reported they were either very likely or somewhat likely to turn to homeopathy if the need arose.

Eisenberg and his associates at Harvard conducted another national survey in 1997,[4] following up on their 1990 data. This time they found that the use of homeopathy increased fivefold to 6.7 million adults—3.4% of the adult population. They also found that the previous dominance of homeopathic self-treatment over professional care increased to more than 82%. This meant that 5.5 million American adults were using homeopathy without professional supervision.

Assuming that the popularity of homeopathy has continued to grow at the same pace, the number of adult Americans using homeopathy in 2002 would have risen to 12 to 13 million, with 8 to 10 million using it on their own.

Although these projections are impressive, a 1999 survey suggests they might significantly underestimate the popularity of homeopathy.[5] Roper Starch Worldwide conducted telephone interviews with 1000 Americans who identified themselves as the primary grocery shopper for their families; 17% reported using homeopathic remedies to maintain health.

Homeopathy in Children

As with CAM use in general, the use of homeopathy in children is disappointingly mysterious. Many of the most popular homeopathic products in the United States are specifically intended for pediatric use, and a number of studies have been published regarding the use of homeopathy in a variety of pediatric conditions.[6-9] However, we have only limited national data regarding the extent and nature of pediatric use.[10] Studies in other countries suggest that although the use of CAM is less common in pediatric populations than among adults, homeopathy represents a relatively larger portion of that pediatric use.[11-14]

Many who are concerned with pediatric use of CAM therapies are concerned about the children, whose use of CAM therapies is not self-determined. It is possible that children may suffer adverse effects from CAM treatment or from neglect of beneficial conventional treatment. A recent regional study raised this issue in the homeopathic community.

As a part of a survey of professional homeopaths and naturopaths in the Boston area, investigators asked how they would manage a febrile newborn infant.[15] Half of the nonphysician homeopaths reported that they would not immediately refer a febrile newborn to a conventional physician (slightly better than the 60% nonreferral rate among the naturopaths). Although the high incidence of this questionable response creates anxiety about the quality of nonphysician homeopathic care, it is only one small bit of data from a small survey considering one very specific clinical scenario. This finding was surprising because all major homeopathic training programs in the United States include instruction about appropriate medical referrals. Clearly, we need more data about the use of homeopathy among pediatric populations, and homeopathic educational institutions must be certain that graduating students recognize their limitations and the need to cooperate with conventional physicians.

Much of Homeopathy is Self-care

One of the most important facts for conventional health care providers to grasp about homeopathy is the predominance of self-care. This pattern is important, because most of those who use homeopathy are not doing so under the supervision of professionally trained homeopathic practitioners. Thus most homeopathy users are quite likely to receive their medical care from conventional health care providers. Because of the increased time they spend with each patient, classical homeopaths tend to see many fewer patients in a day than do physicians. As a result, in some areas of the United States the average busy primary care physician might see more patients who use homeopathy than does the homeopathic practitioner down the street.

Unfortunately, considerable evidence supports the belief that most patients who use CAM do not tell their physicians.[1,4,16-18] So, not only do many conventional primary care physicians care for a large number of patients who use homeopathic remedies, they are unaware of this usage. For the patient to maximize the benefit from treatment while minimizing adverse effects, the physician must be aware of all elements of that treatment. Homeopathy is especially challenging in this way because of its popularity as a self-care modality.

Patient use of homeopathy unfettered by professional supervision is not a new phenomenon, but rather a long-standing tradition. Since the middle of the nineteenth century, homeopathy's greatest popularity has been among laypeople treating themselves or family members, particularly mothers treating their families. For more than 150 years, until the late 1980s, the largest-selling book on homeopathy was Constantine Hering's *Domestic Physician*. Written initially as a self-treatment manual for Moravian missionaries, the author describes his book in the introduction: "It is intended to be an advisor in many cases of indisposition, when one will not or cannot consult a physician."[19] It was most widely used by "Dr. Moms" throughout North America. Professionally administered homeopathy has always been the exception rather than the rule.

CAM Demographics

More specific information, although still quite limited, is just now becoming available about users of homeopathic medicine. Again, because the bulk of data we have pertains to the larger population of CAM users, let us first consider that information and then use the meager homeopathy-specific data to differentiate the homeopathic subpopulation. The best quality data come from Eisenberg's most recent U.S. survey.[4]

CAM users had more education and higher incomes than Americans who did not use CAM. CAM use was most common among females, adults in the 35- to 49-year-old age-group, and Americans living in the Western states. All ethnic groups used CAM, although it was least common among African-Americans (33.1%).

These distinctions are only a matter of degree. CAM practices are so common that essentially all populations in all parts of the United States use them often.

Homeopathy Demographics

Demographic information about homeopathic patients is largely confined to data from two studies, Goldstein and Glik's survey of patients seeking professional homeopathic care in the Los Angeles area[20] and a national sample of physicians practicing homeopathy conducted by Jennifer Jacobs and associates.[10] Both studies surveyed the subset of professional American homeopathy rather than the more prevalent self-care. Although both surveys are limited in scope, the data appear meaningful and useful in our attempts to understand professional homeopathic practice.

Goldstein's regional study found a pattern of demographic characteristics that was much the same as the one seen in general surveys of CAM users. Homeopathic patients had above-average incomes and were highly educated, even more so than average CAM users. More than two thirds of the patients surveyed had completed a college degree, and 95% had attended college.

Jacob's survey, like Eisenberg's, found significant differences in the financial aspects of the homeopathic encounter compared with conventional medicine. Jacob's survey was conducted in 1992, which may alter interpretation of some of the data. Although both Eisenberg surveys found that well more than half of the expenses for professional CAM treatments were not reimbursed by health insurance, Jacobs found that less than 20% of homeopathic visits were not reimbursable by insurance. Given the recent growth in insurance plans that restrict the panel of providers and the rarity of homeopaths practicing within such restrictions, a new survey is likely to reveal significantly different insurance figures. Homeopathic practitioners commonly report that many of their patients with health insurance pay out-of-pocket for homeopathic services because their insurance does not cover visits to a homeopath.

Jacobs learned that the ages of patients seeking homeopathic treatment diverged significantly from those seeing conventional physicians. The portion of conventional patients who were elderly was twice that of homeopathic patients. Similar differences were seen in the 15- to 24-year-old age-group (5.2% of homeopathic patients versus 11.6% of conventional

patients). Patients aged 25 to 64 represent a somewhat larger percentage of homeopathic practitioners' patients.

Finally, given our limited data about CAM use in children, the data in this study add significantly to our understanding. Jacobs found that 23.9% of homeopathic patients in the sample were 14 years or younger compared to only 16.6% of conventional patients. Two of the three conditions most commonly treated by homeopaths (asthma and otitis media) are quite common in the pediatric population. Jacob's data and the popularity of homeopathic over-the-counter (OTC) products specifically intended for use in children suggest that the strength of the homeopathic presence in pediatrics may distinguish it from other CAM therapies.

Age	Homeopathic Physicians (%)	Regular Physicians (%)
>64	10.5	20.5
45-64	27.8	22.8
25-44	32.6	28.5
15-24	5.2	11.6
<15	23.9	16.6

Homeopathic Practice Patterns

Jacob's survey disclosed other highly important differences in the practice patterns of homeopaths compared with conventional physicians. Visit length, number of medications prescribed, and use of laboratory testing all contrasted markedly. These differences could certainly account for some of the appeal of homeopathy to patients who are concerned about overuse of prescription medication and frustrated by the increasingly limited time they have to discuss their concerns with their physician.

Homeopaths spent more time with their patients. Nearly 75% of homeopathic visits were more than 15 minutes in length, compared with 23.2% of conventional visits. Similarly, the mean duration of a homeopathic visit was 30 minutes, but only 12.5 minutes for a conventional practitioner. Given the great amount of clinical information required for classical homeopathic diagnosis and treatment, this dissimilarity is easy to understand.

Another distinction, which is obvious given the historical roots and philosophic impulses of homeopathy, is that homeopathic physicians prescribed much less conventional medication. Conventional physicians prescribed pharmaceutic medications in 68.7% of visits, whereas homeopaths did so only 27.5% of the time.

A final variation, which could prove interesting in this climate of economic restraint in medical practice, was that homeopathic physicians used much less diagnostic testing (39.9% versus 68.3% for conventional physicians). This finding may reflect nothing more than the high frequency with which homeopathic patients had already sought conventional treatment and already received diagnostic tests. This possibility was not investigated in Jacob's survey, and further study is necessary to determine the real meaning of this finding.

Why Homeopathy?

Why Do Patients Turn to CAM?

Astin[21] confirmed many of Eisenberg's demographic findings and also found that CAM users reported poorer health and viewed health holistically, encompassing body, mind, and spirit. They sought caregivers sharing this attitude. People who viewed themselves as culturally creative (i.e., culturally unorthodox), a term coined by sociologist Paul Ray,[22,23] and those who had an experience that transformed their view of the world were even more likely to use CAM. A significant percentage of CAM users become so because they find the philosophy of CAM therapies more congruent with their own values and world-view.

Although these attitudinal differences were significant, safe and effective results were still the patients' primary concern. While Astin found that many CAM users valued the health-promoting effects of such therapies, they rated the superior effectiveness of CAM therapies as more important reasons for their choosing them. The desire to avoid the adverse effects of conventional medicine and the belief that CAM therapies offer an ideal balance of effectiveness and health promotion was an attractive feature for people seeking CAM services.

A London survey[24] of CAM patients reached similar conclusions. These patients sought CAM treatment primarily because conventional medicine had been ineffective or produced adverse effects. In addition, communication issues and philosophic considerations came into play. Many patients chose CAM because of perceived communication difficulties with their conventional physicians. CAM users in this London survey, like those in Astin's survey, attached great importance to psychological factors in disease

and sought out practitioners who shared this perspective.

Rather than set us adrift, Astin's survey and others throw a lifeline to those of us who have invested years of our lives in conventional medical training. That is, patients seldom choose CAM therapies *instead of* conventional medicine, but rather choose CAM *in addition to* conventional medicine. *Complementary medicine*, or even the recently vogue term *integrative medicine*, more accurately describes patient use patterns than does the term *alternative medicine*. It appears that patients recognize roles for a variety of healing approaches, and want to use each of them as seems most appropriate to their health concerns.

Why Do Patients Turn to Homeopathy?

As with the general population of CAM users, most homeopathic patients use homeopathy *in addition to* conventional medicine. Goldstein[20] found that nearly 80% of homeopathic patients tried conventional medicine before turning to homeopathy, and more than 91% tried some other treatment before homeopathy. These figures echo those of Vincent and Furnham's London study,[24] which found that 80% of homeopathic patients had previously accepted conventional treatment for their disease and 96.5% had already seen a physician for the problem.

Goldstein's subjects sought homeopathic treatment primarily to cure a problem that conventional medicine had not. However, nearly one quarter of patients sought homeopathic treatment for general wellness, and others wanted relief that would allow them to avoid toxic medications.[25] This desire to avoid toxic medication echoes Astin's findings[21] regarding the motivations of patients seeking CAM therapies.

Vincent's study[24] gives us additional information on the motivations of homeopathic patients. Those seeking homeopathic treatment were, generally speaking, much like those seeking the two other forms of CAM studied (acupuncture and osteopathy). One exception was that homeopathic patients were more likely to believe that complementary treatment was more natural than conventional medicine. Another striking difference was that homeopathic patients expressed more desperation and a willingness to try anything to get better, which is probably connected to the finding that conventional medicine had been uniquely ineffective for the homeopathic patients. The remaining difference was that homeopathic patients were drawn by the belief that complementary medicine allowed them to take a more active role in their health care. Given the preponderance of homeopathic self-care evident in the United States, this finding is not at all surprising.

Although homeopathic patients tend to have different values from those of conventional patients, they do not reject conventional medicine. They are attracted to homeopathy's philosophy and patient empowerment, and their enthusiasm for conventional medicine has been cooled by their personal experience of its ineffectiveness or by adverse effects that came with its success.

For What Problems Do Patients Seek Homeopathic Treatment?

To analyze patient use of homeopathy, we must consider two categories: professional care and self-treatment. On the professional side, our data come from Goldstein's 1994-1995 Los Angeles area survey[20] and Jacob and associate's 1992 national survey.[10]

Goldstein's subjects sought homeopathic treatment for chronic complaints, with more than 75% having the primary complaint for more than 6 months. Although the problems (patient-defined) were understandably diverse, the most common were chronic pain, anxiety, back problems, chronic fatigue syndrome, addictions, headaches, and arthritis. Astin, too, found that use of homeopathy was common among patients with arthritis and rheumatism, ranking behind only exercise and chiropractic treatment.[21]

Jacob's data on the diagnoses of homeopathic patients are the most extensive we possess. Table 4-1 provides frequency data for diagnosis categories defined by the medical professionals surveyed in the 1990 National Ambulatory Medical Care Survey conducted by the National Center for Health Statistics and the U.S. Bureau of the Census[26] and in Jacob's survey.

Swayne reported similar data in a 1987 survey of homeopathic medical doctors in the United Kingdom.[27] Although the paper contains less specific diagnostic data in its comparison of homeopathic physicians with conventional physicians, similar patterns are evident. Most notable is that homeopaths diagnose twice as many of their patients with mental disorders than do conventional physicians.

The data gathered from these studies are congruent with information gleaned from discussions among homeopathic physicians. It appears that patients seek professional homeopathic treatment primarily for chronic health problems, possibly influenced by the limited number of homeopathic professionals or perhaps because many patients elect to self-treat acute conditions. In addition, many of the professional homeopaths practicing without a medical license refuse patients with acute conditions and treat only patients with chronic diseases.

Information about self-treatment is understandably difficult to come by. Perhaps the best data are sales information from manufacturers of homeopathic pharmaceutics. As of late 1999, 94% of U.S. health food stores, 72% of chain pharmacies, and 30% of independent pharmacies carried homeopathic medicines.[27a]

TABLE 4-1

Ten Most Common Principal Diagnoses of Patients Seeking Care from Physicians Using Homeopathic Medicine Compared with Physicians Using Conventional Medicine[10,26]

Homeopathic Medicine (n = 1177)	Cases (%)	Conventional Medicine (n = 11,614)	Cases (%)
Asthma	4.9%	Hypertension	6.4%
Depression	3.5%	Upper respiratory infection	3.9%
Otitis media	3.5%	Otitis media	3.1%
Allergic rhinitis	3.4%	Diabetes mellitus	2.9%
Headache/migraine	3.2%	Acute pharyngitis	2.6%
Neurotic disorders	2.9%	Chronic sinusitis	2.6%
Allergy (nonspecific)	2.8%	Bronchitis	2.6%
Dermatitis, eczema	2.6%	Sprains/strains	1.7%
Arthritis	2.5%	Back disorders	1.4%
Hypertension	2.4%	Allergic rhinitis	1.4%

Traditionally, homeopathic remedies used by professionals consisted of a single homeopathically processed chemical or biological component. Many products now used by laypeople, however, are combinations of several individual homeopathic remedies deemed helpful for a specified condition. They are labeled appealingly by indication, thus simplifying the selection process for the consumer. The product Calms Forte is currently the fifth-largest-selling OTC sleep aid in the United States. Hyland's Teething Tablets are currently the third-largest-selling OTC product for mouth pain (primarily teething) in the United States.[28] In 1998, the number of Americans who chose the homeopathic flu preparation *Oscillococcinum* to treat their illness equaled the total of all prescriptions for conventional influenza medications.[27a]

These snippets suggest a few conclusions. Combination homeopathic products are highly popular. They appear to outstrip sales of classically prepared individual homeopathic remedies. Their popularity extends to a variety of conditions, some of which are pediatric in nature. Specific products appear to have established a therapeutic identity, which might have little to do with their homeopathic composition. We don't know how many Americans who purchase homeopathic remedies know anything about homeopathic principles or even realize that their purchase is a homeopathic product. For example, a recent British study found that less than 5% of people in a random sample mentioned the idea of using like to treat like when defining homeopathy, although 30% reported they had received homeopathic treatment.[29]

People tend to use homeopathic self-treatment for minor acute complaints. Food and Drug Administration (FDA) regulation of OTC product labeling, including homeopathic remedies, generally discourages self-treatment of chronic conditions. Homeopathic tradition and principles also discourage self-care for chronic or serious conditions because of the complexity of collecting the detailed information needed for these conditions. The self-assessment required is at best extremely difficult. On the other hand, homeopathic tradition strongly supports self-treatment for minor acute conditions and FDA regulations do not discourage this tradition.

It seems fair to conclude there are two distinctive patterns in the clinical application of homeopathy. Most widespread is patient use of homeopathy to treat minor acute conditions independent of professional advice. It appears that this application of homeopathy is not founded on any significant amount of homeopathic expertise among the users. The other pattern, entirely different in character, is patients seeking out highly trained homeopathic professionals for treatment of long-standing health complaints that are unrelieved by other therapies. These patient-professional interactions involve lengthy, detailed consideration of the patient's complaints.

Although these generalizations appear to accurately describe the American homeopathic landscape, worldwide the picture is inevitably more complex. In France, homeopathy might be more popular than anywhere else, with more than 36% of the population using homeopathy in 1992. Quite unlike American usage patterns, 80% of homeopathic medicine used in France is dispensed by prescription.[30-32]

The Medical Profession and Homeopathy

Ever since its founding by Hahnemann, homeopathy has usually been in conflict with orthodox medicine. Considering the fevered intensity of many past battles, the present relationship is positively affectionate by comparison. Today, conflict more often takes the form of collegial debate, as exemplified by the gentlemanly correspondence published in the *British Medical Journal*, than the pitched battle of the nineteenth century.[33] Conventional medicine by no means accepts the legitimacy of homeopathic principles, but the homeopathic community has gained respect for its attempts to produce rigorous experimental investigations of the method.

The oppositional attitude historically so common between conventional and homeopathic physicians appears to derive largely from the conventional belief that homeopathy is "obviously" ineffective. This conclusion, which logically proceeds from rejection of the homeopathic principle of dilution, is seemingly obvious, because how could anyone believe that nothing (a postavogadran dilution) can exert any physiologic effect whatever? The erosive influence of positive findings (in homeopathic clinical trials) on this theoretic objection to homeopathic principles should not be underestimated. In view of the seeming impossibility of physiologic effects, positive findings are surprising and make the "obvious" conclusion less so. The positive trials published in major medical journals have attracted a great deal of attention, and each study opens the door between conventional and homeopathic medicine just a little bit wider. Although these trials have not convinced large numbers of physicians that homeopathy is efficacious, they have made it increasingly difficult for conventional physicians to simply reject homeopathy out of hand.

In addition (and somewhat ironically, given the nature of the previous criticism), some believe homeopathy is dangerous because many homeopathic medicines are made from toxic substances. The process of manufacturing homeopathic medicines is largely one of diluting the source material. Because the dosages most commonly used meet or exceed Avogadro's number, toxicity should not be an issue. However, if undiluted doses of raw source material were used, toxicity could become a concern. Fortunately, homeopathic regulatory agencies, in concert with the FDA, have been working for many years to eliminate this possibility.

Another factor that sometimes contributes to conventional medical hostility toward homeopathy is the tendency to confuse homeopathy with other forms of complementary medicine. For example, occasionally publications in the medical literature refer to toxic effects from homeopathic medicines. Further investigation reveals that the suspect treatment was in fact an herbal preparation or some other treatment that was misidentified as homeopathic.[34,35] Hopefully, as editors and reviewers for medical journals learn more about homeopathy, these errors will disappear and we will get more reliable information about adverse reactions to homeopathic remedies.

A survey of Dutch rheumatologists, their patients, and complementary medicine, including homeopathy, found that rheumatologists who reported a dislike of alternative medicine scored lower in all measures of patient satisfaction than did rheumatologists with a positive attitude toward alternative medicine.[36] This was despite patients' inability to recognize their rheumatologist's favorable or unfavorable bias. Rather than simply putting black hats on those "bad guy" rheumatologists, perhaps this instead reflects a tendency for CAM-inclined physicians to be more people-oriented. This hypothesis makes sense given the relationship-intensive quality of many forms of CAM, particularly homeopathy.

Physicians with better interpersonal skills are simply better liked by patients. Physician antagonism toward CAM could therefore be fueled, to an uncertain degree, by competitive jealousy.

Although a minority of physicians currently believe that homeopathy is a useful or legitimate medical practice, this minority represents a significant percentage of physicians. Regard for homeopathy varies significantly by locale. In the Netherlands, for example, 45% of physicians who do not themselves use homeopathy believe it is effective in the treatment of upper respiratory infections and hayfever, and 30% believe homeopathy is effective for chronic joint problems.[37]

In 1997, Astin and associates reviewed the surveys, published anywhere in the world from 1982-1995, of physicians' use of and attitudes toward CAM.[38] At 25%, homeopathy was in the middle of the range of effectiveness ratings assigned to CAM therapies (range 1% to 53%). Although many of these surveys reflected the greater enthusiasm for CAM and homeopathy typical of non-American physicians, it is interesting to contrast the much lower acceptance of the world's most common CAM practice, herbal medicine, at 13%. Most studies reviewed showed the same relative hierarchy of popularity among CAM methods, with chiropractic rated more highly than acupuncture, which is rated more highly than homeopathy.

Also in 1997, Berman and associates[39] surveyed U.S. primary care physicians regarding their CAM training, attitudes, and practice patterns. They found that 18.4% of physicians surveyed believed that homeopathy was a legitimate medical practice, significantly less than the 27% who believed homeopathy was efficacious in Berman and associate's earlier regional survey[40] of physicians in the Chesapeake Bay Area. When Sikand and Laken[41] surveyed Michigan pediatricians about their CAM use and attitudes, 21% felt that homeopathy might be effective, 12.1% believed that homeopathy is safe, and a slightly larger group (13.5%) stated that they believe homeopathy might be harmful. This modest belief in homeopathy's effectiveness is congruent with the modest use figures discussed later. If more physicians believed homeopathy effective, more physicians would use it.

Attitudes toward homeopathy are changing inside medicine and among the general populace. In some ways they go hand in hand. This warming influence in relations arises from the nature of evidence in medicine. Although medicine prides itself as a scientific discipline, physician beliefs appear more readily influenced by anecdotal evidence and personal experience than by research. For example, a survey[42] of the attitudes of 145 British general practitioners in the mid-1980s found that their views about CAM were most influenced by observed patient benefit (41%) and personal or family experience (38%).

The immense variability of clinical medicine makes conclusive research evidence of the "right way" to manage every single patient nearly impossible. Perhaps this real-world uncertainty generates physician mistrust of results from the idealized world of clinical trials. Whatever the reasons for physicians favoring experience over research, the repercussions are clear. With more patients turning to complementary medicine, including homeopathy, more physicians inevitably hear of a patient's or family member's experience with homeopathy. If these stories are predominantly positive—telling how homeopathy helped with a medical problem—the weight of these favorable impressions creates a favorable disposition toward homeopathy. Astin and colleagues' meta-analysis[38] supported this theory, finding a direct correlation between physicians' interest in and favorable attitude toward a therapy and the popularity of the therapy.

All studies we are aware of show that younger physicians are most favorably inclined toward CAM generally and homeopathy specifically. This suggests that even the passage of time alone is likely to improve acceptance of homeopathic medicine within the medical community.

Although there are dissenters, the net result of these shifting attitudes is that some parts of alternative medicine gradually become conventional.[43] Unorthodox practices become the new orthodoxy, as occurred with relaxation therapies and biofeedback. Various forms of dietary supplementation have gone through this process in recent years, including B vitamin supplementation to prevent neural tube defects and cardiovascular disease and raising recommended vitamin C consumption levels above those needed merely to prevent disease. Perhaps the best CAM example is the newly orthodox application of acupuncture for the treatment of acute and chronic pain.[44]

Can we expect homeopathy to become orthodox? Even *asking* this question seems startling, considering the prevailing attitudes of the recent past. Given the pace of recent changes, anything, perhaps even homeopathy becoming conventional in certain circumstances, seems imaginable.

Referral. Once a physician accepts the validity of a treatment such as homeopathy, it is a matter of time before he or she begins to refer patients for the treatment. For the practicing physician, referral is the middle ground; it falls short of committing the time and energy needed to learn to apply the therapy, but it is nonetheless an acknowledgment that the therapy has a legitimate role to play in health care. Also inherent in the referral is recognition of the limitations of the health care the physician is able to provide to the patient. Or, as one local endocrinologist humorously said to me when he referred a patient, "I wondered whether the voodoo you do would work any better than the voodoo I do."

Data from throughout the world show that conventional physicians are often comfortable referring patients for alternative medical treatments. In a 1987 survey[45] of 360 Dutch physicians, 90% referred patients for complementary therapies of one type or another. Referral rates vary by country and specific therapy.

Conventional physicians refer patients for homeopathic treatment at wildly variable rates, depending on their geographic location and the patient's diagnosis. Astin's 1997 review of the literature[38] found that medical referral rates for homeopathy ranged from 3% to 42%, with the higher rates occurring in Europe. The mean rate for homeopathy was 15%, compared with 43% for acupuncture, 40% for chiropractic, and 4% for herbal medicine.

Wharton and Lewith's 1985 survey[42] of British general practitioners found that 42% had referred to homeopathically trained physicians in the previous year. A study of Dutch physicians[46] shows referral rates up to 42% for certain diseases, particularly arthritic conditions.

In American studies,[47,48] referral rates for homeopathy consistently fall below 10%. For example, Berman's Chesapeake Bay Area survey[40] found that 5% of physicians reported some use of homeopathy, and only 6% referred patients for homeopathic treatment. A sample of Michigan pediatricians found that although 50.3% would refer for some form of CAM, only 4% would refer patients for homeopathic treatment.[41]

Use. In these days of growing acceptance of complementary medicine, many conventionally trained physicians offer some sort of complementary therapies to their patients. The old "us against them" attitude fades as dividing lines erode. Medical insurers and many large medical groups are beginning to see knowledge of complementary medicine as a desirable quality in new physicians.

Despite the growing appreciation of complementary medicine in conventional medical practice, a relatively small group of conventionally trained American physicians provides homeopathic care to their patients. The American Institute of Homeopathy (AIH), the homeopathic counterpart to the American Medical Association (AMA), has fewer than 500 members. This number is misleading because AIH membership is much rarer than is the use of homeopathy among American physicians. Sikand and Laken's Michigan survey of pediatricians[41] found that although 37% used some form of CAM in their personal lives, only 5.5% reported that they or their family used homeopathy, and only 1.1% used homeopathy professionally. Although 10.3% used some form of CAM with patients, only 1.1% used homeopathy in a professional capacity. Berman's survey[40] of Chesapeake Bay physicians found that 5% had used homeopathy. His later national survey[39] asked physicians if they "had used" or "would use" complementary therapies. Regarding homeopathy, 5.9% reported they had used homeopathy and another 27.9% reported they would use homeopathy (a total of 33.8%). Total figures by specialty were 26.3% for pediatrics, 29.4% for internal medicine, and 41.2% for family and general practice.

Astin's international review[38] of studies published between 1982 and 1995 found 9% of conventional physicians using homeopathy with patients. The range was enormous. Although many countries had use rates in the single digits, at the other extreme 45% of German physicians reported using homeopathy, along with 40% of Dutch and 37% of British general practitioners. Given the high level of use in France and the required homeopathic training in French medical education, the paucity of data from that country is disappointing.

Although growing rapidly, the use of complementary medicine generally remains a minority practice among conventionally trained physicians in America. Homeopathy is an even rarer tool, seldom found in the medical bag of American physicians. The rarity of American medical homeopathy does not accurately reflect the presence of homeopathy in the world's medical community.

Education. Most studies show that physicians believe they know little about homeopathy. A Canadian study by Verhoef and Sutherland[49] found that 7% of general practitioners claimed they knew a lot about homeopathy compared with 24% for acupuncture. In Wharton and Lewith's English survey,[42] 79% of physicians rated their knowledge of homeopathy as "poor" or "very poor." Understandably then, physician desire for education about homeopathy is disproportionately high. In fact, with physicians' self-perceived lack of knowledge about homeopathy, it is surprising that physicians are as willing as they are to refer patients to homeopaths.

Institutions of medical education set the tone for each new generation of physicians by means of their instructional content and the attitudes expressed by instructors. Although medical education supports established ways of thinking about and practicing medicine, it can also provide the impetus for change. Throughout their careers, physicians experience some evolution in the way they practice medicine, but these changes tend to be incremental. Because most forms of CAM, and certainly homeopathy, are substantially different from conventional medicine, expanding the clinical practice of medicine to include them is *not* an incremental change.

The opinions of academic medicine are the defining truths of the larger medical community. Highly critical thinking is the foundation of academic medicine. In a climate of skepticism, unfamiliar theories are often subject to derision until they have been intently scrutinized. Academic medicine, which is notorious for criticizing even the most commonplace clinical practices for their lack of scientific rigor, is exceptionally dubious of CAM practices. The penetration of CAM into these truth-defining academic institutions is thus a highly significant trend.

Berman's 1997 survey[39] of U.S. primary physicians clearly demonstrated that familiarity with CAM translates directly into acceptance: "Our finding [is] that knowledge of a therapy best predicts its acceptance and usage.... suggesting once again that familiarity with, not necessarily scientific acceptance of, a therapy plays a major role in its acceptance." An important component of this process of acquiring familiarity is the student's conventional training. In the same way that (according to P.T. Barnum, at least) there is no such thing as bad publicity, there is no evidence that increased awareness of any form of CAM discourages physician acceptance. Teaching medical, osteopathic, and other health sciences students about CAM increases familiarity and therefore leads to further acceptance.

A recent Canadian survey of health science students' attitudes toward CAM disclosed several interesting findings.[50] Echoing Berman's findings, this survey found that, compared with other health sciences students, medical students knew least about CAM and were least favorably inclined toward CAM therapies, including homeopathy. Only 18% believed that they knew "a lot" about homeopathy (compared with 39.3% for massage, 37.7% for chiropractic, 32.8% for herbal medicine, and 18% for acupuncture). Despite their relative conservatism compared with other health sciences students, more than 57% of medical students believed CAM therapies were a useful supplement to regular medicine, and 88.5% believed that physicians should have some knowledge about the most common CAM therapies. Nearly half (42%) of medical students wanted training to learn how to practice some CAM therapy with patients.

In the spring of 1995, the Alternative Medicine Interest Group of the Society of Teachers of Family Medicine surveyed[51] all U.S. medical school departments of family medicine and all family practice residency programs to assess instruction in alternative medicine. This survey was the first nationwide survey of CAM instruction within conventional medical institutions. The survey found that CAM was widely taught in U.S. medical schools (34.0%) and family practice residency programs (28.1%). Some interesting information about the characteristics of the instruction also came to light from the survey. Instruction in CAM therapies was primarily elective (72.2%) and varied markedly in both content and format. In addition, marked geographic variation was found, with CAM instruction most prevalent in the Northeast (65.4% of medical schools) and Rocky Mountain states (50.0% of medical schools), but rare in the South Central area (7.1% of medical schools). Of those medical schools teaching some CAM, only a minority (18%) included instruction in homeopathy.

Furthermore, some of the data gave evidence of the growing trend toward CAM instruction in conventional medical education. While 34.0% of medical schools were offering instruction, another 5.2% were starting up courses and an additional 7.2% were considering offering CAM instruction. Roughly one third of those institutions starting or considering

additional CAM education were planning expansion into homeopathy.

More recent data confirm the growing presence of CAM as part of conventional medical education.[52-54] The most recent data from the Association of American Medical Colleges showed that 82.8% offered some CAM instruction to medical students. Most medical schools included CAM instruction as part of required coursework.

Our 1995 survey[51] found that only eight American medical schools offered instruction about homeopathy. The incidence of homeopathic instruction has grown even more rapidly than the impressive figures for CAM generally. A 1997-1998 AMA survey[55] found that 71 medical schools (56.8%) taught medical students about homeopathy. Sixteen of those (12.8% of all U.S. medical schools) included instruction about homeopathy within required coursework.

European medical education about homeopathy defies generalization. Germany and France require training about homeopathy as a part of every medical student's education. On the other hand, a survey[56] of all British medical schools published in 1997 found that only 12.5% were offering some form of CAM instruction, and only two schools (8.3%) made that instruction part of the core curriculum by requiring instruction in homeopathy. Homeopathy is taught, albeit to an unknown degree, in medical schools in Austria, Hungary, Spain, India, and Mexico.[57] We are unaware of any other published or formally presented data regarding homeopathic instruction in conventional medical institutions in other parts of the world.

We know little about the content of homeopathic education in conventional medical schools. As with many forms of CAM, homeopathy requires a significant amount of training to understand its distinctly different principles and their clinical application. It is quite unlikely that any significant number of conventional institutions of medical education offer enough instruction to really train homeopathic clinicians. The Society of Teachers of Family Medicine's Group on Alternative Medicine produced curriculum guidelines for medical schools and family practice residency programs in an effort to ensure proper instruction in the essential concepts of the most common forms of CAM (including homeopathy).[58]

SUMMARY

Although many of the deepest roots of homeopathy are American, it had nearly withered away here until the social reassessments of the 1970s gave homeopathy new life. Since then, homeopathy has been growing at an ever-increasing pace. It is now one of the many health choices routinely available to consumers, although much more commonly as a self-treatment option than as professional care. Homeopathy appears to be one of the most widespread forms of CAM used in the pediatric population. Homeopathic patients are well educated, concerned about overuse of medication, seeking help for chronic health problems unresponsive to conventional treatment, and impressively compliant to instructions from the physician homeopath. Over the past several years, homeopathy has established a presence in American medical schools.

References

1. Eisenberg D, Kessler RC, Foster C et al: Unconventional medicine in the United States, *N Engl J Med* 328:246-252, 1993.
2. Herbal and homeopathic remedies: finally starting to reach middle America? *OTC News and Market Report* 223-238, July 1991.
3. *The Landmark report on public perceptions of alternative health care*, Sacramento, Calif., 1998, Landmark Healthcare.
4. Eisenberg D, Davis RB, Ettner SL et al: Trends in alternative medicine use in the United States, 1990-1997: results of a follow-up national survey, *JAMA* 280:1569-1575, 1998.
5. Roper Starch Worldwide: *The growing self-care movement*, Washington, DC, 1999, Food Marketing Institute.
6. de Lange de Klerk ES, Blommers J, Kuik DJ et al: Effect of homeopathic medicines on daily burden of symptoms in children with recurrent upper respiratory tract infections, *BMJ* 309:1329-1332, 1994.
7. Jacobs J, Jimenez LM, Gloyd SS et al: Treatment of acute childhood diarrhea with homeopathic medicine: a randomized clinical trial in Nicaragua, *Pediatrics* 93:719-725, 1994.
8. Kainz JT, Kozel G, Haidvogl M et al: Homeopathic versus placebo therapy of children with warts on the hands: a randomized, double-blind clinical trial, *Dermatology* 193:318-320, 1996.
9. Friese KH, Kruse S, Ludtke R et al: The homeopathic treatment of otitis media in children: comparisons with conventional therapy, *Int J Clin Pharmacol Ther* 35:296-301, 1997.
10. Jacobs J, Chapman EH, Crothers D: Patient characteristics and practice patterns of physicians using homeopathy, *Arch Fam Med* 7:537-540, 1998.
11. Spigelblatt L, Laine-Ammara G, Pless B et al: The use of alternative medicine by children, *Pediatrics* 94:811-814, 1994.
12. Paterson C: Complementary practitioners as part of the primary health care team: consulting patterns, patient characteristics and patient outcomes, *Fam Pract* 14:347-354, 1997.
13. Witt C, Ludtke R, Weber K, Willich SN: Who is seeking homeopathic care: the spectrum of diagnoses, *Alternative Therapies* 7:S37, 2001.
14. Menniti-Ippolito F, Gargiulo L, Bologna E et al: Prevalence of use of alternative medicine in Italy: a survey of 60,000 families, *Alternative Therapies* 7:S24, 2001.
15. Lee AC, Kemper KJ: Homeopathy and naturopathy: practice characteristics and pediatric care, *Arch Pediatr Adolesc Med* 154:75-80, 2000.
16. Perlman AI, Eisenberg DM, Panush RS: Talking with patients about alternative and complementary medicine. *Rheum Dis Clin North Am* 25(4):815-822, 1999.
17. Anderson W, O'Connor B, MacGregor RR et al: Patient use and assessment of conventional and alternative therapies for HIV infection and AIDS. *AIDS* 7:561-566, 1993.
18. Elder NC, Gillcrist A, Minz R: Use of alternative health care by family practice patients. *Arch Fam Med* 6(2):181-184, 1997.
19. Hering C: *The homeopathic domestic physician*, ed 14, New Dehli, 1984, Jain.
20. Goldstein M, Glik D: Use of and satisfaction with homeopathy in a patient population, *Altern Ther Health Med* 4:60-65, 1998.
21. Astin J: Why patients use alternative medicine: results of a national survey, *JAMA* 279:1548-1553, 1998.
22. Ray PH, Anderson SR: *The cultural creatives: how 50 million people are changing the world*, New York, 2001, Three Rivers Press.
23. Ray PH: The emerging culture, *American Demographics* February 1997. Available at www.demographics.com; accessed April 10, 1998.
24. Vincent C, Furnham A: Why do patients turn to complementary medicine?: an empirical study, *Br J Clin Psychol* 35:37-48, 1996.
25. Goldstein M: Unpublished additional data presented at the Third Homeopathic Research Network Symposium, San Francisco, 1996.
26. Schappert SM: *National ambulatory medical care survey: 1990 summary*, Advance data from Vital and Health Statistics, No. 213. Hyattsville, Md, 1992, National Center for Health Statistics.
27. Swayne J: Survey of the use of homeopathic medicine in the UK health system, *J R Coll Gen Pract* 39:503-506, 1989.

27a. Personal communication with Thierry Boiron, President, Boiron Laboratories, France, November 1999.

28. Personal Communication with Jay Bornemann, Executive Vice president, Standard Homeopathic Company, Los Angeles, April 2000.

29. Furnham A: Ignorance about homeopathy, *J Altern Complement Med* 5:475-478, 1999.

30. *L'Homeopathie en 1993*, Lyons, France, 1993, Syndicat National de la Pharmacie Homeopathique.

31. Fisher P, Ward A: Complementary medicine in Europe, *BMJ* 309:107-110, 1994.

32. *EEC market for homeopathic remedies*, London, 1992, McAlpine, Thorpe and London.

33. Buckman R, Lewith G: What does homeopathy do— and how? *BMJ* 309:103-106, 1994.

34. Benmeir P, Neuman A, Weinberg A et al: Giant melanoma of the inner thigh: a homeopathic life-threatening negligence, *Ann Plast Surg* 27:583-585, 1991.

35. Boisset M, Fitzcharles M: Alternative medicine use by rheumatology patients in a universal health care setting, *J Rheumatol* 21:148-152, 1994.

36. Visser G, Peters L, Rasker J: Rheumatologists and their patients who seek alternative medicine: an agreement to disagree, *Br J Rheumatol* 31:485-490, 1992.

37. Knipschild P, Kleijnen J, ter Riet G: Belief in the efficacy of alternative medicine among general practitioners in The Netherlands, *Soc Sci Med* 31(5):625-626, 1990.

38. Astin J, Marie A, Pelletier K et al: A review of the incorporation of complementary and alternative medicine by mainstream physicians, *Arch Intern Med* 158:2303-2310, 1998.

39. Berman BM, Singh BB, Hartnoll SM et al: Primary care physicians and complementary-alternative medicine: training, attitudes, and practice patterns, *J Am Board Fam Pract* 11(4):272-281, 1998.

40. Berman BM, Singh BK, Lao L et al: Physicians' attitudes toward complementary or alternative medicine: a regional survey, *J Am Board Fam Pract* 8:361-366, 1995.

41. Sikand A, Laken M: Pediatricians' experience with and attitudes toward complementary/alternative medicine, *Arch Pediatr Adolesc Med* 152:1059-1064, 1998.

42. Wharton R, Lewith G: Complementary medicine and the general practitioner, *BMJ* 292:1498-1500, 1986.

43. Ernst E, Resch KL, White AR: Complementary medicine: what physicians think of it: a meta-analysis, *Arch Intern Med* 155:1405-1408, 1995.

44. Acupuncture, *NIH Consensus Statement* 15(5):1-34, 1997.

45. Visser GJ, Peters L: Alternative medicine and general practitioners in the Netherlands: towards acceptance and integration, *Fam Pract* 7:227-232, 1990.

46. Anderson E, Anderson P: General practitioners and alternative medicine, *J R Coll Gen Pract* 37:52-55, 1987.

47. Borkan J, Neher JO, Anson O et al: Referrals for alternative therapies, *J Fam Pract* 39:545-550, 1994.

48. Goldstein MS, Sutherland C, Jaffe DT et al: Holistic physicians and family practitioners: similarities, differences and implications for health policy, *Soc Sci Med* 26:853-861, 1988.

49. Verhoef MJ, Sutherland LR: General practitioners' assessment of and interest in alternative medicine in Canada, *Soc Sci Med* 41:511-515, 1995.

50. Baugniet J, Boon H, Ostbye T: Complementary/alternative medicine: comparing the view of medical students with students in other health care professions. *Fam Med* 32(3):178-184, 2000.

51. Carlston M, Stuart MR, Jonas W: Alternative medicine instruction in medical schools and family practice residency programs, *Fam Med* 29:559-562, 1997.

52. *1997-1998 curriculum directory*, Washington, DC, 1998, Association of American Medical Colleges.

53. Wetzel MS, Eisenberg DM, Kaptchuk TJ: Courses involving complementary and alternative medicine at US medical schools, *JAMA* 280(9):784-787, 1998.

54. *1998-1999 curriculum directory*, Washington, DC, 1999, Association of American Medical Colleges.

55. Barzansky B, Jonas HS, Etzel SI: Educational programs in US medical schools, 1997-1998. *JAMA* 280(9):803-808, 827-835, 1998.

56. Rampes H, Sharples F, Maraghs S et al: Introducing complementary medicine into the medical curriculum, *J R Soc Med* 90(1):19-22, 1997.

57. *Homeopathy in Europe: developing standards for professional practice of homeopathy in the European Union*, Brussels, 1994, European Committee for Homeopathy.

58. Kligler B, Gordon A, Stuart M et al: Suggested curriculum guidelines on complementary and alternative medicine: recommendations of the Society of Teachers of Family Medicine Group on Alternative Medicine, *Fam Med* 32(1):30-33, 2000.

Suggested Readings

Cohen M: *Complementary and alternative medicine: Legal boundaries and regulatory perspectives*. Baltimore, 1998, Johns Hopkins University Press.

Winston J: The faces of homeopathy: an illustrated history of the first 200 years, Tawa, New Zealand, 1999, Great Auk Publishing.

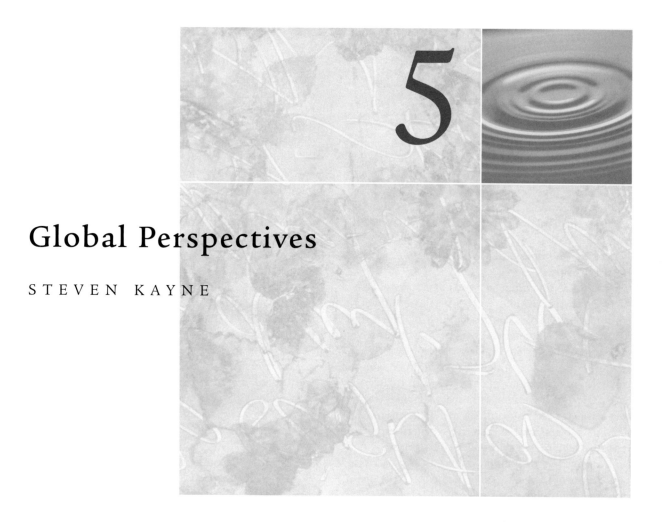

Global Perspectives

STEVEN KAYNE

The popularization of what might be called *modern homeopathy* owes much to international influences. Scotland, Germany, France, and the United States have played major historical roles in its development. Not surprisingly, on the continent where it was popularized by Hahnemann himself, homeopathy is well organized in Europe. Much of this chapter relates to homeopathic practice in Western European countries. Even within this relatively small geographic area, substantial differences occur.

WHY PATIENTS CHOOSE HOMEOPATHY

Homeopathy is one of a large number of nonorthodox disciplines collectively termed *complementary or alternative medicine*. The term *complementary* is preferred in many countries (including the United Kingdom) because it implies that the therapy can be used to *complement* other procedures, rather than to replace them, as inferred by the word *alternative*. However, there is evidence that consumers do buy homeopathic remedies over-the-counter *instead of* orthodox medicines, and the terms are often used interchangeably.[1] It may be that the preferred North American term, *complementary and alternative medicine (CAM)*, could provide a suitable compromise.

The popularity of homeopathy varies in different parts of the world. The most important factors influencing its popularity are public and professional expectations of its effectiveness. Typically, people have more than one reason for switching from orthodox therapies, reasons that vary with their background, culture, and the availability of homeopathy where they live. The balance of this section is devoted to discussion of these varied reasons.

Perceptions of Drug Risks

Many people consider homeopathy and other complementary therapies attractive because they are perceived to have acceptable risk/benefit ratios. Although perceptions are notoriously fickle and are often based on misconceptions, they are important to consider because they influence supply and demand. Perceptions of drug risks have been studied by von Wartburg[2] and found likely to influence patients' treatment choices.

The attitudes and perceptions of a representative sample of Swedish adults with respect to a number of common risks have been determined by Slovic and associates.[3] Respondents characterized themselves as persons who disliked taking risks and who resisted taking medicines unless forced to do so. Unfortunately, homeopathic remedies were not included in the study, but the results for herbal medicines show a very low perceived risk, only slightly higher than with vitamin tablets, and a perceived benefit approximately equal to vitamin pills, contraceptives, and aspirin. On the "likelihood of harm" and "seriousness of harm" scales, herbal medicines were again close to vitamin pills.

Vincent and Furnham[4] examined the perceived effectiveness of acupuncture, herbalism, homeopathy, hypnosis, and osteopathy in the United Kingdom. They showed that conventional medicine was clearly seen by the majority of respondents as being more effective in the treatment of most complaints. Complementary medicine was seen as being most useful in specific conditions, including depression, stress, and stopping smoking (for which hypnosis was perceived as superior to conventional medicine), and in the treatment of common colds and skin problems. Among people with a strong belief in complementary medicine, homeopathy and herbalism were seen as valuable in chronic and psychologic conditions, as well. Overall, herbalism appeared slightly more popular than homeopathy and acupuncture, but homeopathy was favored in the treatment of allergies.

Greater Attention to Symptoms

The great advantage of offering treatment with a holistic discipline such as homeopathy is that attention is paid to the totality of symptoms, not just the physical signs of disease in isolation. This may cause difficulties in countries with socialized medicine. In the United Kingdom, for example, general practitioners conduct their consultations on a 7- to 10-minute appointment scale; many patients believe this is insufficient time to deal with their problem adequately. It has been suggested that homeopathy appeals to patients who like the feeling that attention is being paid to more aspects of themselves than just the symptoms.[5]

Disenchantment with Allopathic Consultation

People who choose homeopathy may do so because of disenchantment or bad experiences with traditional medical practitioners, rather than out of a belief that traditional medicine is ineffective *per se*.[6]

Dissatisfaction with Efficacy of Allopathic Medication

In countries where homeopathy is not considered a realistic adjunct to orthodox treatment, patients may turn to homeopathy out of dissatisfaction with the efficacy of allopathic medicine, according to Avina and Schneiderman.[7] Worries about long-term use of certain medicines (e.g., steroids) also cause some patients to switch.

The "Green" Association

The media often portray homeopathy as "natural," and this approach appeals to the fads and fashions of the "green" lobby in many countries, particularly where the green movement is strong (e.g., Germany). In New Zealand, the fresh green image of the country is used to market "natural" remedies.

Financial Considerations

In the United Kingdom, most homeopathic remedies retail at about half the cost of an average OTC medicine, making them an attractive buy (in other countries, the cost of remedies is rather more expensive). Also, homeopathic medicines are fully reimbursable under the U.K. National Health Service. The net ingredient cost is, on average, substantially below the cost of orthodox medicines for a similar course of treatment, although this figure does not take into account the longer consultation times and does vary widely. Swain carried out a study on the prescribing costs of 21 doctors.[8] The results suggested that physicians practicing homeopathic medicine in the United Kingdom issue fewer prescriptions, and at a lower cost, than their colleagues. Unfortunately, there were several serious limitations to the study, not the least being that the sample was too small to allow generalizations to be made. Further, no account was taken of the extended consultation times involved. However, the survey gained considerable attention in the press. The results were also met with some interest by the health authorities and prompted discussions on widening the availability of homeopathy in the health service. Similar cost advantages have been identified among German dental surgeons.[9]

Even when prescribed, homeopathic remedies offer an advantage to patients. In nearly all cases, the cost of the remedy will be less than the U.K. prescription tax (in effect a flat fee contribution toward the cost of the medicine), but pharmacists will generally invite patients who are subject to the tax to buy the OTC remedies at the lower price.

Influence of Opinion Leaders

Demand for homeopathic remedies in the United Kingdom has been encouraged by the interest of the Royal Family in the discipline, especially the Prince of Wales. This effect has spread to New Zealand and other countries with historic ties to the United Kingdom.

Media Encouragement

More than ever before, patients are being encouraged to question the suitability of existing treatments. In her book entitled *Controversies in Health Care Policies*, the celebrated English rabbi Julia Neuberger states that patients should ask their family doctor a series of questions, including the following[10]:

- What is the likely outcome if I do not have the treatment you are offering?
- What alternative treatments are available?
- What are the most common side effects?
- Would you use this treatment?

Newspapers also encourage patients to ask questions about their treatment and thus make doctors accountable.

Cultural Reasons

A final reason for the increased demand for homeopathic products is increased mobility across national borders of people whose cultural backgrounds demand the use of holistic medicine. People from the Indian subcontinent, China, and Russia take their customs with them when they emigrate to other countries. Either from an inherent mistrust of Western medicine or a misunderstanding of what it can achieve, they look to continue using traditional methods that have proved successful over centuries. The recent influx of Russian immigrants to Israel has caused problems for the authorities in standardizing the remedies being used by their new citizens.

All of these factors have contributed to a significant and steady increase in the number of requests for homeopathic medicines over the past 15 years. In the United Kingdom at least, this increase has been matched closely by a similar trend with homeopathic veterinary practice for the treatment of domestic and farm animals.

INTERNATIONAL DEMAND FOR HOMEOPATHY

If the popularity of homeopathy is compared with three other complementary therapies across several European countries, we find some interesting idiosyncrasies with respect to individual preferences (Table 5-1). In Belgium and France, homeopathy is widely used and is the most popular of the therapies for which data were collected. In Spain and the

TABLE 5-1

Comparative Use of Complementary Medicine
(Percentage of Population Using Complementary Therapies)

Country	Acupuncture	Herbal Medicine	Homeopathy	Osteopathy/Chiropractic
Belgium	19	31	56	19
Denmark	12	—	28	23
France	21	12	32	7
Germany	—	—	—	—
Netherlands	16	—	31	—
Spain	12	—	15	48
UK	16	24	16	36

Data from Fisher P, Ward A: *Complementary medicine in Europe: report from complementary research—an international perspective*, Cost and RCCM Conference, London and Luxembourg, 1994, EU Science, Research, and Development Directorate.
—, Information not available.

United Kingdom, the manipulative therapies appear to be more popular.

Interest in homeopathy does not always translate into use. A survey carried out in Scotland by the *Times of London* in 1989 showed that about 40% of the population in that country considered homeopathy at some time when they were unwell.[11] The figure for the whole of the United Kingdom is likely about 35%. Only about a quarter of the people surveyed, however, actually converted their initial interest into action and used homeopathy. An interesting topic for further study is why so many respondents rejected the therapy. Considerable anecdotal evidence exists that the increased exposure enjoyed by complementary medicine over the past 10 years has helped greatly reduce the traditional worries about effectiveness.

Following heightened interest in the risk/benefit ratios of medicines in the 1960s and 1970s, United Kingdom homeopathy enjoyed a spectacular revival. The market value grew steadily from $25 million in 1994 to $30 million 2 years later. These figures pale in significance compared with those of some other European countries. Figure 5-1 shows the estimated value of markets in other European countries in 1997. France, for example, with a population close to that of the United Kingdom, had a market value of about 15 times the size.[12]

The 1998 market estimate for the United Kingdom is approximately $36 million.[13] This represents a 30% increase over a 4-year period. It compares with market growth of 43% for herbal medicines (to $78 million) and an impressive 100% increase for aromatherapy products (to $32 million) over the same period. Although the homeopathic market is increasing, albeit comparatively slowly, the trends in Figure 5-2 show that homeopathy's popularity is falling behind that of herbalism and aromatherapy. Experience suggests that this is a result of homeopathy's failure to capture new converts to complementary medicine in an overall growing market, rather than as a result of losing loyal followers.

According to Jacky Abecassis[12] of the French homeopathic manufacturer LHF-Boiron, the U.K. market is split nearly evenly between OTC products and prescribed medications. About half of the OTC market (25% of the overall market) is satisfied by pharmacies, the rest by health food stores and other outlets. In the Netherlands, 70% of people taking homeopathic remedies are thought to be self-treating without expert supervision. In France and Germany, the OTC market accounts for a much smaller share—only 20% to 30% and 27% of the total market value, respectively. In the United States, the low rate of prescribed homeopathic medicines has significant implications for the way in which the products are promoted.[14]

The value of the U.K. market for OTC homeopathic remedies is small, accounting for less than 1% of the total pharmaceutic market. Despite its limited value, the market is still considered significant for the following reasons:

1. The growing acceptance of complementary treatments by health professionals and the public
2. The increasing number of people now using such treatments regularly
3. The effect of complementary treatments on health status

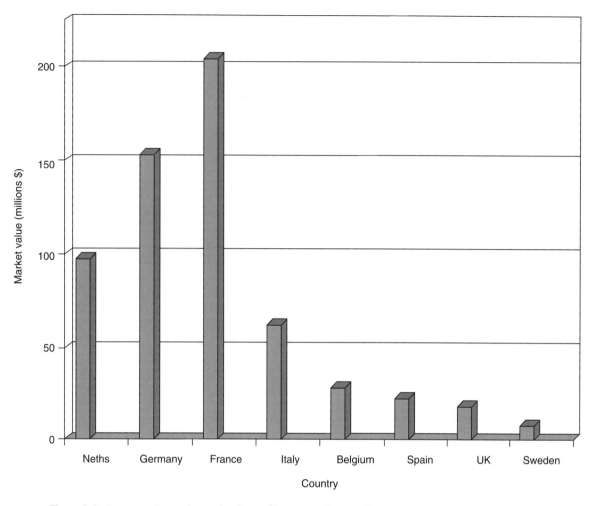

Figure 5-1 Comparative estimated values of homeopathic market in Europe in 1997.

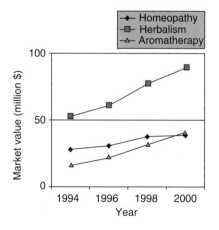

Figure 5-2 Estimated U.K. market trends in complementary medicine 1994-98.

4. The detrimental effect on clinical trials of participants being unwilling to admit using such treatments for fear of admonishment[15]
5. The high rate of use by older people, females, and health practitioners

In the Netherlands, the average per capita expenditure on homeopathy in 1991 was the equivalent of approximately $8.[13] This compares with an estimated 35 to 40 cents in the United Kingdom! The figures are not entirely compatible for a number of reasons, including the fact that citizens of continental European countries tend to buy many more OTC products across all health sectors than people in the United Kingdom. For example, the French and Germans together account for more than half the total European OTC market value of about $12 billion. Even if appropriate adjustments were made, there would still be a large disparity. Homeopathy suffers in most English-speaking countries because of its unexplained mode of action; non–English-speaking countries do not seem to share this concern. There are many examples of orthodox or allopathic medicines whose action is not fully understood; some are not as safe as homeopathic remedies, and they may be potentially dangerous if misused, yet they are freely available in supermarkets, corner shops, and even garages in some countries. Acetaminophen (paracetamol) is one such drug. There have been calls for its restriction in several countries, and recent U.K. regulations reducing the pack sizes that can be sold OTC have gone some way to satisfy these demands.

Buyer Characteristics

In many countries, homeopathic remedies are readily available in pharmacies and health shops, providing consumers with an attractive option. Kayne and associates investigated the characteristics of buyers in the British homeopathic OTC market.[1] In a questionnaire-based study of 407 purchasers in 107 pharmacies, it was found that very few people under age 25 bought OTC homeopathic medicines, and only 12% of buyers aged 25 to 35 years were male. Most respondents bought the remedy for themselves rather than for other members of their family, emphasizing the specific nature of homeopathic medicines. The most popular group of products were polychrests (remedies with a wide spectrum of activity, making them well suited to the OTC environment) and complex remedies (mixtures of remedies, usually with specific uses). There were a small number of branded medicines. The most commonly purchased polychrests were *Arnica* (6.3% of purchases), *Pulsatilla* (3.0%), and *Rhus tox* (2.3%). The predominance of polychrest homeopathic medicines is understandable, because buyers can readily equate remedies with ailments and buy the medicine most likely to be effective for their particular condition, using explanatory leaflets or brochures provided by manufacturers. Retailers also benefit by not having to offer what can be lengthy and complex advice to buyers, given that current legislation precludes giving uses on the label.

Kayne's study showed that the ailments for which OTC homeopathic medicines were bought were very wide-ranging. Many were acute, self-limiting ailments, such as coughs, colds, and minor injuries; others included digestive complaints, skin conditions, and anxiety. In most of these categories, with the exception of anxiety, orthodox OTC products were also available. Most respondents (60%) reported that they took the homeopathic medicine as sole medication for their problem; others (27%) used more than one homeopathic medicine at a time; and some (13%) used homeopathic and allopathic medicines simultaneously.

The excessive length of time for which some respondents took their remedies is a concern. Most homeopathic OTC remedies are designed for short-term administration. Long-term chronic conditions are best treated under the guidance of a practitioner, whose skill should ensure the choice of appropriate therapy, as well as minimize the possibility of adverse effects from taking the correct homeopathic remedy for too long a time. Although taking homeopathic medicines for long periods should not cause any irreversible harm, because the medicines are not in themselves toxic, patients may suffer by not receiving appropriate treatment for their condition.

A similar study by Kayne and Usher in New Zealand produced comparable results.[16] The study documented a high degree of awareness of homeopathy, with 92% of a sample of 503 pharmacy clients claiming to have heard of homeopathy and 67% saying they had used the therapy.

HOMEOPATHIC PRACTITIONERS

In many English-speaking countries, most health professionals have responded reactively to a demand for homeopathy from clients, rather than encouraging its use proactively. With improved access to homeopathic information and training, however, this position is changing.

In the United Kingdom and Ireland, homeopathy may be practiced not only by statutorily registered qualified health professionals, but also, under common law, by non–medically qualified professional homeopaths (NMQPs), who have training in homeopathy but not in conventional medicine, and by lay homeopaths, who have no formal training. NMQPs, and to an increasing extent lay homeopaths, are recognized by the National Health Service in the United Kingdom. Common law permits patients freedom of choice to choose the health care provisions they believe appropriate, and allows people to practice homeopathy if they wish. The main drawback of such a liberal system is that it allows a person to practice as a homeopath with little or no training. Medical homeopathy (together with veterinary homeopathy and other professions allied to medicine) and the NMQPs have separate educational facilities and governing bodies. Despite their substantial training in well-established colleges of homeopathy (and more recently at universities), NMQPs were formerly regarded as second-class practitioners by medical homeopaths, an opinion that continued into the 1980s. However, amicable discussions are now proceeding in the United Kingdom, Australia, and New Zealand, and the two groups are slowly establishing a more solid working relationship.

The incidence of published material on homeopathy in mainstream medical journals is increasing. For example, the *British Medical Journal* has published a series of articles on complementary medicine, including homeopathy.[17]

Professional medical homeopathy in the United Kingdom is controlled by the Faculty of Homeopathy, founded in 1950 by Act of Parliament. National Health Service Homeopathic hospitals are located in Bristol, Glasgow, London, and Tunbridge Wells. Among the health care professions, pharmacy appears to give its undergraduates the best exposure to homeopathy, with 14 of the 16 U.K. schools offering some teaching on the subject. As a result, OTC prescribing is increasing.

The British Association of Homeopathic Veterinary Surgeons has approximately 350 active members and has recently secured specialty recognition from the profession's governing body. Of all the professions allied to medicine, veterinarians have been the most reticent to embrace complementary practice at the highest levels.

Germany has two classes of practitioners—doctors (95% of whom practice some form of complementary medicine) and *heilpraktikurs*. The latter group, literally translated as "health practitioners," developed in the years before World War II, when doctors did not have a monopoly on the delivery of health care. At present, the ratio of practicing heilpraktikers to physicians is about 1:4. Heilpraktikers are not obliged to undertake formal medical training, but are obliged to take a test administered by the local health authority. If a candidate fails, he or she may retake the test until successful. Heilpraktikers'

activities are comparable to those of British NMQPs, except that they tend to use several different therapies concurrently and place more emphasis on diagnostic procedures.[18]

In Belgium, France, and Italy, the law states that only medical doctors may practice medicine or perform a medical act. Homeopathy is fully integrated into the medical system and is widely prescribed. Non–medically qualified practitioners are obliged to keep their activities low-key, otherwise they are likely to be taken to court by medical doctors.

In Denmark and the Netherlands, medical and nonmedical homeopaths can practice. In Greece, Portugal, and Spain, although nonmedical homeopaths are theoretically excluded, they are seldom prosecuted.

APPROACHES TO PRACTICE

In Europe and in other countries where European influence is strong, homeopathic remedies are prescribed in three ways: one remedy at a time, more than one remedy at a time, or in mixtures of two or more remedies at different potencies.

One remedy at a time, in a single or repeated dose, is prescribed by practitioners claiming to be *classical*, or *unicist*, homeopaths, and is generally favored by homeopaths in the United Kingdom. However, Hahnemann changed his ideas several times, especially toward the end of his life, and so the term *classical* could be applied to several prescription methods. The influence of the great American homeopaths has also been significant in shaping current practice. There is no "standard" or "pure" form of homeopathy, because the so-called *classical* homeopathy is really a rather complex mixture of ideas drawn from a variety of sources, some of which were unconnected with homeopathy.[19]

When more than one remedy at a time is prescribed, they may be given in alternation or concurrently. This practice is called *pluralist prescribing* and claims to treat more than one aspect of a patient's condition. It is common in France, Germany, Italy, and where remedies from these countries are available.

Mixtures of remedies at different potencies, selected for their combined effect on particular disease states, can be combined in one container. This method, known as *complex prescribing*, is very popular in France and Germany, where it is not uncommon to have 15 to 20 remedies ranging from very low to high potencies in the same preparation. Classical homeopaths claim that this is not true homeopathy, because the patient's symptoms and the drug picture (a comprehensive review of the symptoms that a specific medicine produces when given to healthy individuals) are not individually matched. Further, no provings exist of the mixtures. Interestingly, this complex approach to prescribing is being adopted in modern orthodox medicine as an element of care plans for the treatment of various diseases, including diabetes.

HOMEOPATHIC REMEDIES

Three main issues should be considered regarding homeopathic remedies, all of which are concerned with obtaining equivalence among international suppliers: nomenclature, methods of manufacture, and licensing requirements to ensure safety and quality.

Nomenclature

When discussing homeopathic remedies with homeopaths from other parts of the world, a serious problem often arises: Are we all talking about the same remedy? The current nomenclature of homeopathic remedies, and the abbreviation system by which remedies are identified, has evolved over 200 years and is full of irregularities and mistakes. Plagued by a multitude of synonyms, different spellings of homeopathic remedy names, and differences in the botanic parts used for the remedy preparation, international confusion is difficult to avoid. Within a particular country, it is unlikely that any conflict will arise. However, the situation is rather different internationally. Patients are well advised to take any prescribed medication with them when they travel.

Difficulties with nomenclature are not confined to remedy names. A group of Latin American and European authors has pointed out that international confusion exists as to the exact meaning of many words used routinely in homeopathy, and suggests that many inaccurate or imprecise terms should be replaced.[20] The idea of seeking a consensus view is not new. In 1990, Bernard Poitevin wrote, "Studies and discussions concerning homeopathic medical concepts are an integral part of homeopathic research and are the cornerstone of its evolution."[21]

The following examples, which illustrate sources of potential confusion, have been highlighted in a report prepared by Dellmour and associates under the auspices of the European Committee for Homeopathy (ECH).[22] Most botanic names used in homeopathy are similar to the botanic nomenclature used for the source material. However, some remedies have synonyms that do not correspond with either the pharmacopoeias or the current botanic names. For example, *Belladonna (Atropa belladonna)*, *Cactus grandiflorus (Cercus grandiflorus)*, and *Chamomilla (Matricaria chamomilla)* are commonly used homeopathic names that are incorrect. Further, the botanic nomenclature used in homeopathy does not indicate the part of the plant that has been used. In some countries the whole plant is used, in other countries it can be the root, the seeds, the leaves, the flower, or the fruit. It would help greatly if the parts were clearly defined and specified in the remedy name.

Most zoologic names used in homeopathy are similar to zoologic nomenclature, such as *Apis mellifica* (honey bee), *Latrodectus mactans* (black widow spider), and *Vespa cabro* (wasp). Some, however, are not. For example, *Cantharis* would be more correctly called *Lytta vesicatoria*, and *Coccus cacti*, *Dactylopius coccus*. Snake venoms present another problem. Often, a third Latin name denotes the different subgenus (e.g., there are four variants of the copperhead snake, each with its own name). Variants of *Cenchris* are probably used from country to country. Similar problems exist for *Naja*, *Vipera*, and *Crotalus*. In addition, some products of plants and animals, like *Ambra grisea*, *Calcium carbonicum (Hahnemanni)*, *Opium*, *Secale cornutum*, and *Resina laricis*, do not represent the whole organism, but are natural products or artificially obtained substances having their own particular identity.

Remedies from *chemical* sources may present problems as well. Compounds with F, Br, IO, or S ions are usually called *fluoratums, bromatums, iodatums,* or *sulphuratums*, respectively. Calcium fluoride is called *Calcarea fluorica* in some countries, and *Calcium fluoricum* in others, which is not consistent (*Calcium fluoratum* would be more logical).

Many of the nosode names used in homeopathy are insufficiently specific (e.g., *Psorinum, Carcinosinum, Tuberculinum, Medorrhinum*). Nosodes from various locales often use different starting materials and are derived through manufacturing methods.

Homeopathy needs a consistent international nomenclature system to ensure the accurate identification of remedies and the logical incorporation of new remedies in the future. The ECH has proposed the development of a more logical system of abbreviations that will ensure international standardization. It seems sensible for the homeopathic community to adopt the International Code of Botanical Nomenclature, which stipulates that single-word names no longer be applied. Thus, for example, one would use the following:

- *Aconitum napellus* instead of *Aconitum* to distinguish the remedy from *A. cammarum, A. ferox*, and *A. lycoctonum*
- *Euphorbium resiniferum* instead of *Euphorbium* to distinguish the remedy from other *Euphorbium* species
- *Pulsatilla pratensis* to avoid confusion with the other *Pulsatilla* species

To leave no doubt as to the source of the remedy, the exact plant part should also be specified. *Rheum palmatum (radix)* or *Cinchona pubescens (cortex)* are examples. I favor the addition of a suffix to indicate which pharmacopoeia is being used; this change would also help identify the source material being used.

Zoologic material can be identified by using the International Code of Zoological Nomenclature. Latin is the accepted language in this reference. The Committee's proposals suggest that the name of zoologic species and the source of the material should be used in the same manner as for botanic species; thus *Lac felinum* should be *Felix domestica (lac)*.

The international *chemical* nomenclature is given mainly in English, but also in Latin. However, the ECH suggests that Latin nomenclature is preferred for its conformity with the botanic and zoologic nomenclature and acceptance by French, Spanish, and Russian homeopaths.

The generally accepted Latin names of elements are no different from homeopathy's current use (e.g., *Aurum, Plumbum*), but sometimes there are slight differences from some old and obsolete English names (e.g., *Barium, Calcium, Kalium, Natrium* instead of *Baryta, Calcarea, Kali, Natrum*). In addition, a few changes are new for homeopathy (e.g., *Stibium* and *Hydrargyrum* for *Antimonium* and *Mercurius*, respectively). Some special homeopathic preparations, such as *Causticum* and *Mercurius solubilis*, should, after standardizing, take names that refer to the method of preparation (e.g., *Mercurius Hahnemanni* [to distinguish from the pure *Hydrargyrums*] and *Causticum Hahnemanni*).

Nosodes constitute a nonhomogenous class of homeopathic remedies. Most nosodes, except in vitro cultures and vaccines, are derived from a diseased host, which means that the composition and quality of the matter used to prepare the nosode depend not only on the infectious agent, but also on the features of the individual host. Such features vary widely across international borders. So many variables influence the symptom picture of nosodes that it would be impossible to arrive at an appropriately comprehensive description in the name of the remedy. For example, *Tuberculinurn* might be called *Mycobacterium tuberculosis pulmonis macerati (sputi resp.) hominis mortis!* There is still work to be carried out in this area to reach some degree of international consensus.

The Manufacture of Homeopathic Remedies

Associated with the nomenclature issue is the problem of differences in method of preparation among manufacturers, depending on which pharmacopoeia is being used. Preparation methods differ between German and French pharmacopoeias, introducing an international variable. For example, the German text states that to make a mother tincture, the source material must be macerated for at least 10 days at a temperature not exceeding 30°C, whereas the French publication specifies a period of 3 weeks. Other pharmacopoeias, notably the Indian, are used elsewhere in the world.

In the absence of a European pharmacopoeia (which has been under preparation for many years), British manufacturers have relied on a selection of foreign reference works for most of their information, particularly with regard to the analysis of starting materials. They used principally the German Homeopathic Pharmacopoeia (HAB) with its various supplements, together with the French and U.S. pharmacopoeias. The first edition of the British Homeopathic Pharmacopoeia (BHomP) was published by the British Homeopathic Society in 1870, with later editions in 1876 and 1882 by E Gould and Son of London. It then went out of print for more than a century. Spurred on by the requirements of the European Parliament's Directive number 92/73/EEC, a new edition of the BHomP was published by the British Homeopathic Manufacturers' Association in 1993, and an updated edition was issued in 1999. In loose-leaf format, the book reflects many of the current practices developed by British manufacturers in adapting German methods.

Little research has been carried out to quantify the variance in active ingredients that may occur, although nuclear magnetic resonance (NMR) techniques can test source materials.[23] The manner in which the first potency is made also varies according to the pharmacopoeia. This has implications for higher potencies. In the French Pharmacopoeia, the 1C potency is made by adding one part of mother tincture by weight to 99 parts of 60% to 70% alcohol, whereas in the HAB it is made by adding 2 parts by weight to 98 parts of 43% alcohol. The U.S. Homeopathic Pharmacopoeia directs that a 1:10 dilution of a 10% mother tincture be prepared in 88% alcohol. Such differences mean that remedies may well differ from country to country even though the potencies appear to be equivalent.

Regulatory Affairs—the Licensing of Remedies

Manufactured homeopathic remedies are subject to careful scrutiny to ensure that they are of the highest quality and safety. In the United Kingdom, they have been treated as medicines since the inception of the National Health Service in 1948, and are available on medical prescription just as orthodox medicines are. As a result, they are subject to rules governing their manufacture and supply.

During the late 1950s and early 1960s, a number of babies were born with deformed limbs as a direct result of their mothers taking the drug thalidomide during pregnancy. Unfortunately, it was not the practice in those days to test new drugs for adverse reactions during pregnancy before putting them on the market. Following these tragic consequences, the Medicines Act of 1968 was implemented in the United Kingdom to protect the public. Thereafter, manufacturers wanting to bring a new medicine to the market were obliged to demonstrate safety, quality, and, in the case of orthodox medicines, efficacy, before their product could be licensed for any given

application. In addition, premises used for manufacturing medicines became subject to regular inspection and approval. About 4000 homeopathic medicines were already on the market before the Medicines Act became law, and were granted Product Licences of Right (PLRs) and allowed to remain on sale.

On September 22, 1992, the European Parliament adopted Directive number 92/73/EEC, designed to establish regulations for homeopathic medicinal products throughout what was then called the European Economic Community, now known as the *European Union* (EU). The Directive is divided into four chapters and eleven articles covering scope, manufacture, control and inspection, placing on the market, and final provisions. It passed into U.K. law on January 1, 1994, and defines homeopathic medicine as any medicinal product prepared from products, substances, or compositions called homeopathic stocks in accordance with procedures described in any recognized pharmacopoeia.

The labeling requirements for homeopathic medicinal products and the provisions for controlling the import, export, and manufacture of homeopathic medicinal products are specified in the European Directive. In addition, Member States are obliged to share with each other the information necessary to guarantee the quality and safety of homeopathic medicinal products within the EU.

The Directive acknowledges the difficulty in applying established scientific methods of demonstrating efficacy to homeopathy by adopting a special licensing scheme for homeopathic medicines based on safety and quality only. The main provisions are as follows:

1. The remedies must be intended for oral or external use only (i.e., not injections).
2. The remedies must be sufficiently dilute to guarantee safety. A minimum dilution of 4X (a homeopathic dilution made by serially diluting a mother tincture 1:10 four times) is specified for most remedies. Mother tinctures are covered by other means.
3. No claims for therapeutic efficacy can be made. The remedy must be sold without specific indications (e.g., "for back-ache" or "colds and flu"). Despite this requirement, when seeking a license, manufacturers are obliged to submit evidence from authoritative repertories and textbooks that the remedy has been recommended for a particular use in the

past. The customer is obliged to choose the correct product, by whatever method he or she can. Advice from health professionals, the media, and leaflets in the retail outlet are the main sources of information.

4. The phrases "Homeopathic medicinal product without approved therapeutic indications" and "Consult your doctor if symptoms persist" must be on the label.

5. Brand names and names that indicate possible uses (sometimes called *fantasy names*) are officially banned, but there appear to be areas where the Licensing Authorities will allow some latitude in the regulations with respect to the naming of homeopathic products containing a number of different remedies. Following representations from some manufacturers regarding safety, some complex remedies containing several ingredients are being licensed with names of the type "Remedy X Co" to obviate the necessity of remembering a long list of ingredients when requesting an OTC remedy or writing a prescription. There is a potential source of confusion here, because some products that were on the market before the new legislation was adopted are still allowed to use brand names and even make limited claims of effectiveness. The Licensing Authorities have not announced a date by which the products licensed under the old regulations have to be relicensed under the new EU regulations. Until they do, both types of medicine will be sold, although many manufacturers are beginning to register their products voluntarily. There is provision for one other national route of registration under the Directive. Individual Member States can introduce a set of national rules. National rules allowing limited claims of effectiveness to be made (based on bibliographic evidence) are being developed in several countries.

A multidisciplinary expert committee, the Advisory Board on the Registration of Homeopathic Products, was established in the United Kingdom in 1993 to advise the Medicines Control Agency, the government body responsible for assessing the safety and quality of homeopathic remedies before they are licensed. The committee comprises a number of practicing doctors, pharmacists, veterinarians, and academicians. Similar bodies exist in other European countries.

Directive 92/73/EEC has been implemented across European Member States to varying degrees. For example, it has been implemented into Dutch law as *Besluit Homeopathische farmaceutische producten*. This law establishes two procedures for acquiring marketing authorization for homeopathic products in the Netherlands. First, when the homeopathic medicinal product is intended for oral or external use, no therapeutic indication appears on the labeling. Second, if there is a sufficient degree of dilution to guarantee the safety of the medicinal product (diluted to at least 1:10,000), the registration will be applied for according to Article 4 of the regulations. Homeopathic medicinal products that do not comply with the above-mentioned Article 4 criteria have to be authorized according to the assessment criteria of Article 6, corresponding to the implementation of Article 9.2 of Council Directive 92/73/EEC.

In the Netherlands, homeopathic medicinal products are authorized by the Medicines Evaluation Board on the basis of quality and safety, much the same as the U.K. Medicines Control Agency. Authorized homeopathic medicinal products are recorded in a register that may be inspected on the Internet. For every product to be evaluated, a company must submit a dossier comprising a number of specified documents.

It is generally accepted that the United Kingdom interprets Directive 92/73/EEC strictly and this has traditionally presented a barrier to foreign companies wishing to bring their products to this country. In particular, the inclusion of certain nosodes and other biologic material, the purity of which is thought difficult to prove, has not been viewed favorably by the Advisory Board on the Registration of Homeopathic Products. A few foreign remedies have been licensed, however, and this trend will likely continue in the future.

None of the regulations discussed heretofore preclude experienced homeopathic practitioners and pharmacists from continuing to recommend and supply remedies compounded for individual needs. When a professional is involved, the guarantee of quality and safety is the integrity and skill of the operator—as it always has been.

In France, remedies for sale and use are restricted to potencies below 30C. Homeopaths have to purchase higher potencies from abroad, usually Switzerland, Germany, or the United Kingdom.

In October 1998, the French authorities suspended the license of a number of nosodes, including *Medorrhinum*, *Morbilinum*, and *Psorinum*, and 170 remedies of animal origin for safety purposes. The authorities were dissatisfied with the dossiers on microbial safety submitted by the laboratories producing these remedies. In Germany, sterilization of the starting materials for nosodes has been obligatory since 1985, according to HAB monographs. We don't yet know how sterilization may alter the effectiveness of the remedy. Recently, French manufacturers were asked to submit their dossiers on nosodes for approval to the registration authorities. If the dossiers are not approved, the market authorization for nosodes will be withdrawn.

Some manufacturers are apparently considering the use of allopathic vaccines as starting material for certain nosodes. This action would have substantial implications for the material media and would necessitate new provings.

The German authorities have recently made changes to the sterilization methods required for the licensing of remedies of zoologic origin. There was some concern that the high core temperatures stipulated (133 degrees for 20 minutes) might denature the remedies.

In countries outside Europe, the licensing regulations vary from absolutely nothing to requirements for the adoption of good manufacturing procedures.

HOMEOPATHY WORLDWIDE

Homeopathy is found in many countries worldwide, and outside Europe each has its own particular way of dealing with the therapy. The following is not meant to be comprehensive, but is offered as a brief survey and an indication of how widely homeopathy is practiced.

Africa

The new South Africa provides an environment in which homeopathy can make considerable progress. The ongoing war between medically qualified doctors and dentists and NMQPs has been resolved and the two factions are working amicably, each under its own code. Homeopaths are able to request medical tests, receive referrals from other health professionals, hospitalize patients when necessary, and visit hospitals. A comprehensive training course is offered by the Technikons of Natal in Durban and Witwatersrand in Johannesburg. This course was set up in association with the statutory body with whom homeopaths must register. Approximately 450 homeopaths are registered in South Africa.

Training for health professionals (physicians, dentists, and pharmacists) has been provided by the British Faculty of Homeopathy with local assistance. Students have taken both the Primary Care Certificate and the more advanced Member of the Faculty of Homeopathy (MFHom) examinations. However, veterinary homeopathy is in its infancy.

Homeopathy has been practiced in Nigeria for at least 40 years. The first formal organization, the All Nigeria Homeopathic Medical Association, was founded in 1961, shortly after Nigeria gained independence from Britain. Dr. Peter Fisher visited the country in 1989 and found it difficult to identify the number of practicing homeopaths, partly because of the problem of defining exactly what constituted a homeopath.[24] There were about 50 to 100 homeopaths with an acceptable level of training at that time. Generally speaking, the standards of training were below what would be expected in developed countries. Dr. Fisher reported that there were a number of homeopaths in and around the federal capital, Lagos, and in the eastern part of the country, particularly in the states of Imo and Anambra. By 1991, some progress had been made, and the acceptance of the medical and dental professions had been secured.[25] Further advances have been hampered by political pressures.

Asia

Homeopathy in India is widespread, with an estimated 150,000 practitioners. According to Julian Winston, in his fascinating chronicle of the history of homeopathy,[26] 110 institutes teach the subject as a basis for degrees and doctorates in homeopathic science. A substantial book publishing industry exists, and several manufacturers produce remedies of varying quality.

The influx of Jewish refugees from countries of the former Soviet Union to Israel has caused a substantial increase in demand for homeopathy. A large number of the immigrant practitioners are preparing their own remedies (as indeed Hahnemann and his followers did), but there are no official standards. Contact with Europe (mainly through visiting lecturers from France, Germany, and the United Kingdom) has helped to establish trained practitioners, and discussions are in progress to regulate homeopathic practice and manufacture.[27] The Israel Association of Classical Homeopathy is active in promoting homeopathic practice and maintains contact with the Israeli authorities.

Homeopathy was introduced to Malaysia during World War II by Indian soldiers who were fighting for the British Army, and influence from the subcontinent is still strong. Teaching began in 1979 under the auspices of the Faculty of Homeopathy Malaysia. There were four homeopathic medical centers in the country in 1988.[28] Although the government allows complementary medicine, there are no formal registration procedures for practitioners. An organization called the Registered Malaysian Homeopathic Medical Practitioners Association was established in 1985 to unite qualified homeopathic practitioners. Without standards, it is uncertain as to exactly what constitutes qualification. The group has about 500 members.

Singapore recognizes homeopathy, but there is no legislative framework to control its practice. Few if any practitioners are medically qualified.

Australia

Approximately 150 medical homeopaths practice in Australia, of whom about 20 may be considered committed to using the discipline. An outpatient clinic operates in Sydney at the Balmain Hospital. The split of medical and nonmedical homeopathy seen in the United Kingdom is present in Australia as well. The state societies for nonmedical homeopaths eventually merged to form a national organization known as The Australian Homeopathic Association. The medical homeopaths' organization, which contains a number of British-trained practitioners, is known as the Australian Faculty of Homeopathy. One active Australian homeopathic manufacturer is situated in the Barossa, a renowned wine-producing area of South Australia.

In New Zealand, nonmedical homeopaths outnumber medical homeopaths. Physicians appear to have an open mind, with various surveys showing that upward of 80% of family doctors do not object to their patients consulting professional homeopaths. Regulations for the licensing of homeopathic remedies are being developed, and most pharmacies stock homeopathic medicines.

Caribbean

Cuba, a republic of 20 million people, has a well-organized homeopathic presence.[29] Some Mexican doctors helped reintroduce homeopathic practice to Cuba in 1992, when it was incorporated into the National Health Service. A year later, some Brazilian homeopaths offered the first formal medical training. Other health professions—pharmacy, dentistry, and veterinary surgery—followed shortly after. There are now a total of 922 homeopaths in Cuba, including 320 physicians, 220 veterinary surgeons, 161 pharmacists, and 141 dentists. Instruction uses a national homeopathic curriculum and leads to the award of a diploma after 1 year of study. Unfortunately, further development is being hampered by a shortage of literature and remedies, particularly in hospitals.

All the municipalities around Havana and many elsewhere in the island offer homeopathic treatment through family doctors and clinics. Many pharmacies, including a magnificent new homeopathic pharmacy in Havana, dispense homeopathic prescriptions. They are state owned. The 48 homeopathic dentists in the capital have performed 667 extractions collectively with the aid of homeopathic anesthesia, achieved with the remedy *Hypericum* 200C given by mouth. Gathering statistics about consultations is difficult because homeopathy is officially included with other therapies, under the heading Traditional Medicine, by the health authorities, but there is considerable sympathy for the discipline at high levels within the government. I was privileged to meet with the Minister of Health, who reiterated a commitment to providing homeopathic facilities. Homeopathy is used by the medical facilities at Havana International Airport. Almost all the 200 patients who used this these facilities last year improved within 20 minutes of receiving their medicines. Of the 49 different remedies used, the most popular were *Baryta carbonica* and *Nux vomica*.

A considerable amount of homeopathic research is being carried out, particularly with animals. For example, homeopathic veterinary surgeons have reported that homeopathy can be used as a growth promoter for animals in the food chain, especially cows, pigs, and chickens, and also to treat mastitis. A recent congress in Cuba received delegates from Jamaica, but the general status of homeopathy in that country is unknown.

Eastern Europe

Although officially allowed only in Russia in 1992, homeopathy had been widely available unofficially in the republics of the former Soviet Union, where many practitioners prepare their own remedies. In Russia, homeopathy is taught in medical schools and minimal standards have been introduced to try and standardize remedies, many of which are now being prepared by pharmacies. International congresses are held by the Russian Homeopathic Association on an irregular basis.

Occasional correspondents in Bulgaria, Hungary, Poland, and Romania have indicated that homeopathy is available in those countries. Although generally restricted to medical doctors, some pharmacists are also involved. Small, active communities are working hard to establish its popularity, and with increased contact with the West following the fall of communism, progress is being made.

Latin America

Homeopathy is popular in Costa Rica, where more than half the population uses the therapy regularly. Training is available for both medical doctors and practitioners who are not medically qualified.

Homeopathy is also practiced in Argentina, Brazil, and Mexico. Of the three, Mexico is the best organized.[30] Training to become a medical doctor and homeopath is available from two facilities in Mexico City. Three other institutions offer postgraduate training. In 1996, the National School of Medicine and Homeopathy (Escuela Nacional de Medicina y Homeopatía) celebrated its hundredth anniversary.

Homeopathy in Mexico dates back to 1850, when migrating physicians from Spain taught local physicians.[31] One of the first successes was attributed to a Dr. Carbo, who, in 1854, treated 45 patients during a yellow fever epidemic on the island prison of San Juan de Ulúa. His success was rewarded by President Antonio López de Santana, who granted Dr. Carbo a certificate to practice medicine in Mexico. In 1867, the first homeopathic pharmacy was founded, followed by the first homeopathic hospital at San Miguel de Allende Guanajuato 4 years later.

Many pharmacies now stock remedies, and several others manufacture remedies. Although only medical practitioners are supposed to practice homeopathy, many active practitioners are not medically qualified. One state in Mexico allows training for such practitioners.

In Brazil, homeopathy as a therapeutic option became a politically tenable possibility only in the 1980s, in spite of the presence of homeopathic medicine in the country since 1840.[32] Overcoming resistance from academic and clinical sources can be difficult. Only medical doctors, dental surgeons, and veterinarians are legally able to prescribe homeopathic remedies. However, supplies may be purchased from pharmacies and "Drogeries," whose exact status is difficult to identify. Drogeries appear to sell most of the items found in pharmacies, but without a qualified pharmacist on the premises. The small but active group of homeopaths in Brazil uses a variety of approaches to prescribing.

Argentina also has a modest number of homeopaths (approximately 1500), but little is known about the methods being used to treat patients or the distribution of the services they offer.

SUMMARY

The practice of homeopathy varies throughout the world. The global distribution of homeopathic practice is encouraging, especially because it appears to be spreading further. The problems associated with the lack of international standards make it rather confusing for the traveling practitioner and patient. It is important that the potential difficulties are acknowledged and appropriate steps taken to minimize the possibility of untoward outcomes.

References

1. Kayne SB, Beattie N, Reeves A: Buyer characteristics, *Pharm J* 263:210-212, 1999.

2. Von Wartburg WP: Drugs perception of risks, *Swiss Pharma* 6(11a):21-23, 1984.

3. Slovic P, Kraus NN, Lappe H et al: Risk perception of prescription drugs: report on a survey in Sweden, *Pharmaceut Med* 4:43-65, 1989.

4. Vincent C, Furnham A: The perceived efficacy of complementary and orthodox medicine: preliminary findings and development of a questionnaire, *Complement Ther Med* 2:128-134, 1994.

5. English JM: Homeopathy, *The Practitioner* 230:1067-1071, 1986.

6. Furnham A, Smith C: Choosing alternative medicine: a comparison of the beliefs of patients visiting a general practitioner and a homoeopath, *Soc Sci Med* 26(7):685-689, 1988.

7. Avina RL, Schneiderman LJ: Why patients choose homeopathy, *West J Med* 128:366-369, 1978.

8. Swain J: The cost and effectiveness of homeopathy, *Br Homeopath J* 81:148-150, 1992.

9. Feldhaus H-W: Cost-effectiveness of homeopathic treatment in a dental practice, *Br Homeopath J* 82:22-28, 1993.

10. Neuberger J: *Controversies in health care policies*, London, 1994, BMJ Books.

11. Anon: Take a little of what ails you, *The Times* (London), November 13, 1989.

12. Abecassis J: *Homeopathic OTC medicines in Europe*, Proceedings of International Conference, Royal London Homeopathic Hospital, London, January 23-24, 1997.

13. *Mintel report on complementary medicine*, London, 1999, Mintel International Group Limited.

14. Borneman JP: Executive Vice President, Standard Homeopathic Company, Los Angeles, personal communication, April 1997.

15. Vickers A: Use of complementary therapies, *BMJ* 304:1105-1107, 1994.

16. Kayne SB, Usher W: Homeopathy: attitudes and awareness amongst pharmacy clients and staff in New Zealand, *N Z Pharm* 19:32-33, 1999.

17. Vickers A, Zollman C: ABC of complementary medicine: homoeopathy, *BMJ* 319:1115-1118, 1999.

18. Ernst E: Towards quality in complementary health care: is the German 'Heilpraktiker' a model for complementary practitioners? *Intl J Qual Health Care* 8:187-190, 1996.

19. Campbell A: The origins of classical homoeopathy? *Complement Ther Med* 7(2):76-82, 1999.

20. Guajardo G, Bellavite P, Wynn S et al: Homeopathic terminology: a consensus quest, *Br Homeopath J* 88:135-141, 1999.

21. Poitevin B: *Introducion a la homeopatia*, (nueva ed), Mexico City, Mexico, 1990, Medico Homeopatica Mexicana.

22. Dellmour F, Jansen, Nicolai T et al: *The proposal for a revised international nomenclature system of homeopathic remedies and their abbreviations*, Brussels, 1999, European Committee for Homeopathy.

23. Kayne SB: Homeopathic pharmacy: an introduction and handbook, Edinburgh, 1997, Churchill Livingstone.

24. Fisher P: Homeopathy in Nigeria, *Br Homeopath J* 78:171-173, 1989.

25. Okpokpor SO: Homeopathy: Nigerian update, *Homeopathy* 41:140, 1991.

26. Winston J: *The faces of homoeopathy*, Tawa, 1999, Great Auk Publishing.

27. Moschner A: Homeopathic pharmacist, Tel-Aviv, personal communication, October 1999.

28. Nasir N, Zain M: A brief history of homeopathy in Malaysia, *J OMHI* 1:26, 1988.

29. Kayne SB: Homeopathy today, *Br Homeopath J* 89:99-100, 2000.

30. Guajardo G: Instituto de Investigaciones en Ciencias Veterinarias, University de Baja California, Mexico, personal communication, October 1999.

31. Oceguera JA: Sección de Estudios de Posgrado e Investigación, Escuela Nacional de Medicina y Homeopatía Mexico DF (translated by Germán Guajardo-Bernal), personal communication, October 1999.

32. Luz, MT: The incorporation of homoeopathy into public health, *Br Homeopath J* 81:55-58, 1992.

Suggested Readings

Kayne SB: *Complementary therapies for pharmacists*, London, 2002, The Pharmaceutical Press.

Mitchell A, Cormack M: *The therapeutic relationship in complementary health care*, Edinburgh, 1998, Churchill Livingstone.

Stone J, Matthews J: *Complementary medicine and the law*, Oxford, 1996, Oxford University Press.

Vincent V, Furnham A: *Complementary medicine. a research perspective*, Chichester, UK, 1998, John Wiley & Sons.

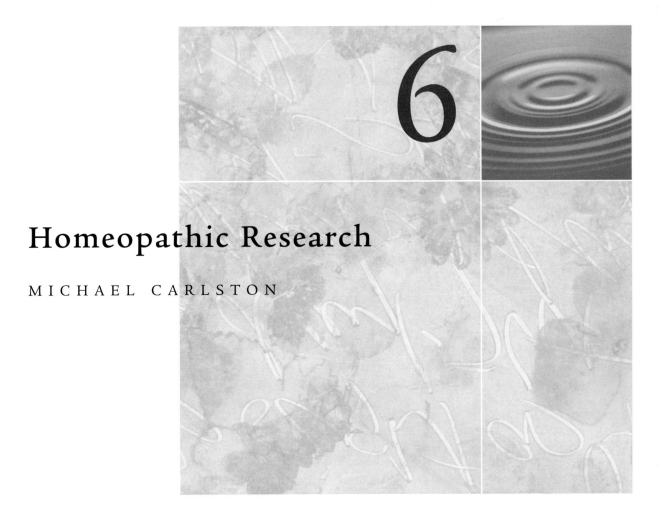

Homeopathic Research

MICHAEL CARLSTON

INTRODUCTION AND FUNDAMENTAL ISSUES

"There are three kinds of lies: lies, damned lies, and statistics."

BENJAMIN DISRAELI

Medical research and the scientific method have been an integral part of homeopathy since its inception. Hahnemann's experimentalist temperament led him to reject conventional wisdom and medical practices because he observed the harm they caused while providing little benefit to the patient. As a result of this observation, he developed an alternative approach and tested it methodically. Ever since, the homeopathic scientific community has spent much of its time attempting to prove that he did not go astray.

The customary means of developing that proof has been through scientific experimentation. As early as 1833, clinical trials instigated by homeopaths compared conventional and homeopathic treatments.[1] Throughout the second half of the nineteenth century, the American Institute of Homeopathy annually challenged the American Medical Association (AMA) to compare treatment effectiveness in a scientific study. The AMA ignored the challenge. When homeopaths were finally accepted into the AMA early in the twentieth century, the challenge was dropped in the new, less contentious social climate.

Research is an extremely important tool for evaluating the merits of any medical therapy. Certainly, we should respect the clinical wisdom of any experienced health care provider. However, the complexity and variety of human experience can lead to incorrect conclusions. Experience and common sense can be inadequate or even misleading at times when we study complex living organisms.

One of the classic examples of research disproving a "common sense" treatment was the famous study of internal mammary artery ligation for angina pectoris.[2] Because angina is caused by inadequate blood flow to the heart, in the late 1950s surgeons attempted to divert blood flow to the heart by ligating the internal mammary artery. Many physicians thought the treatment effective until the publication of a study that would never be approved by a human subjects committee today. In this study, the surgeon performed either the usual mammary artery ligation procedure or a fake operation. The highly invasive placebo proved as effective as the real surgery.

Formalized research, particularly human clinical research, can help bring objectivity to the analysis of healing interventions. This ritualized investigation process is particularly important when the intervention is controversial. Although a double-blind randomized placebo-controlled trial (RCT) does not automatically produce truth, it does lend credibility.

Several types of studies are currently in use, some of them observational and others experimental. Ideally, for the sake of credibility and comparison, experimenters should use conventional research designs. However, as we will discuss in the following section, homeopathy, like acupuncture and some other forms of complementary medicine, does not lend itself well to many conventional research designs. Unfortunately, this is particularly true of the double-blind RCT design.

Although consensus is difficult to achieve when the topic is homeopathy, most of the medical community agrees that research is important. It is wise to keep Disraeli's caution in mind, but research support for the controversial theories of homeopathy is essential. Homeopathy does have research support. Furthermore, this support has had an important effect on increasing physician awareness and acceptance of homeopathic medicine.

When conventional physicians and the conventional medical community are asked to consider any form of complementary medicine, the first response is asking to see the research. Questions about patient safety are also important, but scientific evidence of efficacy is the foundation for credibility. This demand for research evidence is reasonable and customary in modern medicine. The worth of a conventional medicine is proved by research evidence that it is superior to placebo or, better still, clinically effective (i.e., the treatment has an effect on the disease that is meaningful to the patient) in a rigorous trial.

Achieving such standards can be difficult, expensive, and time consuming. Some observers believe that when homeopathic medicine is being studied, the standard must be higher than for conventional medicine, because the ability of extreme dilutions, or perhaps the "memory" of the therapeutic agent, to generate physiologic effects would fly in the face of current scientific understanding. Supporters of homeopathy respond by claiming that the scientific evaluation of a treatment is based on its effectiveness, not on our understanding of the mechanism of its effect. In this view, the focus is on *whether* it works, not *why* it works. Our failure to understand *why* something works is not an indication that it does *not* work. Is it hypocritical—or prudent—to demand more than proof of effectiveness for an intervention whose mechanism of action we do not understand?

The Nature of Proof

I may have taken liberty depicting my fellow physicians as more scientifically objective than we truly are. Is credibility synonymous with scientific proof? Studies of physicians find that we do not customarily rely on research findings when we make decisions about complementary and alternative medicine (CAM) therapies or even in our use of conventional medicines.[3-16] Noncompliance with formal guidelines for clinical practice is common, and its causes are many.[17-26]

Although the reasons for our ambiguous relationship with scientific evidence are complex and poorly understood, our recommendations are clearly more arbitrary than the average patient believes. Too often it appears that some physicians selectively recognize research evidence supporting their preexisting opinions and ignore studies that contradict those opinions. This is as true of physicians who use CAM as of those who use only conventional medicine. Such bias is most unfortunate. Although we might prefer to categorize evidence in terms of simple dichotomies (e.g., *wonderful* or *worthless*), the complexity of contradictory or seemingly contradictory findings often leads to greater understanding. Reality is seldom so black and white.

Two examples from nutritional medicine might be helpful. We have good evidence that high dietary consumption of beta carotene is associated with many health benefits, including decreased risk of lung cancer. We also have evidence that supplementation with synthetic beta carotene actually increases this risk. Why? Also, high levels of urinary calcium are associated with increased risk of kidney stones, so for many years patients were told to restrict dietary calcium. The medical literature of those years contained articles supporting the efficacy of this intervention.[27,28] However, we now believe that high calcium intake does not lead to calcium-containing renal calculi—but rather *prevents* them.[29,30] The instances when common sense conflicts with observed facts or when research data are inconsistent are precisely when we can learn the most. It is foolish and unscientific to blind ourselves to contradictions or data that make our world a little less tidy than we formerly believed it to be.

Although an argument could be made that the statistical methods employed by medical researchers serve only to find falsehood and not truth, the impetus for research is the search for proof, proof of efficacy and proof that an intervention works. We can collect survey data or conduct case control studies or clinical trials in our efforts to answer this question. Survey data are seldom convincing because of uncontrolled confounding factors. To establish credibility, investigations of homeopathy and other forms of CAM must be of the very highest quality. Is it fair to require higher standards of CAM therapies than would otherwise be necessary? Probably not, but present political realities of medicine necessitate the very highest standards.

The most highly regarded study design is the double-blind, placebo-controlled RCT. RCTs, whether single-blind or double-blind, are costly and laborious. The requirements of a well-designed RCT can make the results difficult to generalize to less-precisely defined circumstances (i.e., "the real world"). RCT design can be extremely difficult to apply in therapies like homeopathy or acupuncture, which make blinding the patient nearly impossible (discussed later in more detail). Although these factors limit the practicality of RCTs, they remain important because they are the gold standard of today's medical research.

Stages of Proof

Usually these trials are "ideal-world" studies in the sense that investigators select the problem, practitioners, and patients to maximize the chances of a positive finding. If the initial ideal-world scenario shows promise, further research follows. If subsequent research, most commonly investigations of other ideal-world circumstances, is similarly positive, the medical community might conclude that the method works. Besides being somewhat premature, this conclusion is also naïve, for reasons discussed later. Proof is relative, and there are different levels or stages of proof along the path to integrating an unfamiliar system of therapy into conventional medicine.

The first investigation stage is to consider whether the entire therapeutic system is faulty. This initial process is extremely dependent on making optimal investigative choices. For example, we know that surgery is a useful technique under the correct circumstances. A study of a surgical intervention for appendicitis will show positive outcomes. A single study, or even a series of studies, of surgical treatment for viral gastroenteritis would lead investigators to the conclusion that surgery does not work. If a fanatical supporter of surgery with an unlimited budget persisted and conducted trials investigating surgical treatment of anxiety and hay fever, the cumulative negative findings would make it difficult to argue the case that surgery has a legitimate role within modern medical practice. Similarly, assuming that surgery can successfully treat any problem based upon a single positive finding is naïvely optimistic.

The first stage of investigation is much like sending out a scouting party for a quick glimpse of the terrain. The information obtained at this level of investigation is quite inadequate and very frustrating for patients and clinicians, because while a positive finding can raise hopes, it does not give us the practical information necessary in clinical practice—we need to know for what it works and when. On the other hand, this stage is a necessary screening hurdle that a therapy must jump before more energy is dedicated to the investigation process.

After demonstrating a pattern of apparent effectiveness, investigations proceed to the next level. This next stage has two components. The first is building an evidence base for the use of a treatment in specific clinical conditions. The second is conducting more real-world investigations of the treatment as applied in the average community setting. Real-world studies are important because they most truly reflect the average patient's clinical experience. Eventually the focus of study can move to other matters, such as delineating differences between treatment approaches and evaluating the therapy's cost effectiveness for example.

The recent National Institutes of Health (NIH) Panel Consensus on Acupuncture is a good example of the early stages of this process. After critically reviewing MedLine's indexed studies, the panel concluded that there was promising evidence of acupuncture's efficacy in certain clinical conditions. They also determined that there was suggestive but inconclusive evidence about a number of other conditions. They reached these positive conclusions despite an admitted lack of understanding for the mechanisms behind acupuncture's effects.[31-34]

Outcomes Research

"The patient's opinion is the ultimate outcome measure."

IAN CHALMERS

I would be remiss not to include some discussion of outcome measures, because this issue strikes very close to the heart of the philosophic differences between many CAM therapies and conventional medicine. Many conventional medicine practitioners would argue that this division exists within conventional medicine as well.

What do you measure to determine a treatment response? Clearly the most acceptable and perhaps the most objective way to measure response is via physiologic parameters that can be measured by laboratory tests. We have a great deal of experience with such measures, and precise information about the reliability of the testing procedures themselves. These procedures can be costly, always an issue in clinical trials, but more importantly the information may not tell us what we hope it will. Although we use these tests as surrogate disease markers, very few tests indisputably quantify a patient's disease state. Most importantly, these tests do not tell us whether the patient feels better and is more fully able to function. A good example of this deficiency is found in clinical cancer research, which increasingly includes valuation of the *quality* of a patient's life, as well as the traditional method of simply tracking the length of a patient's survival.

We are in the infant stages of developing reliable measures to answer the very simple question, the one most crucial to the patient, "How do you feel?" Many CAM therapies, homeopathy more than most others,

espouse a philosophy of health based on *all* aspects of a human being: physical, mental, emotional, and even spiritual. It is therefore essential to attempt to measure patients' health just as broadly. Homeopathic principles sometimes define even the *worsening* of some physical symptoms as an improvement in a patient's condition, provided this decline is linked to improvement in other, more important, facets of the patient's health. Patients often share the homeopathic perspective, recognizing that they feel better because of their improved mental state, for example, although their skin condition may have worsened.

The current state of homeopathic research is ambiguous and complicated. We do not have simple answers about clinical homeopathic medicine or the basic science questions its efficacy would pose. Homeopathic research is a conundrum—fertile ground for questions about homeopathy and the process of scientific research. Although it is not easy to use conventional scientific protocols to examine homeopathy, the attempt teaches researchers a great deal about homeopathic principles. A researcher must overcome considerable challenges if he or she is to simultaneously respect homeopathic principles and conventional research methodology. Designing homeopathic clinical trials can be more than a little challenging; however, with great understanding and effort, it is possible.

Methodology Issues

"A poorly or improperly designed study involving human subjects is, by definition, unethical."

SCIENCE, 11/18/1977

Because a clinical trial must inevitably expose subjects to some risk of adverse effects, a study that does not lead to an answer needlessly places subjects in harm's way. The essential principles of homeopathy must be respected for research investigations to produce meaningful answers.

Mistakes do occur and they are an inevitable part of the learning process. If we do not learn from our research mistakes we only compound them and act irresponsibly.

First, let us consider the most essential homeopathic principle, using like to cure like. In practical terms, this principle necessitates highly individualized prescriptions for each patient. The intense and usually lengthy homeopathic interview, which is a necessary step toward providing highly individualized prescriptions, may be an ideal setting to maximize placebo effects. The interview also makes *blinding* uniquely difficult. The practitioner carefully considers the patient's words and expressions as she draws conclusions about the nature of the patient and the correct homeopathic prescription. The patient becomes an important party in the decision-making process as questions and answers pass back and forth confirming or denying the practitioner's suspicions. Subtle indications of the practitioner's certainty about the prescription are likely to affect the patient's expectations about the response to the treatment. Interpersonal perception and interaction is central to the homeopathic clinical process.

Although these interpersonal elements might be controlled by a dispassionate third party actually administering the medicine, other issues arise. Most obvious is the certainty that, in an unknown percentage of cases, the interaction between practitioner and patient *is* the cure. The placebo effect may be even more important to the success of homeopathy than to conventional medicine. Taken to the extreme, if the effects of homeopathy were predominantly the result of placebo, it would not mean that homeopathic treatment is worthless, but that the most important element is the interaction, that the person was more important than the pill.

Several years ago, I had an interesting discussion with a European homeopathic researcher in which we lamented the vanishing opportunity to test this hypothesis by conducting a "homeopathic trial" with American patients whose only treatment would have been the homeopathic interview. Americans were starting to learn enough about homeopathy to expect more from a homeopath than only an interview, no matter how insightful.

Most homeopaths believe that the success of homeopathic treatment is almost entirely dependent on the accuracy of the practitioner's prescription. A trial of classical homeopathy cannot be credible, therefore, unless it is based on accurate prescriptions. A trial design not meeting this requirement that leads to a negative finding would generate a loud chorus of complaint from the homeopathic community about the inadequacy of the homeopath who chose the homeopathic remedy. Negative findings from poorly designed trials are meaningless, because an informed advocate or critic would expect that failure was the only likely outcome.

One means of overcoming this difficulty is for a *panel* of homeopaths to select the correct homeopathic remedy for each patient. This method makes it necessary for each panelist to independently interview every patient, or for the panel as a group to examine each patient (a circumstance that would very likely significantly alter patients' behavior), or for the panel to watch videotaped cases. A videotaped case does not allow for interaction between the patient and the panelists, thus changing the dynamic and each practitioner's perception of the patient. The practitioners viewing the videotape could not question the patient, thus limiting the information on which they based their prescriptions. On the whole, the process of prescription by committee is very time consuming and potentially contentious.

Another research-complicating factor involved in providing highly individualized prescriptions is that every disease must be treated with one of a large number of homeopathic remedies. For example, one of the classic texts in homeopathy, Kent's *Repertory of the Homeopathic Materia Medica,* lists more than 120 different homeopathic medicines for asthma. No classical homeopath believes that all of them would be useful for any one patient with asthma. To the contrary, the classical homeopath believes that there is one best choice for each patient. Other remedies may be of limited benefit, but *one* will be uniquely helpful. It is worth emphasizing—the choice of the homeopathic remedy is crucially important.

Another issue was brought to my attention a decade ago during a research meeting in the Department of Family and Community Medicine at the University of California, San Francisco. After I proposed a trial and explained some of the methodology issues, one of the two department research specialists insisted that any homeopathic study must use only one homeopathic remedy for proper statistical analysis. She argued that every different remedy was a different treatment. The other disagreed. If "correct design" in a trial of classical homeopathy means using only one single remedy, homeopathic clinical research would be so impractical it would be essentially impossible. Although we might reach a point where we can compare the effectiveness of various homeopathic remedies in certain disease conditions, at this point we have yet to produce incontestable research evidence settling the more fundamental question of homeopathy's effectiveness as a system of medicine.

Clinical trials using classical homeopathic principles represent only a small fraction of homeopathic clinical research. Given the foregoing difficulties, it is easy to sympathize with researchers who choose not to try to pick their way through this Gordian knot complicating homeopathic clinical research. Unfortunately such expediency is unacceptable when we must be consistent with homeopathic principles to get meaningful answers.

Like the many-headed Hydra, a new series of problems arise to take the place of each one conquered by the researcher. Ignoring the demands of classical homeopathy simplifies the problems; however, the requirements posed by more simplistic versions of homeopathy are still formidable. Each challenge demands careful consideration from a conscientious researcher. Overlooked, they can easily negate any conclusions derived from what will surely be a poorly designed study.

Response Expectations Change with the Passage of Time

Patient response varies with time. Once a patient takes the correct homeopathic remedy, he is expected to improve after a certain interval (Figure 6-1). That interval is dependent on several factors, among them the patient's disease severity, duration of illness, general health, and age. In addition, homeopaths expect a short-term intensification of a patient's symptoms (aggravation) before long-term improvement sets in.

Homeopaths expect the correct remedy to make the patient worse at time B but better at time C. Choosing the correct time to measure response is one of the arts of combining homeopathic clinical experience with research methodology. Some studies creatively used the homeopathic aggravation as an outcome measure, identifying a temporary decline in patients' condition as a successful intervention.

A correct homeopathic prescription should lead to persistent improvement in the patient's clinical condition. This process should continue long after the patient stops taking the homeopathic remedy. Theoretically, the long-term effect of homeopathy would be expected to confound the response of a study group changing from active treatment to placebo. This effect makes it very difficult to perform crossover studies.

Provings Make the Patient Worse

A patient who takes too much of the correct homeopathic remedy for too long a time will get worse. Healthy people test homeopathic remedies by taking them for a time, hoping to develop a reaction to the medicine (proving) and thereby learn what symptoms suggest its use. In the same manner, patients who take a remedy repeatedly will pass the point of improvement and get worse from taking too much of what would otherwise be a beneficial remedy. In addition, patients who overmedicate often temporarily develop symptoms of the remedy they did not previously suffer.

Dosage

Questions about dosage may be homeopathy's not-so-secret Achilles' heel. Although dosage is the most obvious sticking point, it is separate from and secondary to the principle of using like to treat like. Perhaps like to treat like will prove useful for certain conditions only if certain doses are administered. Homeopaths often argue among themselves, sometimes heatedly, about appropriate dosage regimens, whereas conventional critics seldom investigate homeopathy any further than the dilution controversy. There are many different points of view on this issue, which is a question of interest to all parties debating the worth of homeopathic medicine.

REFLECTIONS ON PLACEBO

Why Talk About Placebo?

The use of placebo controls in research is an important component of the effort to develop a foundation of evidence on which to base the clinical practice of medicine. Unfortunately, the term *placebo* has pejorative connotations in clinical medicine.[35] Considerations of

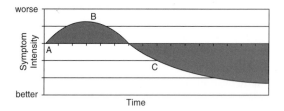

Figure 6-1. Response to homeopathic treatment. *A,* Start of treatment; *B,* homeopathic aggravation; *C,* long-term improvement.

alternative forms of medical care, for example, inevitably rouse cries of, "Placebo!" from the most skeptical corners of the medical community.[36-38] *Placebo* is too often a term of disparagement, not discussion. Given homeopathy's marked difference from conventional medicine—its extreme "otherness"—the placebo issue naturally arises and must be examined when considering homeopathy as a medical science.

Homeopathy as "Other"

Homeopathy is nearly archetypal in the numerous challenges it poses to conventional medical thinking. Metaphors of battle often appear when an author on one side writes about the other side. The differences between the systems are so profound that the use of such metaphors is understandable.

The following passage (in my opinion, one of the finest in homeopathic literature) is a beautifully clear depiction of the philosophic battleground from the homeopathic side. The author, John James Garth Wilkinson, was introduced to homeopathy through his friend, Henry James, Sr. Wilkinson is famous in homeopathic history for spreading the therapy among the upper class in England, in no small part because of his gift for communicating homeopathic ideas. One of his friends, Ralph Waldo Emerson, praised his "rhetoric like the armory of the invincible knights of old." The following quotation is from a letter to Henry James:

The matter of doses depends upon the fineness of the aim. In everything there is a *punctum saliens* so small, that if we could find it out, a pin's point would cover it as with a sky. What is the meaning of that invisible world which is especially versed about organization, if there be not forces and substances whose minuteness excludes them from our vision? We have not to batter the human body to pieces in order to destroy it, but an artistic prick—a bare bodkin—under the fifth rib, lets out the life entire. Nay had we greater skill of delineation, a word would do it. The sum of force brought to bear depends upon precision, and a single shot, true to its aim, or at most a succession of a few shots would terminate any battle that was ever fought, by picking off the chiefs. If our gunnery be unscientific, the two armies must pound each other, until chance produces the effects of science, by hitting the leaders; and in this case a prodigious expenditure of ammunition may be requisite; but when the balls are charmed, a handful will finish a war. It is not fair to count weight of metal when science is on the one side, and brute stuff on the other; or to suppose that there is any parallel of well-skilled smallness with ignorance of

the most portentous size. The allopathic school is therefore wrong in supposing that our "littles are the fractions of their mickles"; the exactness of the aim in giving the former a new direction, takes them out of all comparison with the unwieldy stones which the orthodox throw from their catapults.

But again there is another consideration. Fact shows that the attenuation of medicines may go on to such a point, and yet their curative properties be preserved, nay, heightened, that we are obliged to desert the hypothesis of their material action, and to presume that they take rank as dynamical things. A drop of *Aconite* may be put into a glass of spirit, a dreg of this latter into another glass of spirit, and so on, to the hundredth or the thousandth time, and still the *Aconite*-property shall be available for cure. Here then we enter another field, and deal with the spirits of things, which are their potential forms, gradually refining massy drugs, until they are likened to those sightless agents which we know to be the roots of nature, and feel as the most powerful in ourselves. How such delicate monitors be looked at from the old point of view, as assimilated to the violence that is exercised by materialist physic? If the latter would stir the man, it does by as much main force as it dares to use; whereas the former moves him by a word, through the affinities and likings of his organization.[39]

Although homeopathy has changed from the days of Wilkinson, a gulf remains between the medical philosophies of the average homeopathic physician and the typical conventional physician. The differences between these understandings of patient health continue to create a great deal of mistrust on both sides.

There are points of contact. A homeopath looking at conventional medicine will recognize that homeopathy's primary principle, like cures like, has unwittingly been used to a limited degree in conventional medicine and in many forms of traditional healing. However, this principle is far from being generally accepted.

Homeopathic and conventional opinions about the effects of a specific treatment on a specific patient are often diametrically opposed. These disagreements are a daily event in the practice of clinical medicine. In some instances, viewing the patient's clinical response to conventional treatment through the lens of Hering's Laws of Cure leads to the conclusion that the conventional medical treatment harmed the patient. This interpretation is usually at odds with the conventional interpretation of the same experience.

The matter of homeopathic dilution is quite disturbing to most scientifically trained professionals.

How could any physiologic effect possibly result from ingesting such fantastic dilutions? It is so unsettling that some find it impossible to seriously consider the possibility that there may be something of value in the other elements of the homeopathic approach to patients.

I recall an incident years ago when I presented a proposal for a homeopathic study to a research group at the University of California, San Francisco. After hearing my proposal and learning I was a homeopath, a physician with whom I had earlier been having a very friendly discussion became quite agitated and refused to consider the proposal in any way. When another faculty member asked him what he would do if the study were perfectly designed and found homeopathy effective, he replied, "Design another study." The proposal, which was for a trial of homeopathic treatment for pediatric diarrheal disease, was very similar to a study later completed by Dr. Jennifer Jacobs and associates finding homeopathy statistically superior to placebo.[40]

Another factor heightening the belief that homeopathy's effects could result solely from placebo is the homeopathic interview. The classical homeopathic interview, with its carefully detailed, respectful inquiry into the patient's medical and life history, appears ideally suited to maximize the placebo effect.

These many fundamental questions about homeopathic medicine demand attention. It is important to consider the possibility that *homeopathic treatment* is synonymous with *placebo treatment*.

Some within the homeopathic community are offended when this issue is raised. They are threatened by the derogatory implications of the word *placebo* and consider raising the question of placebo tantamount to impugning their honesty or intelligence. They point out that homeopathy has continued in much the same form for nearly 200 years, with a large cadre of enthusiastic patients. Surely this lengthy track record of satisfied patients must prove efficacy and therefore disprove the supposition that homeopathy is placebo.

Other homeopaths take a broader view. They are not frightened by the complicated questions growing out of our ignorance about the nature of the placebo effect. They consider discussion of the placebo issue fascinating and potentially laden with vitally important information about the healing process—information from which all health care providers can learn. Their view is that homeopathy

has survived because it appears to have some degree of clinical efficacy and therefore considerable implications for medicine. This is true regardless of whether homeopathy is entirely or only partially placebo.

This second group of homeopaths agrees with the opinion, widely accepted within conventional medicine, that alternative forms of medicine must be subjected to scientific examination. Just as conventional medical practices need to be critically evaluated, this age of evidence-based medicine demands nothing less of alternative medical treatments. The gold standard of research in clinical medicine is the double-blind placebo-controlled RCT. Because RCTs often use placebos as controls, understanding the placebo is essential to the process of understanding medicine, including alternative medical practices such as homeopathy.

Homeopathy is Placebo, But . . .

Is homeopathy then placebo? The brief and misleading answer is certainly *yes*. Every patient encounter generates placebo effects, whether the treatment is homeopathy, psychiatry, or surgery (interestingly, surgical procedures appear to create some of the most powerful placebo effects known[41]).

A better question is this: How much of the benefit derived from homeopathic treatment is *exclusively* the result of placebo? The answer to this question is much more difficult and likely to change with differing circumstances. Unfortunately, despite the routine use of placebo in clinical trials, few in the medical profession have any clear understanding of the nature of placebo. Because of the limited amount of research and its inconsistent results, even placebo experts debate the nature or even existence of placebo. One of the few points of agreement is our ignorance; we do not understand placebo as well as we should, given its omnipresence and its apparent power as a healing force.

What Is Placebo?

"Placebos, in other words, are not only puzzles to be 'solved,' but—to the extent that they elude ready solutions—they also teach us how far we still are from closure on the question of what it will mean to create a science subtle and complex enough to encompass all that is entailed in being human."[42]

ANNE HARRINGTON, Harvard University

The word *placebo,* literally translated, means "I shall please." Defining placebo is far more difficult than simply translating the word from Latin. In fact, it is reasonable to argue that there is no satisfactory definition of placebo at this time. Nearly every author on the subject has devised a different definition. Each definition is at odds with some part of what we know about placebo. Some academicians recommend abandoning the concept entirely because of the immense confusion about what placebo is.[43,44]

One of the most commonly accepted definitions in clinical research defines placebo as an intervention believed to lack a specific effect (there is no empirically supported theory for its action) on the studied condition, but which has been demonstrated better than no intervention. By this definition, placebo is something that works when we believe it should not. This is most unsatisfying because it merely highlights our ignorance—we do not understand it, therefore it is placebo.

In clinical practice the deficiencies of this definition are even more apparent. The definition does not encompass the circumstance that is the crux of the placebo–alternative therapy question. The following example may illustrate this point. A patient receives a treatment from an individual who believes it will help the patient. Later, a placebo-controlled trial shows no difference between the treatment and placebo. Despite the research finding, using the definition in the previous paragraph, the practitioner's belief that the treatment would have a specific effect on the patient's disease would mean the treatment was not a placebo.

A historical example of this circumstance in conventional medicine might be helpful. In the late 1970s, Benson and McCallie reviewed various treatments for angina, treatments that were later found ineffective.[45] They learned that many of these ineffective therapies showed response rates up to 100% in early open and double-blind trials (mean response 82.4%) involving 1187 patients. Several patients who were improved by these interventions continued to be well for more than a year (unfortunately, few patients had such extended follow-up). Benson's analysis was a dramatic demonstration of the effectiveness of "ineffective" treatments. The clinicians did not realize that their interventions were merely placebo.

Most definitions of placebo require that the physician believe that the treatment is ineffective. By these definitions, placebo is at some level a deceit.[46]

Traditional treatments acquire the placebo label when the medical community acknowledges that they were ineffective. Although the past errors of conventional medicines are recognized, no one seems eager to label those misguided practitioners as quacks. Similarly if practitioners of homeopathy and other forms of CAM are making clinical errors, these mistakes are most likely the result of well-intentioned ignorance rather than deliberate deceit. Muddling these uses of the term *placebo* (placebo equals trickery, as opposed to placebo equals error) may contribute to physician mistrust of alternative medicine.

Placebo Theories

Many theories have been proposed to explain the mechanism of placebo action. The popularity of each theory waxes or wanes as new information comes to light, and the relative importance of each is open to debate. Placebo effects most likely derive from a variety of causes unified only by the patient's experience of improved well-being.

The placebo-reactor theory maintained that certain individuals were susceptible to placebo and others were not. Research in the 1970s proved otherwise.[47] No correlation between clinical placebo effects and suggestibility exists. The sole personality characteristic consistently associated with a greater likelihood of placebo response is anxiety. We also learned that everyone is a placebo-reactor at one time or another. Placebo reactivity varies more from one time to another in an individual than it does from person to person. Unfortunately many physicians are unaware of the inaccuracies of the placebo-reactor theory. Sadly, some of these confused physicians view a placebo reaction as an indication that the patient is hysterical.[48]

Another theory that has impeded our understanding of placebo is the misattribution theory. This theory argues that the patient would have gotten better anyway and wrongly attributed improvement to an inactive intervention. Most acute illnesses and minor complaints do tend to go away with the passage of time, and the symptoms of many major chronic diseases vary in intensity over time. We know that a positive benefit from placebo is more likely in conditions that have a variable natural history. Also, because of the phenomenon of regression toward the mean (i.e., extreme states are unusual, and change is therefore likely to be in a beneficial direction), repeated measurements or patient contacts are likely to show improvement. However, a significant accumulated body of research demonstrating reproducible physiologic changes following placebo administration in human being and animal experimental models exists. It does appear that something "real" happens from placebo.

Pain appears particularly responsive to placebo treatment.[49] The discoveries of endorphin biochemistry and its importance in the central nervous system, stimulation by placebo, and blockage of placebo pain relief by naloxone were very exciting to placebo researchers. However, the answers we gained chiefly succeeded in multiplying our questions.[50] Although placebo-induced endorphin release can account for placebo effectiveness in pain control, how does placebo induce endorphin release? Even more importantly, what could placebo-induced endorphin release have to do with non–pain-related placebo effects?

There is much to learn from the conditioning model of placebo. Essentially this theory maintains that associating an intervention with an outcome leads to a persistent linkage. Patients then achieve the identical response even if the active part of the intervention is missing. For example, people who believe they are drinking alcohol will develop symptoms of alcohol intoxication even if the drink is entirely alcohol-free. Building on Ader's earlier work (see discussion of nocebo later in this chapter), Olness and Ader reported on a patient for whom they were able to use this linkage of expectation to the patient's benefit.[51] A child undergoing chemotherapy had difficulty tolerating cyclophosphamide treatment for lupus. The cyclophosphamide was routinely administered with cod liver oil. The researchers then gave the child cod liver oil alone for half of the chemotherapy sessions, resulting in the same benefit as the cyclophosphamide but without the same degree of adverse effects.

Placebo theories include societal factors as well. The theory of ritualized healing recognizes the potency of cultural elements. Shamanic rituals, for example, typically require participation of the patient's family and community in the healing process. Of course, our own system of clinics, pharmacies, and hospitals can be viewed as an alternative form of ritualized healing.

The most often repeated example of one placebo theory is of great interest to homeopaths. This theory is that placebo effects logically follow expectations about the treatment. Patients respond because they have, in some way, been told they should respond. Unlike the conditioning theory, patients need not have any prior experience with an active agent associated with the treatment. In 1950, Wolf reported that ipecac was a successful means of treating disabling nausea in a pregnant woman.[52] He even documented the physical effects of the ipecac through gastric pressure monitoring. The use of ipecac in conventional medicine is limited to its emetic effects—precisely the opposite action sought in this pregnant patient. Of course, when ipecac is used in homeopathy, the patient is expected to suffer from nausea that the ipecac is expected to relieve, giving this classic example an alternative explanation.

The most appealing placebo theory to many clinicians is the interpersonal theory. Patients who perceive their physician as warm, caring, attentive, and positive are more likely to enjoy the benefits of the placebo response than are other patients. Some have said that the most powerful placebo is the physician. The idea that healing can happen just by listening and attending to the patient is a powerful concept, one distinctly at odds with the weaknesses of modern technologic medicine. Interesting, isn't it, that the qualities so valued by patients are also highly valued by homeopaths?

None of these theories can account for all instances and aspects of placebo. Each of them provides some information, helping us get a sense of the bounds of our understanding of placebo—much like the tale of four blind men describing an elephant by the part each was touching. Perhaps the best way to understand placebo is by its effects—what it can do and when it does it.

Characteristics of the Placebo Response

"You should treat as many patients as possible with the new drugs while they still have the power to heal."

TROUSSEAU

The response of patients to placebo varies. The patient's anxiety, perception of the physician, expectations, and prior experience of the treatment affect his or her response. As Trousseau wrote long ago, enthusiasm for a new or unfamiliar treatment can accentuate the reaction. Interestingly, patient compliance is also associated with a positive placebo response. In a study of patients taking a drug to lower cholesterol, those who took their pills regularly had a reduced mortality rate in both the active and placebo treatment arms of the trial.[53]

Most published placebo research suggests that every human ill responds to placebo, at least transiently. Pain is particularly responsive to placebo, as are diseases that have an erratic clinical course. Human case reports and animal studies indicate that even serious diseases appear to respond to placebo. Unfortunately, some misguided physicians have erroneously convinced themselves that a patient's response to placebo is proof that the patient did not have a "real" medical illness. Few doctors believe such reasoning has any role in the ethical practice of medicine.

The placebo response occurs in every clinical encounter. The evidence suggests that every clinical interaction has the potential for an entire spectrum of patient response, ranging from wonderfully beneficial to extremely harmful. Clinicians have a professional obligation to recognize this potential. We must carefully avoid interactions that harm the patient as we strive to help to the best of our ability.

Some research supports the idea that transience is a characteristic of placebo response. Benson and McCallie's angina work[45] and a few other studies suggest otherwise. To those who prefer a world ruled by common sense, proof that placebo effects are transient would provide a mind-settling confirmation of placebo's ephemeral nature. In addition, a pattern of fleeting response could become the key to distinguishing placebo effects from the "real" effects of active treatment. Only time and further research will tell.

Adverse Effects of Placebo

Another false belief about placebo, a belief that is particularly relevant to homeopathy, concerns adverse effects. Some have claimed that one of the proofs that the effects of homeopathic treatment are not solely attributable to placebo is that homeopathic remedies can cause adverse effects. Homeopaths accept that the correctly chosen homeopathic remedy for a chronic condition is likely to create a transient exacerbation of symptoms. The term *aggravation* is used to describe this process. The aggravation concept is so well accepted that homeopaths sometimes express concern that the correct remedy was not given if an aggravation does not take place.

However, the ability to produce adverse effects does not prove that homeopathy is more than placebo, because placebos can generate adverse effects. Before discussing adverse effects created by placebo, it is important to distinguish adverse placebo effects from nocebo effects. *Nocebo,* which means "I shall harm," is the true opposite of placebo. Nocebo effects are those that result from negative expectations. In other words, a patient expects some damaging effect from an inactive treatment and the expectation leads to the undesired outcome. One of the most famous studies in placebo literature is an example of the power of nocebo. In 1975, Ader and Cohen released a study regarding the administration of cyclophosphamide mixed in saccharin water to rats.[54] While tracking the rats' death rate following ingestion of this combination, Adler and Cohen discovered that even when cyclophosphamide was no longer administered, rats receiving saccharin alone continued to die as if they were still suffering the ill effects of the cyclophosphamide.

Rats are not alone in their vulnerability to placebo or nocebo. Conditioned nocebo effects also occur in human beings. Various reports, usually unsubstantiated, of "voodoo death," in which a person dies after having been the subject of a curse placed by a powerful member of the community, have been a part of the lore of placebo for generations. There have been a number of recent reports of mass hysterical-symptom outbreaks following perceived (but subsequently disproved) exposures to toxins.

Adverse effects from placebo are unexpected, undesired reactions to treatment. The patient's high hopes are disappointed or accompanied by additional unforeseen unpleasant effects.

The previously cited study by Shapiro and associates[47] found that more than half of a group of patients taking placebo to improve their general health experienced adverse effects of some sort. Interestingly, Shapiro also found that patients who did not benefit from the placebo also did not experience any adverse effects. In other words, not only do adverse effects occur, but they often appear to be an integral part of the placebo response.

Another viewpoint considers the issue of placebo irrelevant. The patient's beneficial response to a treatment is important. The means to that end is not. This view is most commonly that of clinicians and, of course, patients themselves. A recent *Lancet* editorial advocated more research into this aspect of the placebo:

Second, perhaps there should be more investigations into the role of placebo, not as a confounding factor interfering with study design, but as a method of enhancing the efficacy of and reducing the variable response to analgesics and other methods of pain control.[55]

Carrying the idea of patient benefit as the physician's primary ethical duty further, some believe that raising the specter of placebo might have unethical repercussions. Discussing the concept of placebo could be harmful to the patient, because acknowledging the possibility of placebo treatment alters the interaction with the patient. The possibility that the treatment might be placebo can reduce the response to an effective nonplacebo treatment.[56]

Placebo effects are not restricted to inactive treatments. They also augment effective ones.[57] In a study by Skovlund, women who had just given birth were treated for postpartum uterine pain.[58] In the first phase, following an informed consent procedure, they were given either paracetamol or placebo. In the second phase, conducted immediately afterward, a new group of patients on the same hospital ward were randomly given paracetamol or naproxen knowing they might receive either medication. Interestingly, the effect of the paracetamol in the second trial was markedly enhanced, apparently by the patients' knowledge that they were certain to receive active treatment (Figure 6-2).

Although complementary medicine is certainly not entirely placebo, placebos appear to be a form of complementary medicine, because their effects augment the effectiveness of conventional medicine. Conversely, the knowledge that he or she might not be receiving an effective treatment diminishes a patient's expectations and therefore the clinical response. One could argue that it is the ethical duty of the physician to set aside doubts about the effectiveness of a treatment and administer treatment with a full measure of conviction to maximally benefit the patient.

Limitations of Placebo in Research

Although these concepts have many repercussions for clinical medicine, the challenges created for researchers are no less significant.[59] Distinguishing a treatment from placebo is the usual objective of clinical trials. Although this is a difficult task, it is often by itself insufficient to meet the needs of patients and clinicians.

Time	2 Hours	4 Hours
Paracetamol 2	0	40	38
Paracetamol 1	0	30	29
Naproxen 2	0	20	18
Placebo 1	0	3	2

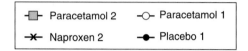

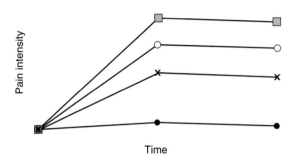

Figure 6-2. Effect of expectation on pain relief.

Because placebo can be effective treatment for many patients, its power must be recognized and respected. When placebo's power is respected, comparing a treatment to placebo becomes a consideration of the degree of effect as well as the frequency and nature of adverse effects.

Statistical superiority over placebo can be misleading. Some homeopathic trials have been criticized on this basis. A difference that is statistically significant but not clinically meaningful to the patient is irrelevant to that patient and his physician unless there is some other compelling advantage, either in the adverse effect profile or cost of the treatment.

It is clear that an important limitation of RCTs is the issue of clinical relevance—sometimes the patient is forgotten in clinical research. Researchers who are primarily interested in measuring quality of life have come to believe that the patient's well-being is the ultimate outcome measure.[60] In addition, there is some evidence that the patient's opinion might be the best discriminator between placebo and active treatment.[61] It is essential that the patient never be forgotten in research as well as in clinical medicine.

Lessons from Placebo and Homeopathy

"Homeopathy may bring benefit, as do so many other forms of alternative medicine, because its practitioners are friendly and unhurried, taking into account the patient's values and teaching that illness is a part of life, to be overcome when it cannot be eliminated."

HOWARD SPIRO, *The Power of Hope: A Doctor's Perspective*

There is evidence that homeopaths were the first to use placebo controls as a consistent part of clinical research; placebos have been used in homeopathic provings since 1828.[62] Hahnemann used placebo routinely in his clinical practice as early as 1819 to establish a symptom wash-out period for new patients and to provide them with otherwise needless daily treatment. There is also evidence that placebo controls were used in attempts to challenge and to prove the efficacy of homeopathy, perhaps as early as 1834 but certainly by 1846 (despite the rather lengthy investigation conducted in the years hence, we still do not have clear answers).[63]

Although there is ample reason to believe otherwise, if homeopathy is solely placebo, studying such a popular therapy could help teach us a great deal about the nature of placebo. Similarly, an exclusively placebo homeopathy could teach us about the deficiencies of current medical practice. Why favor a conventional treatment that is no more effective than a homeopathic placebo? If the adverse effects produced by conventional treatment outweigh those produced by a similarly effective placebo, does it follow that the placebo is the better prescription? The first line of the Hippocratic Oath—*primum no nocere* ("first do no harm")—leaps to mind and suggests so.

One of the greatest truths to be gained from placebo research is that the most powerful placebo is the physician. Our demeanor has considerable effect on patients' well-being. A reasonable summary of placebo research regarding patient-physician interaction is that the effect of physicians can be range from extremely positive to extremely negative.

Perhaps another of the lessons conventional physicians can learn from homeopathy has to do with the attention a homeopath gives to the patient. The interview must be conducted with careful and respectful attention to the patient's complaints and to the patient as a unique individual. The great homeopaths have always taught their students about the tremendous importance of the interview process. When properly conducted, the homeopathic interview appears ideally suited to maximize placebo effects. We must approach each clinical encounter thoughtfully if we hope to provide the best possible care to our patients.

Modern medical practice has become increasingly technological, and many believe we have neglected the relationship aspect of the healing process. Bernard Lown, MD, Professor Emeritus at Harvard University, recently wrote:

Medicine's profound crisis, I believe, is only partially related to ballooning costs, for the problem is far deeper than economics. In my view, the basic reason is that medicine has lost its way, if not its soul. An unwritten covenant between doctor and patient, hallowed over several millennia, is being broken.[64]

The covenant Dr. Lown believes is being broken is the physician's respectful commitment to the patient, unsullied by arrogance, selfishness, or ridicule of the patient's concerns. Homeopathy, through the interview, represents one pathway back toward a healthier relationship between physician and patient.

Just as patients are increasingly displeased with the medical care they receive, physicians are increasingly disenchanted with the system of medical care in which we find ourselves immersed. Time constraints often force the hurried conventional physician to view the patient as a runny nose that must be treated and sent back out the door as quickly as possible. Homeopaths learn that the story of every patient is in some way interesting. The richness of the homeopathic interview enlivens the patient-physician interaction. Perhaps this interaction, which can heal the patient, can also heal the physician in a certain way.

Whenever I find myself struggling with a challenging patient, a bit of advice from one of my favorite homeopathic teachers comes to mind. His advice was, "Always remember that you must be there with the patient. Do not worry about which remedy the patient needs while you are taking the case. If you attend to the patient, he will get better and you will find the remedy." Sage advice, it seems, for a healer of any therapeutic persuasion.

PUBLISHED HUMAN TRIALS OF HOMEOPATHY

Now that we have completed our preparatory consideration of methodology issues, let us move on to the research itself. The following review will not be exhaustive; far too much work has been completed to give due consideration to the entirety of homeopathic research. Although there are earlier bits of data about homeopathic effectiveness in various epidemics and for patients exposed to mustard gas in World War I, homeopathic clinical research has really blossomed in the past two decades.

For the sake of clarity, we should review a few bits of statistical terminology used to identify significance. The "*p*" value is an indicator of the probability that a difference is due to chance. Customarily a *p* value less than .05 is accepted as meaningful. This means that there is one chance in 20 (1/20 = .05) that this finding was an accident. The lower the *p* value the less likely this is a chance finding. Relative risk (RR) provides a ratio of the incidence of a variable (disease, symptom, abnormal laboratory value) for treated subjects as compared to an untreated population. In case-control studies the odds ratio (OR) is used and is roughly equivalent to the RR used in cohort studies. Confidence intervals (CI) are usually expressed as "95% CI" followed by a numerical range. Using a CI recognizes that the true value cannot be determined, but we can determine that it is within a certain range with a specific degree of certainty. A 95% CI (range, x-y) means there is a 95% chance that the true value is between x and y. In a simplistic way, we can say that the wider the CI, the less reliable the results of the study. A meaningful result will have a CI that does not include identity between the groups (0 change or 1 when used with RR or OR to differentiate between groups). Confidence intervals are also useful in that they are readily compatible with meta-analysis techniques and help lead to estimates of the size of the treatment effect, not only whether one occurred.

1980-1984

The first homeopathic study published in a major clinical journal was a trial of homeopathic treatment of patients with rheumatoid arthritis.[65] Two homeopathic physicians examined 46 patients meeting American Rheumatism Association diagnostic criteria for rheumatoid arthritis; the examinations were conducted at The Centre for Rheumatic Diseases, Royal Infirmary, Glasgow, Scotland. The two examining physician-homeopaths categorized the patients by the clarity of their homeopathic cases. This is one means of controlling for the uncertainty of response attributable to errors in remedy selection. The patients were then divided equally between treatment and placebo groups by a third physician not otherwise involved in the clinical assessments. The physicians then used a matching strategy to assign patients to placebo and control groups by the conventional medications they were taking to treat their disease. The investigators also attempted to equally divide the subjects by disease severity. The 23 patients in the treatment group received 20 different homeopathic medicines. The article contains no information about the concentration of the homeopathic remedies used in the study. The placebo powders were indistinguishable in appearance from the homeopathic remedies, and both were dispensed by double-blind protocol. The treatment period was 3 months. During that interval the patients were seen four additional times and the homeopath was allowed to change the homeopathic prescription if indicated by the patient's condition.

Assessment criteria were laboratory data (complete blood count, sedimentation rate, serum biochemistry, and serology) collected at the beginning and end of the study, a pain rating along a visual analog scale (VAS), articular index of joint tenderness, grip strength in both hands, digital joint circumference, duration of morning stiffness, and functional index. An independent assessor who routinely performed these tasks for the clinic conducted the clinical assessments. Although the results of laboratory tests were unchanged at the conclusion of the study period, all clinical measures excepting digital joint circumference were statistically favorable to homeopathy, with *p* values less than .005. Improvement was most marked in patients with clear homeopathic symptoms (i.e., those with the most obvious homeopathic prescriptions). There were no significant outcome differences between the examining physicians.

This trial would be a powerful landmark finding for homeopathy if the data were incontestable. They are not. The differences in disease severity and ongoing medication use were inadequately controlled by the design. The small sample precluded random subgroup assignment. Variability among outcome measures is found in all subsequent homeopathic trials and is normal in clinical trials. The lack of variability in this study is surprising. These flaws make it difficult to draw meaningful conclusions.

A study by Shipley and associates[66] was the next trial of note. For this study, 24 adult females and 12 adult males with osteoarthritis of the hips or knees by clinical and x-ray examination were enrolled in a double blinded RTC published in *Lancet* in 1983. Previous use of either study medication (fenoprofen and homeopathic *Rhus toxicodendron*) excluded patients from the trial. Patients who did not meet the most essential homeopathic characteristics of *Rhus toxicodendron* (aggravation from initial movement with improvement from continued motion and exacerbation of pain from cold and damp) were excluded from the trial.

Two sets of patients were recruited. The 15 constituents of one group were specifically referred for homeopathy at the Royal London Homeopathic Hospital. The other group of 21 entered the study through two conventional hospital departments of rheumatology.

The trial was a crossover design comparing fenoprofen (600 mg tid), *Rhus toxicodendron* 6X dilution (1:1,000,000 or 1×10^{-6}) tid, and placebo. Patients received each treatment for 2 weeks in random order. Visual analog scales (VAS) and a four-point pain score were used to measure pain outcomes. Subjects were also asked which of the three treatments they preferred.

Two of the three patients who dropped out apparently did so as a result of the aggravation of symptoms they experienced (customary while receiving homeopathic treatment). The other drop out occurred because a patient rose to the top of the waiting list for a hip transplant during the course of the trial.

On nearly every measurement fenoprofen was statistically superior to *Rhus toxicodendron* and placebo. The only significant adverse effects experienced by the subjects occurred during the fenoprofen treatment phase. Despite the side effects, patients preferred the fenoprofen over both *Rhus toxicodendron* and placebo, each by a 4:1 margin. There was no difference in response among patients who had contact with the study's homeopaths.

Surprising to no one, homeopathic advocate or critic, this study found that improperly used home-opathy did not work for osteoarthritis. Although this study appeared to be well designed to the conventional investigators, it was not from a homeopathic perspective and so brought down a rain of protest. Despite the experimenter's cursory effort to screen for appropriate patients, the idea of using one of 1600 homeopathic medicines for a common a problem like osteoarthritis ignores basic homeopathic reasoning. Similarly, a treatment interval of just 2 weeks is likely to document only the initial homeopathic aggravation of symptoms common in chronic conditions. A decline consistent with this expectation was clearly documented in five patients. Although the decline could have resulted from terminating effective treatment, it could also have been the short-term homeopathic aggravation without sufficient observation time allotted to document subsequent improvement. Also, the delayed effects of homeopathy make the crossover design of this trial untenable.

One of the homeopathic investigators wrote the following in response to criticism of the study's methodology:

One cannot logically extrapolate from this any conclusions about other potencies of *Rhus tox.*, other homeopathic remedies, or homeopathic medicine in general. The most important lesson that we have learned from this study is that a double-blind crossover trial of short duration using a single potency of a remedy prescribed on local features is unlikely to be a fruitful method of seriously studying homeopathic medicine.[67]

1985-1989

There have been a series of small but interesting trials of the use of a homeopathic preparation made from the topical plant *Galphimia glauca*. The first was published in 1985.[68] In this trial Wiesenauer and Gaus compared a 6X homeopathic preparation (1×10^{-6}) with placebo and with a nonhomeopathic 1×10^{-6} simple dilution. Although the study was too small to achieve statistically meaningful results, they found strong trends toward efficacy of the homeopathic preparation and equivalency of the placebo and simple dilution. This study is especially interesting because of the suggested differences between the homeopathic remedy, with its process of succussion and dilution, compared with the simple diluted material.

Homeopaths have long been at the forefront of medical science in allergic disease. The physician who demonstrated that pollens cause hay fever was a homeopath, and his findings were published in several issues of a homeopathic medical journal.[69-75] Homeopaths also introduced low-dose allergen desensitization.[76] Perhaps, then, it should not be surprising that the next important trial involved homeopathic treatment of airborne pollen reaction.

The publication of a study by Reilly and associates[77] marked the emergence of a series of investigations by Reilly that only recently concluded. The study involved 158 patients over age 5 with a history of at least 2 years of seasonal rhinitis. The patients came from two hospital-based homeopathic clinics and 26 National Health Services general practitioners' offices across Britain. Recent use of allergy medication or immune suppressant drugs was one of the exclusion criteria.

Following randomization, the patients went through a 1-week run-in period to develop a symptom baseline, then received 2 weeks of treatment and a final 2 weeks of observation. Patients recorded the intensity of the entirety of their symptoms on a 100-mm VAS. They also scored certain specific symptoms on a 0 to 3 scale and logged the use of any of the escape medication (chlorpheniramine). These data were recorded daily. At week three (end of the treatment phase) and again at the study's end at week five, a physician assessment was also documented. The study medication was a 30C dilution (1×10^{-60}) of mixed grass pollens most commonly associated with seasonal rhinitis in the United Kingdom.

The homeopathic treatment group showed a clear symptomatic improvement. The response began in earnest in the second week of treatment and progressed as the study continued. VAS scores improved by 17.2 mm in the homeopathy group and 2.6 mm in the placebo group (difference = 14.6 mm, 95% confidence interval [CI] 2.5-26.5 mm, $p = .02$). Although the drop in symptom scores for the homeopathic group was significant ($p = .02$), the drop in the placebo group was not significant. Differences between the patients' prestudy and poststudy clinical condition by physician assessment also achieved statistical significance ($p = .05$). Use of antihistamines was significantly higher in the placebo group. The data were analyzed after correction for pollen counts, disproving local pollen levels as a significant confounding factor. The classic homeopathic pattern of initial aggravation followed by long-term amelioration emerged from these corrected data.

The investigators cleverly applied homeopathic principles to develop another outcome measure. They used the run-in week to develop a baseline to more clearly assess the initial response to the homeopathic remedy. There was a statistically significant difference in the frequency of symptom aggravation during the first week in the homeopathy group compared with placebo ($p < .05$). Furthermore, the patients who experienced an aggravation were markedly improved compared with the placebo group ($p = .0004$; 95% CI 18.4-52.6 mm).

There were two notable weaknesses in this trial. The first was that the principal outcome measure, the VAS, is not an objective instrument. However, this method of assessment is relatively common in certain studies, particularly of allergic and rheumatologic disease. It has the advantage of generally reflecting patients' perceptions of their disease state, whereas specific symptom ranking might mislead us regarding the patient's appreciation of the treatment or lack thereof. Given the controversial nature of homeopathy, highly objective data are most desirable. Laboratory data were collected but not reported.

The other flaw is a homeopathic matter. The investigators used a homeopathic preparation made from material allergenic to most of the patients. They did not select a treatment specific to each patient's pattern of symptoms. We do not know if any of the patients had a traditional homeopathic interview elucidating their symptoms. Therefore this was not a trial of classical homeopathy. This more superficial approach was a reasonable compromise given the nearly nonexistent body of homeopathic research literature of the time. In addition, although many assume that classical methods are superior, final judgment on this matter awaits research confirmation. If the approach used in this study (isopathy, as it is often called—using something in homeopathic potency to treat reactions to material doses of the same substance) is effective, it would be much easier to apply clinically than classical homeopathic practice.

In 1989, Lancet published an editorial entitled "Quadruple-blind."[78] Posing the question "Can blind discussion remove bias from the reader?" the writer went on to describe a trial of an unspecified influenza treatment. After the description and a brief discussion of the respectable positive findings, the editorialist closed with, "Now let the code be broken—the active treatment was a homeopathic preparation."[78]

The *Lancet* editorial referred to a study of 478 patients with a clinical diagnosis of influenza, enrolled from the offices of 149 general practitioners in France.[79] In this double-blind placebo controlled RCT, the homeopathic remedy was a preparation made from duck heart and liver in the 200C potency (1×10^{-400}). Worldwide this product is one of the most popular over-the-counter products for relieving the symptoms of influenza.[80]

In the first 48 hours, patients in the active treatment group recovered at a rate nearly 70% greater (RR 1.67, 95% CI 1.1-2.7, p = .03) than those receiving placebo. The difference in recovery rate was strengthened by data adjustment for covariates, including age, intraepidemic timing of disease onset, treatment delay, symptom severity, and the use of antibiotics or other drugs for symptom control (RR 1.9, 95% CI 1.1-3.4, p = .02). Patients who received active treatment also required less medication for symptom relief (p = .04). A significantly greater number thought their treatment was effective (p = .02).

Although the design of this trial was generally thought excellent, it was not perfect. Using the clinical diagnosis of influenza as the main admission criteria would be more acceptable for a later round of research. Initial studies customarily involve rigorously defined parameters (usually defined by laboratory measures). The fact that this trial took place in a setting more typical of the average patient-physician encounter confuses interpretation somewhat. On the other hand, because a "real world" setting usually tends to weaken the treatment effect, it might actually strengthen the finding for homeopathy. Also, during the study, independent government immunologists working in the region identified an epidemic influenza virus (A H1N1), thus supporting the belief that the patients did have influenza.

In 1989, the *British Medical Journal* published Peter Fisher and associates' study of homeopathic treatment of fibromyalgia.[81] Fibrositis, or *primary fibromyalgia* as it called in the United States, frustrates patients and physicians alike because of the limited effectiveness of conventional treatments. A useful alternative treatment would be welcome. The investigators also hoped to overcome the errors of previous studies by designing a study that was truer to homeopathic principles and yet methodologically sound. To a great extent they accomplished their objectives. They had previously learned that a great number

(42%) of their patients with this disease matched the symptom pattern of the homeopathic remedy *Rhus Toxicodendron*. This unusual congruence between homeopathic and conventional diagnoses would allow the investigators a reasonably large pool of patients satisfying conventional and homeopathic eligibility requirements. In addition, the nature of this disease should lead to a more rapid response than would be expected in the arthritic conditions previously studied. These factors should make the study results more reliable.

Patients were recruited through the rheumatology department of St. Bartholomew's Hospital in London. The screening process excluded patients who did not meet conventional criteria for fibrositis or homeopathic criteria for *Rhus toxicodendron*. Thirty adult men and women were selected and randomly divided into placebo and active treatment groups. Each patient received *Rhus toxicodendron* 6C (1×10^{-12}) or identical-looking placebo three times a day for 1 month and then crossed over to the other treatment. The choice of potency (low potencies are believed to act for a shorter period of time than higher dilutions) and the characteristics of this disease minimize (but do not eliminate) errors created from the crossover design. Outcomes were to be the number of tender spots, VAS measurement of pain and sleep, and overall assessment of treatment.

Although patients showed a preference for the homeopathic treatment, the difference was not statistically significant; the other outcomes were significant. The number of painful spots was reduced by about 25% (p < .005). After completing the trial, the investigators simplified the VAS data to "worse" or "better" and lumped the sleep and pain data together. Analyzing these data showed a significant improvement with the homeopathic treatment (p = .0052).

Although this study represented an improvement, it still had some problems. The crossover design could be problematic, but if it were, the duration of the study would most likely bias the results against a finding for homeopathy. The VAS data processing may be more of a problem. *Post hoc* alterations are always open to criticism, as is the practice of combining disparate information (the sleep and pain scores). Although it might be reasonable to attribute the sleep disturbance suffered by fibromyalgia patients to pain, it might not.

1990-1994

In the 1990s, the pace of homeopathic research rapidly accelerated. A number of important trials were published in many of the most prominent medical journals. As the meta-analysis came into vogue, academicians applied these tools to homeopathy with meta-analyses of the entirety of homeopathic research and of specific diseases.

Kleijnen, Knipshild, and ter Riet wrote a paper titled "Clinical Trials of Homeopathy," published by *Lancet* in 1991.[82] The Dutch government funded their evaluations of many different forms of alternative medicine. Before writing this article, they had issued negative reviews of iridology, acupuncture, and herbal medicine research. In addition to their conventional research expertise, these investigators clearly understood the issues raised by homeopathy's unique theories. Their favorable assessment of homeopathic research surprised many, including the authors themselves.

This group's effort to uncover the maximum number of homeopathic clinical trials was impressive and necessary given Kleijnen and Knipschild's[83] later publication demonstrating the limitations of searching computer databases for studies of homeopathy and other CAM topics. In addition to searching MedLine indexed publications (1966-1990), they tracked down articles referenced in those publications and in textbooks. They scoured most homeopathic journals and the records of the proceedings of homeopathic conferences. They also contacted homeopathic researchers, manufacturers, and libraries. Their diligence led them to 107 controlled trials worldwide.

The researchers demonstrated their knowledge of homeopathy with comments like, "Virtually no evidence exists about the correct choice of remedy and the potency to be used (different potencies or homeopathic substances should be compared in controlled trials)."[82] And another: "[Homeopathy] is not just another therapy but a distinct outlook in medicine, and several interpretations have developed, often contradictory to one another"[82] They pointed out that trials of classical homeopathic methods were a small minority (14 of 107), with isopathy (like Reilly's rhinitis study) used in 9 trials and combinations of homeopathic remedies used in another 26. The most common approach (58 of 107) was to give one homeopathic medicine to all subjects with the same conventional medical diagnosis.

The investigators excluded two trials from the analysis because those trials merely compared one homeopathic treatment with another. The trials were ranked by total scores derived from the following rating categories: adequate description of patient characteristics (10 points), number of patients analyzed (30 pts), randomization (20 pts), well-described intervention (5 pts), double blinding (20 pts), relevant and well-described effect measurement (10 pts), and results presented in such a way that the reader could recheck the analysis (5 pts).

Kleijnen and associates found that the quality of the trials was generally not very good. For example, patient characteristics were adequately described in just more than half of the studies, and only 17 studies described the method of randomization. Only one of the trials considering classical homeopathy rated above 60 on the 100-point scale. To be fair, most conventional research from this time span was not a great deal better methodologically. Still, the quality of homeopathic research is clearly an important issue that deserves the full attention of future investigators.

Another problem was that the studies were typically small. More than half of the trials involved subject groups of 25 or less. Recruiting an adequate of subjects is usually problematic for any researcher. Given the controversy and lack of financial support for homeopathic research, performing larger trials has been extraordinarily difficult.

Only 2 of the best 15 studies found against homeopathy. In no specific disease category did sufficient evidence exist to claim that homeopathy offered effective treatment for the condition. The authors considered the possibility that a greater proportion of positive trials had successfully navigated the review process through to publication. Although they did not evaluate this possibility systematically, their intensive efforts to discover unpublished trials as well as published ones should mitigate publication bias to an uncertain degree.

They summarized their findings as follows:

The amount of published evidence even among the best trials came as a surprise to us. Based on this evidence we would be ready to accept that homeopathy can be efficacious, if only the mechanism of publication were more plausible. . . . The evidence presented in this review would probably be sufficient for establishing homeopathy as a regular treatment for certain indications. There is no reason to believe that the influence of publication bias, data massage, bad methodology, and so on is much less in conventional medicine and the financial interests for regular pharmaceutical companies are many times greater. Are the results of randomized double-blind trials convincing only if there is a plausible explanation? Are review articles of the clinical evidence only convincing if there is a plausible mechanism of action? Or is this a special case because the mechanisms are unknown or implausible?[82]

In 1991, the *Scandinavian Journal of Rheumatology* published a report by Andrade and associates of a 6-month trial of nonclassical homeopathy in the treatment of rheumatoid arthritis.[84] The investigators used clearly defined clinical and laboratory inclusion criteria to select 33 patients. Patients using steroids equivalent to a dose greater than 10 mg of prednisone were excluded. One homeopath saw all patients and initially selected two homeopathic remedies for each patient. Homeopathic remedies were administered twice daily. One was prescribed based on the specific features of joint symptomatology, whereas the other was selected by more general patient characteristics. Although the homeopath could change the prescribed remedy during the study, both practitioner and patient were blind as to the substance actually administered to patients (i.e., whether it was active or placebo).

The study's results were mixed and confusing. Homeopathy achieved statistically significant improvement in 15-meter walking time, Ritchie articular index, functional class (Steinbrocker criteria), and prednisone dosage. The placebo group achieved statistically significant improvement in Ritchie articular index, prednisone dosage, and NSAID daily use. The homeopathic improvement was superior to placebo in 15-meter walking time and functional class. Physician observers assessed the improvement attributable to homeopathy as superior to improvement attributable to placebo (59% vs 44%), but this was not statistically significant.

Careful review of the data suggests the possibility of a type II error. In other words, there were consistent trends favoring homeopathy but the number of subjects may have been too small to demonstrate a statistically meaningful difference. The authors did not mention a power calculation to help them predetermine the requisite number of subjects needed to demonstrate their anticipated effect size. It would be incorrect to claim that these data would certainly support homeopathy if the study were larger. If a larger study were to demonstrate statistical superiority over placebo, the lack of a clear difference in this trial (small effect size) might suggest that that superiority would not be clinically meaningful. Another important homeopathic criticism of the study (in addition to the nonclassical homeopathy used) is the absence of global outcomes to measure changes in patients' well-being in addition to disease severity.

European medical journals have published the lion's share of homeopathic research. In 1994, *Pediatrics* published the first homeopathic trial in a major American medical journal, a study by Jacobs and associates of the treatment of acute childhood diarrhea with homeopathic medicine in Nicaragua.[40] Worldwide, the leading cause of death in children is acute diarrhea. Homeopathy is popular worldwide, including many third-world countries where this problem is most devastating. Homeopathy is well-suited for use in third-world countries for a number of reasons, including its independence from laboratory testing and its inexpensive medications. For these reasons and others Jacobs has conducted a series of trials using homeopathy to treat acute pediatric diarrhea in underdeveloped countries.

Building on the experience of an earlier pilot study,[85] children between age 6 months and 5 years received homeopathic treatment in Leon, Nicaragua, in a double-blind placebo-controlled RCT. The patients were enrolled through government-funded clinics in impoverished neighborhoods. Children within this age range who presented with a history of three or more unformed stools in the previous 24 hours were screened for the study. Exclusion criteria included diarrhea over 1 week; receiving more than one dose of an antibiotic, antiparasitic, or antispasmodic medication within 48 hours before the study; and World Health Organization (WHO) type C (most severe) dehydration. Type C patients were transferred to the hospital for treatment, as was the custom of these clinics.

Each child was examined according to conventional standards (including anthropomorphic data) and homeopathic standards. Stool specimens for each child were analyzed for pathogenic organisms at a local hospital. At each data-collection point, investigators graded the patients based on a previously established diarrhea score combining vomiting (0-2), abdominal pain by mother's report (0-2), temperature (0-3), unformed stools in past 24 hours (0-6), and WHO dehydration classification (0-2).

Experienced physician homeopaths conducted the homeopathic evaluation, augmented by a computerized homeopathic expert system to maximize prescribing consistency.

Individualized homeopathic remedies in the 30C (1×10^{-60}) dilution or an identical placebo were distributed to each patient's family. They were to give the child one dose after every unformed stool and record the stool characteristics on a card. Community health workers made daily home visits with each patient during the treatment. During these visits the workers reexamined the patients, answered questions, and reviewed the completed cards. They left a new card for the parents to complete during the following 24-hour period. Children whose condition deteriorated were referred back to the clinic. The homeopaths were not allowed to change their prescription during the course of each patient's 5-day treatment. Patients also received customary antidiarrheal measures per WHO guidelines, including oral rehydration therapy and continuation of the child's normal diet.

Of the 87 patients enrolled, 6 dropped out of the study (3 each in the treatment and control groups). Workers were unable to find the homes of 4, and the patients' parents wanted some other treatment in 2 cases. The homeopaths prescribed 18 different remedies.

Jacobs found statistically significant differences favoring the treatment group for three of the five principal outcome measures: days to 2 consecutive days of fewer than three unformed stools (1.5 days, p = .048); days to 50% improvement in unformed stools (1 day, p = .036); and mean diarrhea index score (0.4, p = .037). The intergroup difference in days to first formed stool (2.5 days, p = .054) and weight/height percentile change (5%, p = .30) did not achieve significance.

The data were also analyzed based on the presence or absence of a pathogenic agent on culture (several strains of pathogenic *E. coli*, *Rotavirus*, *Entamoeba histolytica*, and *Giardia lamblia*). For all but the weight/height percentile change, patients infected by a pathogenic organism were much more likely to respond to homeopathic treatment than placebo, with p values ranging from .003 to .034.

I criticized the use of the diarrhea index score because the WHO criteria were not weighted heavily enough.[86] Although type A patients did not have any symptoms of dehydration and type C patients were quite severely dehydrated (10% or more), the point range for this part of the scale was only 0 to 2. Less important symptoms were assigned greater weight. Because the sickest patients responded most strongly to the homeopathic treatment, correcting this bias in the scoring system would have probably led to an even more favorable outcome for homeopathy.

Another criticism was that the principal outcome measure—number of days to achieve 2 consecutive days of fewer than three unformed stools—only narrowly achieved statistical significance with a p value of .048. A p value of .05 or less has become a magical boundary between truth and falsehood. Although it is an accepted demarcation, in reality it is an arbitrary division. The difference between .048 and .051, although practically ephemeral mathematically, is psychologically massive. More recently, the same investigators conducted a similar trial in Nepal; this trial's similar results add further weight to the belief that homeopathy effectively treats acute childhood diarrhea.[87] In this study, they arranged to have random samples of the study medication analyzed by an independent laboratory, thereby short-circuiting criticism that the homeopathic remedies used in the first trial could have been adulterated.

1994 was a landmark year for homeopathic clinical research. In addition to Jacob's study, two other major homeopathic trials were published that year. In November, the *British Medical Journal* published de Klerk and associates' highly labor-intensive trial of classical homeopathic treatment as a preventive measure in children prone to upper respiratory infections.[88] Many homeopaths believe that treatment strengthens patients, thereby making them more resistant to many health problems, including infectious disease. This study formally tested that assumption.

Children between 18 months and 10 years of age who had at least three upper respiratory infections in the prior year, or a history of two upper respiratory infections in the prior year and otitis media with effusion at the time of the entry examination, were candidates for this trial. Children who had had a tonsillectomy, adenoidectomy, any of a large variety of chronic health conditions, or recent homeopathic treatment for chronic health problems were excluded, as were children for whom the prescribing homeopath was unable to confidently choose a homeopathic remedy.

There were two elements to the treatment intervention. Parents received written instructions about dietary interventions to help improve their child's health. The homeopathic intervention was individualized, classical homeopathic treatment prescribed in every case by the principal investigator. The investigator/clinician managed each patient's care for up to 1 year.

The study ran for a bit less than 5 years. Although visits typically occurred at 2-month intervals, de Klerk was personally available every day of the trial by phone and was able to change the homeopathic prescription at any time. However, she did not know whether the patient was receiving active or placebo treatment. Each patient remained in either the placebo or homeopathy group for the duration of their participation in the trial.

Every 2 weeks investigators retrieved a variety of symptomatic and behavioral data from parental diaries. They used these data to develop a daily symptom score (DSS) weighted toward respiratory symptoms (range 0 to 56, with respiratory symptoms accounting for up to 42 points). The predetermined principal outcome measure was the calculated mean of the DSS for individual patients and the treatment group as a whole. In addition, investigators collected information about other medical care. Data were analyzed from the 170 patients who completed more than 26 weeks of care (five participants dropped out: two from the homeopathy group, three from the placebo group).

The incidence rate of possible confounding factors (including family history of allergic disease, smoking in the home) was the same in each group. The difference in mean DSS favored homeopathy in each of the three age groups (18 months to 2 years, 2 to 5 years, and 6 to 9 years) for both the 1-year study and for the other data split, which used only the data from the last 9 months of the trial. None of these six comparative advantages for homeopathy achieved statistical significance; *p* values ranged from .06 to .09. The mean percentage of symptom-free days also favored homeopathy, but again to a degree less than statistical significance.

The antibiotic usage data are worthy of further discussion. The number of antibiotic courses favored homeopathy in all but 1 of 15 group comparisons and in total antibiotic courses, 77 to 59. Again, this trend was not statistically significant. Compared with pretrial history, the number of children taking antibiotics dropped markedly in both treatment (73 to 33) and placebo (69 to 43) groups, but the difference between the groups was not significant (*p* = .38).

The rate of surgical interventions (e.g., adenoidectomy, tonsillectomy, pressure equalizing [PE] tubes—also known as grommets, paracentesis, and sinus drainage) favored homeopathy. Once again, these results did not reach the point of statistical significance.

This study is one of the most interesting homeopathic clinical trials to date because of the numerous discussion points it raises. A few months after publication, the principal investigator presented the results of the study at the Second Homeopathic Research Network Symposium, held that year in Washington, D.C. The presentation engendered a lively discussion. One criticism was that a single homeopath (the principal investigator) treated every patient; thus the question of her homeopathic skill is vitally important. Although this particular criticism is important and has been heard many times (the first study criticized on this basis was published in 1835), the greatest controversy centered on the investigators' conclusion that homeopathic medicines produce no clinically relevant improvement in recurrent upper respiratory tract infection.

The authors themselves pointed out that the difference in mean DSS could have been reduced by the difference in antibiotic usage. Because the placebo group used more antibiotics, the antibiotics might have altered the clinical course of those patients (as was undoubtedly the intention of the prescribing physicians), thus reducing the DSS and the difference between placebo and homeopathy groups. This expected reduction could easily have prevented a statistically significant finding in favor of homeopathy.

If the DSS scoring were reliable, there would be another statistical issue. Many statisticians believe that best way to look at data like the DSS data is to compare the change in DSS in each patient and then compare changes in the weighted group mean. This is conventional procedure in studies using a continuous variable such as peak expiratory flow in asthma studies.

As a clinician, one of the most striking aspects of this study is the significant improvement experienced by the placebo group. This improvement could be the result of a declining rate of upper respiratory infection in children as they age. It could also be a result of the broader components of the homeopath's treatments in this study. In addition to prescribing remedies, the classical homeopath traditionally counsels patients about health-promoting lifestyle changes and helps the patient avoid needless medication use by education. The principal investigator decided to compare the entirety of the homeopathic approach with all of homeopathy, *except* the remedy. The placebo group experienced the intensive questioning and decision-making process all the way through remedy selection. Both homeopathy and homeopathy-without-the-remedy appeared helpful, but the importance of the remedy hovered at the threshold of respectability. As a clinician, my primary goal is helping my patients get better. Both patient groups in this study achieved that goal and improved impressively. Sharing this clinical bias and considering the study's other problems, the consensus of the group of homeopathic researchers at our meeting was that the authors' conclusions were unwarranted, over-simplified, and probably misleading.

De Klerk's study was an attempt to look at the effects entirely attributable to the homeopathic remedy itself. Although this was a laudable attempt, unfortunately the methods were seriously flawed. Because this was, in many ways, a good study, the controversy surrounding it highlights the complexity of homeopathic research and even the more fundamental question, "What is homeopathy?" Is homeopathy the remedy, the entire classical home-opathic clinical process, or something in between?

Also in 1994, *Lancet* published another install-ment in the Reilly and associates' homeopathic immunotherapy series, including a meta-analysis of the series to date.[89] An asthma clinic in west-central Scotland served as the recruitment center for this trial. Eligible patients were bronchodilator-responsive adults with more than 1 year of asthma who reacted to inhaled allergens and had positive allergic skin tests. After being screened by a homeo-path and one of the asthma clinic physicians, the patients received skin and pulmonary function test-ing followed by a 4-week single-blind placebo run-in period. The conventional and homeopathic physi-cians excluded unsuitable patients.

Investigators randomized the subjects into groups stratified by their daily dose of inhaled steroids and the allergen to which their skin reaction was most pronounced. In a double-blind protocol, subjects received a homeopathic remedy in the 30C dilution (1×10^{-60}) prepared from the allergen to which their skin test reaction was the most pro-nounced. The study period continued another 4 weeks (except for patients who wished to extend their treatment even longer with an additional 4 weeks). Although investigators collected a variety of data (e.g., pulmonary function testing, symptom diaries, rescue medication use, IgE antibody titers), the prin-cipal outcome measure was a VAS worded identically to the VAS used in the previous trials.

Although many data sets showed trends favorable to homeopathy, they did not generally achieve statis-tical significance. The blinded homeopathic physi-cian and patient rated homeopathic treatment more effective ($p = .04$). The homeopathic doctor was more likely to correctly identify which patients had received placebo than the nonhomeopath. The VAS results strongly favored homeopathy ($p = .003$), with a difference of 33%.

The authors then performed a meta-analysis by combining the VAS data from this trial with the same information from the two previous studies. The com-posite p value from the pooled data was $p = .0004$, leading to the conclusion that "either answer sug-gested by the evidence to date—homeopathy works, or the clinical trial does not—is equally challenging to current medical science."[89]

Although some trials have been quite favorable to homeopathy, few of them have been replicated. Reilly's series is exceptional in this regard. However, the subjectivity of the principal outcome measure, the VAS, dims the achievement in the eyes of some. Although the diseases Reilly studied were all atopic, the symptomatic manifestations of the immunologic disturbance differ. This difference calls into question the decision to combine the trials in a meta-analysis. It also makes it difficult to find a unified measuring scale, thus Reilly's use of the VAS.

Had other, more traditional measures achieved significance, this would not have been an issue. For example, the most common measure of clinical bene-fit in asthma is the forced expiratory volume in one second (FEV_1). In this latest trial, the change in FEV_1 favored homeopathy, but not significantly ($p = .08$). Although there is little reason for such a concern, theoretically this disparity between a patient's subjec-tive sense of improvement and possibly unimproved clinical condition could lead to inappropriate under-medication. Given the small size of this study, a type II error could easily account for the insignificant change in FEV_1.

1995-1999

One of the most popular applications of homeopathy is for postinjury healing. Homeopathic *Arnica*, administered following trauma, may be the most common first experience of homeopathy. Kleijnen's 1991 meta-analysis[82] found that the outcomes of 18 of the 20 trials of homeopathy in trauma were favorable to homeopathy. To test the efficacy of homeopathy as a treatment for acute trauma, a group of Norwegian investigators recruited a group of healthy young adults facing surgery for impacted wisdom teeth.[90] Of the 24 patients who participated in the study, 14 were students at the Norwegian Academy of Natural Medicine and were therefore enthusiastic about participating in a trial of homeopathy.

The experimenters standardized the surgical procedures and anesthetic for the patients. Each patient had two surgeries, one for each side of the mouth. One surgeon performed all of the surgeries. Both procedures for each patient took place at the same time of day (with two exceptions). Each patient's procedures were performed on the same day of the week. Two homeopaths treated the patients with homeopathic remedies selected by classical symptomatic indications. The article is unclear as to whether the homeopaths discussed the choice of the patients' homeopathic remedies. The patients received homeopathic remedies at uniform intervals regardless of clinical response. Codeine pain medication was available to those patients who needed it.

The trial design included subjective and objective outcome assessments. One measure was a series of 28 VAS ratings of pain. Observers measured facial swelling and ability to open the mouth with mechanical devices. They also recorded complications, most notably postoperative bleeding.

Most patients received homeopathic *Arnica*. The next largest group was patients receiving phosphorus. There was no significant crossover effect. The only statistically significant difference in favor of homeopathy was a reduction in trismus (inability to open the mouth). The authors criticized their own study design because a previous trial had shown *Arnica* ineffective at the same concentration used in this trial.[91] They also noted the surprisingly low pain levels experienced by the placebo group: "The physicians believe that the low pain scores and satisfaction of the patients may at least partly reflect the clinical skill of the two homeopaths."[91] Although

this interpretation, if correct, would support the benefits of the homeopathic process, and although the significant reduction in trismus might be meaningful, it is difficult to interpret this trial as favorable to homeopathy. The studies' lack of power due to the small number of subjects might be a significant problem because intergroup differences of 30% to 40% would have been needed to achieve statistical significance.

The *Journal of the Royal Society of Medicine* published another study of homeopathy in surgical trauma in 1997.[92] A total of 73 patients completed this trial of homeopathic *Arnica* as a specific preventive for postoperative pain and infection following total abdominal hysterectomy. The patients received two doses of *Arnica* 30C in the 24 hours preceding surgery, and three doses every day for the subsequent 5 days, or an identical placebo regimen.

There was no difference between the active and placebo groups in pain, medication use, hospital stay, or rate of complications. When the means were adjusted by analysis of covariance, patients in the *Arnica* group might have recovered more rapidly. This difference could have been a result of the younger average age and simultaneously longer surgical times among the *Arnica* patients. Because of the longer surgical times, this group may have felt worse immediately following the procedure, and younger patients are known to recover more rapidly.

As have other studies, this investigation produced data suggesting support for the expectation of homeopathic aggravation. Pain scores rose in the 12 hours following treatment with *Arnica*, although not to a statistically significant degree.

The acupuncture literature appears to show that general anesthesia might block acupuncture's effectiveness in certain circumstances.[93] This has yet to be investigated in homeopathy but could have been a confounding factor in this trial because of the difference in anesthetic usage between study groups.

The other weaknesses of this study involve the homeopathic dose. The correct homeopathic dose is almost entirely speculative; it is seldom researched and is the source of many disagreements among homeopathic clinicians. Theoretically, the clinical effects of different doses should vary. Although more modest, the effect of an imperfectly chosen dose should still be demonstrable. If not, how could homeopathic clinicians reliably help patients to any significant degree?

Another dose-related issue is the prophylactic administration of homeopathic remedies. The indications for homeopathic medicines are a pattern of clinical symptoms, such as bruising or pain after trauma. Some homeopaths argue that using *Arnica* prophylactically before symptoms are present runs counter to homeopathic theory and therefore should not work.

The authors suggested that further trials of homeopathic *Arnica* focus on tissue trauma and bruising rather than pain and wound healing. They based their recommendation on the findings of their trial and others. Even this adjustment of expectations, incompletely rejecting the efficacy of *Arnica* in the context of postsurgical trauma, runs counter to customary use of homeopathic *Arnica*, which is practically unchallenged as the correct initial treatment following physical trauma. Perhaps homeopaths have scuttled homeopathic principles in the routine use of *Arnica*.

There have been a series of trials of the use of homeopathic *Arnica* in distance runners. Two were conducted at the Oslo marathon in 1990 and 1995.[94,95] These studies were small, and although all of their outcome measures demonstrated positive trends, only one of these measures was statistically significant. That advantage for homeopathy was the runners' pain measurement immediately after the marathon ($p = .017$).

A much larger English study of runners, including 262 marathon runners, was designed to duplicate the Oslo trials.[96] The only outcome favoring homeopathy in this larger trial was a 2% to 3% improvement in runners' times. There was a similar reduction in homeopathically treated runners' times in both Oslo trials. In those trials the difference was not significant, possibly because of a type II error with the small effect size coupled with a small study population. The sole significant finding in Oslo, the immediately postmarathon pain level, was not assessed in the English study.

Although the English trial adds some additional evidence against homeopathic *Arnica* generally, the matter is clearly unsettled. The favorable findings—enhanced performance and immediate pain reduction—bear further investigation. Are these findings an indication of homeopathy as an athletic performance-enhancer or merely a result of the laws of probability leading from multiple measurements to a solitary positive outcome?

In 1997, a German medical journal published a meta-analysis of 11 trials using a single homeopathic remedy, *Galphimia glauca,* for relief of eye symptoms caused by airborne pollens.[97] All of these trials had been conducted by the authors of the meta-analysis over a 10-year period. The trials included a total of 1038 subjects. Seven of the trials were double-blind placebo-controlled RCT design (752 subjects). Patients in the treatment group were 1.25 times as likely to improve as those in the placebo group (95% CI 1.09-1.43).

Lancet published another meta-analysis of the entirety of homeopathic clinical trials in 1997.[98] Linde and associates searched the conventionally published literature as well as conference proceedings and books. They also contacted researchers, publishers, and manufacturers in search of homeopathic RCTs published in any language. They found 189 trials, 119 of which met inclusion criteria. Of those meeting inclusion criteria, 30 were excluded because of inadequate information to conduct the meta-analysis.

Linde calculated an odds ratio favoring homeopathy over placebo of 2.45 (95% CI 2.05-2.93). Limiting the meta-analysis to the 26 good quality studies reduced the odds ratio to 1.66 (95% CI 1.33-2.08). Publication bias tends to favor positive findings. Applying a statistical technique called *funnel plotting* (which is used in meta-analyses to eliminate the effects of publication bias) to the high quality trials, they found an odds ratio of 1.78 in favor of homeopathy (95% CI 1.03-3.10). In addition, they found good support for homeopathic effectiveness in certain conditions (seasonal allergies and postoperative ileus), but the data were not strong enough to constitute convincing evidence of efficacy.

This meta-analysis had an ambitious reach. Although 189 RCTs would have been an unimaginable sum a decade ago, it is still a small number. As a consequence of the relatively small number coupled with the lack of any organized effort to selectively research certain clinical conditions, this meta-analysis had to combine data from studies of entirely unrelated medical conditions. This approach is not unreasonable, but results must be interpreted cautiously. Some argue that pooling unrelated positive trials could erroneously add up to a conclusion that homeopathy is an effective therapy across the range of medical conditions. As usual, there is another side to these arguments. Pooling data from multiple clinical conditions might obscure the value of homeopathic treatment if homeopathy is effective for certain of the conditions studied but not for others.

Repeating trials with closely parallel designs is an important step in the process of proving efficacy. Seeking out more uniform data sets, Linde[98] also clustered and evaluated the trials by disease-specific criteria. Unfortunately, the data were too limited to reach definitive conclusions. To more fully appreciate the tenuous state of the research, consider the two areas of homeopathic practice with the clearest research support. Every trial of postoperative ileus has been positive—except one. That one study was the largest and best designed. It found homeopathy no better than placebo. *Pollinosis* (hay fever) studies offered another disease-specific research cluster. Four studies were sufficiently similar to allow data pooling with a reasonable expectation of accurate interpretation. Although these pooled data were impressive, and were collected at multiple sites with different clinicians, the same principal investigator supervised all four trials. The authors believed it necessary that at least two independent groups of investigators replicate positive studies to confirm an original finding. So once again, the reliability of many homeopathic studies is not as incontestable as would be ideal.

Linde and associates concluded that their findings were "Not compatible with the hypothesis that the clinical effects of homeopathy are completely due to placebo."[98] They advocated continued research but only if that research were of high quality: "We believe that a serious effort to research homeopathy is clearly warranted despite its implausibility."[98] Specifically, they recommended that researchers attempt to develop laboratory models to explore possible mechanisms, replicate trials, and research clinical effectiveness rather than placebo differentiation.

Linde's recommendations deserve further comment. Because the absence of a well-accepted mechanism of action is an insurmountable intellectual barrier for many, discovering one would affect attitudes toward homeopathy immeasurably. It is essential that favorable clinical trials be confirmed through replication by independent researchers.

Linde's final recommendation that future studies focus on clinical effectiveness rather than placebo differentiation may be the most important recommendation to come out of this study. It is certainly congruent with the growing movement toward outcomes research. Although demonstrating a difference

from placebo is scientifically important, the question of the treatment's ability to relieve the patient is far more important to the patient and to health care providers. If the benefit is statistically significant but clinically imperceptible, no one will be satisfied.

Weiser, Strosser, and Klein investigated a specific homeopathic treatment for vertigo. The results of their investigation were published in *Archives of Otolaryngology—Head and Neck Surgery* in 1998.[99] Subjects were diagnosed with acute or chronic vertigo and must have had three or more attacks of moderate to severe vertigo in the week before entering the study. Exclusion criteria were newly treated chronic vertigo, vertigo caused by tumor or drug use, and history of a recent myocardial infarction or other disease contraindicating the use of betahistine.

This was a double-blind RCT using treatments that were identical in appearance and taste. Three times a day for 42 days the subjects received 15 drops of a homeopathic combination or oral betahistine. Betahistine is considered an effective and standard treatment for this condition in Europe. Investigators made the decision to compare the homeopathic intervention with active treatment rather than placebo because denying an effective conventional treatment for an illness that creates significant morbidity would have been unethical. The homeopathic treatment was a proprietary combination of homeopathic remedies that are commonly used individually to treat vertigo or motion sickness. Each was prepared as a homeopathic dilution to various degrees (1×10^{-3} to 1×10^{-8} [*Ambra grisea* 6X, *Anamirta cocculus* 4X, *Conium maculatum* 3X, and *Petroleum rectificatum* 8X]).

Predefined outcomes measures were the frequency, duration, and severity of vertigo episodes and, secondarily, health-related quality-of-life measures. Both groups experienced adverse effects; nausea and tremor of the hands in the homeopathy group and headache in betahistine group. There were nine dropouts. Of the seven participants who dropped out as cured, four were from the homeopathic group. In addition, two patients from the betahistine group quit because of intolerance of the medication.

All measures were improved in both groups. There was no difference in patient outcomes between the groups. Although patients in the homeopathic group had a 60% greater reduction in the frequency of their attacks, this difference did not achieve statistical significance.

Limitations of the study are common to many clinical trials. Because many clinicians are not overly impressed with the effectiveness of conventional treatments for vertigo, a placebo group would have been scientifically desirable but ethically unacceptable. 90% of participants did not have a definitive diagnosis for the cause of their symptoms, thus it is possible that disparate clinical conditions were compared. However, initial empiric treatment of patients with new-onset vertigo is customary in primary care medicine. Because more than 70% of the study patients had never before been treated for vertigo, the study reasonably mimicked standard clinical practice.

These imperfections are not significant. This study suggests that homeopathy is as good as one widely used conventional medication for vertigo. Given the absence of dropouts from the homeopathic group because of adverse effects, the equality of clinical benefit found here argues that homeopathic treatment may be superior to conventional treatment for vertigo.

In 1997, two studies of classical homeopathy as a treatment for chronic headaches were published. These trials followed a highly positive trial reported by Brigo[100] at an international homeopathic conference. Although the initial trial was positive and relatively well designed, the follow-up trials were negative and better designed than the original.

Walach and associates' trial incorporated a design element that has been a topic of discussion at a number of homeopathic research meetings.[101] Because classical homeopathic treatment demands individualized treatment, it is difficult to study. However, classical homeopathy is generally considered the ideal model of homeopathic practice, so this method *should* be tested despite the inherent difficulties. A study of classical homeopathy that uses a single prescribing homeopath is always open to criticism on grounds that the homeopath's skills are subpar and therefore his or her treatment is likely ineffective. To overcome this uncertainty, a panel of homeopaths, which prescribed by consensus, treated Walach's subjects. There was no difference in response between homeopathic medicine and placebo. One flaw in the study was unbalanced randomization; there was a large numerical difference between placebo and homeopathy groups.

Later the same year, Whitmarsh, Coleston-Shields, and Steiner's trial of classical homeopathy as a prevention for migraines was published.[102]

Investigators excluded patients if the homeopathic remedy believed to be their chronic remedy (*simillimum*) was not one of the 11 medicines preselected for use in the study. Although the risk ratio was 2.13, favoring homeopathy, the 95% CI included *1;* therefore both groups *could* be identical, thus precluding significance. As did Walach's trial, this well-designed study found no difference between homeopathy and placebo. There were questions about intergroup disparities in the baseline status of patients, but this difference was of questionable significance.

At the end of 1997, I was part of an international group of human and animal researchers that gathered under the sponsorship of *Commonweal,* the Harvard Center for Alternative Medicine Research, the John E. Fetzer Institute, the Geraldine R. Dodge Foundation, and the StarFire Fund to develop a consensus statement on the current state, problems, and prospects of future research in homeopathy.[103] The following comments from that statement are relevant to our discussion.

The first comment arose out of our recognition of the tantalizing yet frustratingly inconclusive nature of both human and animal clinical research at the time.

Anecdotal reports in veterinary clinical practice using homeopathy mirror the results in human medicine. While veterinary clinical research in homeopathy has resulted in hundreds of citations in the veterinary literature, there have been few high quality controlled trials.

Several hundred experimental animal studies have demonstrated positive results but much of the research is of low quality. The areas of study include toxicology and biochemistry in the modulation of in vivo and in vitro enzymatic activity using preparations at homeopathic levels of dilution. Increased excretion of toxic substances have been enhanced by homeopathic preparations.[103]

What follows is our comment regarding mechanism of action:

Theories have been proposed for a mechanism of action for homeopathy, yet results of basic sciences research have been inconclusive. No current mechanism of action for ultra-high dilutions is known today and there are inconsistent research strategies being pursued at the present time.

On the other hand, fundamental principles of homeopathy such as the biological action of the micro-dose, hormesis, and the similia principle are consistent with recognized mechanisms of action of treatments that are used therapeutically in some areas of conventional medicine.[103]

In closing, the group made the following recommendations:

Further scientific exploration of homeopathy and its effectiveness should be evaluated in relation to many of the challenging issues in health care today. These include efficacy, safety, toxicity, prevention, cost-benefit, quality of care and outcomes research.[103]

Classical homeopathy is often considered the "holy grail" of clinical homeopathy. Homeopaths expect classical homeopathy to be the most effective treatment for patients. The classical method is the most time-consuming and difficult to implement. Studies of classical methodology are similarly difficult and are therefore relatively rare, despite the expectation that classical homeopathy would be optimal for investigating the pinnacle of homeopathic effectiveness. In 1998, the *Journal of Alternative and Complementary Medicine* published Linde and Melchart's meta-analysis of clinical trials of classical homeopathy.[104]

The authors included all studies published up to May 1998 in their meta-analysis. They found 32 studies, with 6 "likely to be have good methodological quality" and another 6 "unlikely to have major flaws."[104] Overall the findings were favorable to homeopathy (pooled rate ratio 1.62, 95% CI 1.17-2.23). Because the CI range is greater than 1, this was a significant finding. However, restricting the pool to the best studies did not demonstrate superiority of classical homeopathy over placebo (rate ratio 1.12, 95% CI 0.87-1.44). Although four of the six best studies found a rate ratio higher than 1, thus favoring homeopathy, in five of the six the 95% CI included 1. Definitive answers are elusive.

When the U.S. Congress created the Office of Alternative Medicine within the NIH, one of the purposes was to encourage research in CAM therapies. In 1999, the results of the first homeopathic trial funded by this office (now the National Center for Complementary and Alternative Medicine) were published.[105]

Mild traumatic brain injury (MTBI) affects 750,000 Americans annually, and 5% to 15% of patients with MTBI experience persistent symptoms and disability for more than 3 months after a traumatic injury to the brain. Although the pattern of short-term recovery from MTBI is unpredictable, complete recovery is rare when symptoms persist beyond 6 months. The social and economic costs of MTBI are estimated at $3.8 billion annually.

Investigators studied 61 Boston-area adult patients meeting standardized criteria for MTBI with symptoms persisting more than 3 months (mean 2.93 years, range 4 months to 16 years). Most of these patients continued to suffer deficits that impaired their functional ability. Investigators selected 18 homeopathic remedies suitable for symptoms experienced by MTBI patients. The remedies were selected based on case reports and symptoms documented in the homeopathic literature that paralleled complaints of MTBI patients. The principal investigator was an experienced homeopathic physician. He chose the remedies for each patient in consultation with a psychiatrist on the staff of the rehabilitation hospital through which the study was conducted. There is no reference in the article regarding the psychiatrist's homeopathic training, if any. The patients received either placebo or the selected homeopathic remedy in the 200C potency (1×10^{-400}). Most patients received this dose three times at 12-hour intervals at the outset of the study. Patients who were using conventional medication took the study medication (or placebo) daily for 7 days. Every patient, even those from the study medication group, then received a daily placebo for the duration of the study (4 months). The homeopathic physician was allowed to change the prescriptions of patients who were not responding adequately, but did not know which group (active or placebo) the patients were assigned to.

The principal outcome measure was a scale traditionally used by the staff at the study hospital to assess patients' clinical condition. Patients in the treatment group improved significantly compared with those in the placebo group. The greatest improvement occurred in the group of patients with the lowest expectation of improvement, those with the longest-standing symptoms.

Only one patient experienced the classical homeopathic aggravation of symptoms. Approximately 10% of homeopathic patients experienced some "minimal" adverse effects, including one patient with nausea and another with depression. Concurrent use of conventional medicine did not augment, interfere, or apparently interact with homeopathic treatment in any way.

The authors point out that the compromises they made to adapt homeopathy to their research model, by restricting the number of homeopathic remedies allowed and limiting follow-up to 4 months, probably reduced the effect of the homeopathic treatment. They recommended a larger and longer trial allowing the use of all homeopathic remedies. A longer trial would also satisfy critics because placebo-induced improvement tends to be short-lived. This positive finding is heartening because we lack effective treatment for MTBI in conventional medicine. Further examination of homeopathic treatment of this condition appears justified.

In 1999, Linde and associates, authors of the 1997 *Lancet* meta-analysis,[98] revisited the data to consider the effect of various indicators of methodological quality on study outcome.[106] They found a clear trend toward smaller effect sizes among the most rigorous trials. Double-blinding was the most influential factor. They concluded that this evidence of bias, coupled with the high-quality negative trials published following the 1995 cut-off date for their meta-analysis, meant that they likely had "at least overestimated the effects of homeopathic treatments."[106] Although the tendency for more rigorous trials to yield more modest effect sizes is customary in conventional medicine as well, this article serves as a cautionary reminder of the hazards of interpreting meta-analyses.

2000-2001

In 2000, Jacobs and associates repeated their earlier study of acute childhood diarrhea, this time in Nepal.[87] Again they found significant reduction in the duration of pediatric diarrhea in response to homeopathic treatment. Although the reduction was modest, any positive effect on an illness that is the leading cause of pediatric mortality in much of the world should be respected and replicated by independent researchers.

In August of 2000, the *British Medical Journal* published Taylor and associates' study of homeopathic immunotherapy, the final installment in the series of Reilly's studies).[107] As in the three previous trials, patients with atopic inhalant allergy received treatment with a 30C dilution (1×10^{-60}) of their principal allergen. Patients with allergic rhinitis for more than a year who passed a variety of exclusionary criteria

(including mechanical nasal obstruction, respiratory infection, pregnancy, breast feeding, recent corticosteroid use, serious illness, and recent conventional allergic desensitization) were skin-tested to determine the allergen to which they were most sensitive. Patients received three doses of placebo during a 2-week run-in period. Qualifying patients were then randomized to receive three doses of active or placebo treatments taken within the initial 24 hours of the study.

Investigators measured several outcomes. Patients used an instrument recognized as a valid measuring device for nasal inspiratory flow. Previous conventional studies have established a range of 13 to 18.5 L/min increase as an indication of significant clinical improvement. Consistent with previous trials, the patients graded their general condition every day on a VAS. As with previous trials, random samples of the study medication were analyzed for contamination with conventional allergy medications or house dust mite antigen. The placebo was indistinguishable in taste, smell, and packaging. Although the placebo did not contain the starting allergen, it was diluted and shaken in the same manner as the active preparations.

Patients in the placebo group averaged 2.5L/min improvement in nasal inspiratory peak flow compared with 22.3L/min in the homeopathy group ($p = .0001$, 95% CI 10.4-29.1). This improvement was comparable to that achieved by nasal steroids. Unlike previous trials, the VAS data did not show a significant difference ($p = .82$, 95% CI 9.8-7.8). A greater percentage of homeopathic patients (29%) experienced the classic homeopathic aggravation of symptoms by 48 hours than did placebo patients (7%). This difference was statistically significant ($p = .04$). The investigators speculated that the high percentage of homeopathic aggravations adversely colored the perceptions of the subjects, leading to disappointing VAS scores in contrast with the positive objective outcome measures.

Because the ultimate outcome measure of a clinical intervention is always the patient's perception, the meaning of this final chapter in the series is open to debate. Does an objective finding that is of questionable health significance (nasal inspiratory peak flow) have meaning when the patients did not report feeling better? This is not an example of a *post hoc* favorable analysis. The nasal inspiratory peak flow measurement was predefined as one of the principal outcome measures. This measure favored homeopathy strongly, but would such a treatment satisfy patients and clinicians in daily practice? Although this question was not the subject of this investigation, it and similar questions regarding other clinical conditions must be answered in the future to determine the true worth of homeopathic treatment.

Continuing their ongoing meta-analysis, the investigators pooled the VAS data from this trial with those of the three previous trials. Although there was no significant difference between the mean active and placebo VAS scores in this trial, pooling VAS data from all trials nevertheless showed homeopathy strikingly superior to placebo (p = .0007, 95% CI 4.2-15.4). Reasonably, the authors concluded that it was more likely that homeopathy was having some effect than that they had made a series of errors grand enough to falsely achieve such impressive statistical results.[107]

In Jacob's 1992 survey, otitis media was the third most common diagnosis among patients of American physicians specializing in homeopathy.[108] Stimulated by this finding and by the growing controversy surrounding customary use of antibiotics for this condition, Jacobs and associates examined classical homeopathy as a treatment for acute otitis media (AOM) in 75 children from 18 months to 6 years of age.[109]

Children with clinical characteristics of AOM (i.e., middle ear effusion with fever or pain) for less than 36 hours were recruited from a conventional pediatric practice. The study compared individualized homeopathic remedies (selected in the classical homeopathic method) with placebo three times a day for up to 5 days. Treatment was stopped earlier if symptoms resolved, per traditional homeopathic practice. The treating homeopaths prescribed a total of eight different remedies in the 30C dilution (1×10^{-60}). It is interesting to note that only four remedies covered 88% of the cases, and one of them (*Pulsatilla nigricans*) was used in more than 60% of the cases. In addition to having symptoms for more than 36 hours, exclusion criteria were antibiotics in the previous week, a homeopathic remedy in the prior 72 hours, any other current medication, ear discharge, perforated tympanic membrane, history of PE tubes, tonsillectomy, adenoidectomy, cleft palate, or Down syndrome. Patients were allowed the use of analgesics.

Assessment criteria were both objective and subjective. Parents kept a diary of patients' symptoms, which were scored for evaluation, as well as a log of medication used. Treatment failure was identified by persistent fever or pain as early as 24 hours into the trial. An independent clinical audiologist evaluated the patients' tympanograms. To eliminate questions about contamination or adulteration of the study medication, samples were independently analyzed (using gas chromatography and bacterial inhibition techniques) by the Departments of Medicinal Chemistry and Laboratory Medicine at the University of Washington.

The rate of treatment failure was higher in the placebo group than in the treatment group at every measurement point. At 5 days 19.4% of the homeopathic patients had failed treatment, compared with 30.8% of the control group (11.4% difference). At 2 weeks the homeopathic group had 18.4% fewer treatment failures and at 6 weeks the difference was 19.9%. Despite the consistency of these figures, the difference was not statistically significant. Based on the difference in the failure rates at 5 days, the investigators calculated they would need close to 500 subjects to achieve statistical significance.

Patients in the treatment group experienced a statistically significant decrease in pain scores at the 24-hour and 64-hour evaluations (p < .05). No significant adverse effects were reported in either group. Compliance with the study medication and placebo was good. Analgesic use was nearly twice as common in the placebo group (10 of 39 vs 5 of 36). There were no significant differences in the rate of middle ear effusion following the intervention. However, the subgroup of patients with documented effusion at the time of study entry had the highest rate of response to the homeopathic treatment with differences in failure rate of 14.7% at 5 days, 29% at 2 weeks and 33.7% at 6 weeks.

Although the design of this study reflected the realities of clinical practice, the accuracy of diagnosis in studies of AOM is often controversial and a source of some question here. The placebo recovery rate was lower than in the placebo group of many other studies of AOM. The authors reasonably suggest this was probably the result of the stringent treatment-failure criteria they used, as required by the human subjects committee. Although the statistically significant improvement in pain scores at two measurement points was encouraging, the other seven points before and afterward did not achieve significance. At each point the trend favored homeopathy, so the lack of significance could be the result of the effect size relative to the number of subjects. A larger study should follow, both to determine whether a statistically significant result is achievable and if that difference is clinically meaningful for the patients.

Treatment of AOM may be a very important example of a good role for homeopathy. It is a common problem for which the efficacy of conventional treatment is limited.[110-113] Questions about the consequences of conventional treatment persist, especially regarding the adverse effects of antibiotics—GI problems, allergic reactions, and rising bacterial resistance. Other long-term concerns are coming to the fore, particularly the growing epidemic of asthma and other atopic disease and the possibility that overuse of antibiotics in young children may be contributing to this rise in immune dysfunction.[114-116,118] Although the study group here was older than the population seemingly most susceptible to interference with developing immune maturity, there is no reason to presume that younger children would respond any differently to homeopathic care. Homeopathic clinical practice customarily includes the treatment of infants.

OTHER RESEARCH

Although clinicians (and patients) prefer proof of efficacy in human clinical investigations, most practitioners believe that if homeopathy works, it should produce demonstrable effects on animals and on portions of living organisms (tissues and cells). There have been a number of studies of homeopathy in tissue and cellular research published over decades. Just as in human clinical research, the sum of these investigations is both encouraging and ultimately uncertain. Although some homeopathic clinical trials have received a fair amount of attention, undoubtedly the biggest stir was created by one of these cellular investigations.

Benveniste

A team of investigators, including Dr. Jacques Benveniste, a French immunologist and an employee of France's National Institute of Health and Medical Research (INSERM), conducted a trial, the results of which were published in *Nature*.[117] This trial has become a landmark in the scientific literature, chiefly because of the manner in which the journal handled the publication and subsequent investigation.

Following along the lines of an earlier pilot study[119] Benveniste's group prepared homeopathic dilutions of anti-IgE antiserum and measured their effects on degranulation of human basophils. They found that dilutions far beyond Avogadro's numerical limit appeared to cause degranulation in human basophils. In addition, they found that violating certain physical conditions that are considered essential in the production and care of homeopathic medicines prevented the degranulation effect. For example, if they did not vortex the dilution; used a homeopathically unorthodox solvent; or heated, froze, or exposed the highly diluted product to ultrasound, the solution produced had no effect on the basophils.

Because these effects were so remarkable and unexpected, the editorial staff of *Nature* insisted that other laboratories replicate the experiment. Benveniste selected four other laboratories, two in Israel and one each in Italy and Canada, which then participated in the trial and final publication. *Nature* made publication contingent on Benveniste's acceptance of a team of independent investigators visiting his laboratory to observe a replication. *Nature* also ran a sidebar "Editorial reservation" on the last page of the article, promising a report on that investigation in a future issue. An editorial, "When To Believe the Unbelievable," ran in the issue containing Benveniste's original article. The editorial described the challenges raised by this research and cautioned against accepting the results as published.[120]

Unfortunately, the tenor of the debate, prominently including *Nature*'s manner of response, was seldom either polite or scholarly. The initial editorial included comments such as, "there can be no justification, at this stage, for an attempt to use Benveniste's conclusions for the malign purposes to which they might be put." The article reviewing the findings of the investigative team was titled, "High-dilution Experiments a Delusion."[122] The entire process almost immediately degenerated to finger-pointing and name-calling.

Nature's three investigators were the journal's editor, James Maddox, who had a background in theoretical physics; an organic chemist, Walter Stewart, an NIH employee notorious for his aggressive hunt for scientific misconduct; and James Randi ("The

Amazing Randi"), a professional magician.[121] This investigative team acknowledged their own lack of expertise in immunology research: "We acknowledge that we are an oddly constituted group.... None of us has first-hand experience in the field of work at INSERM 200."[122] *Nature*'s editor described his team as "self-appointed keepers of the scientific conscience . . . with no substantial scientific published record."[123]

Depictions of the investigators visit to Benveniste's laboratory sound like scenes from a poorly scripted movie. Under the direction of the *Nature* investigators, laboratory staff and the investigators themselves conducted 5 days of trials that would have normally taken the experienced laboratory workers 2 to 3 weeks. Although results of three of the first four batches were consistent with the published data, the investigators insisted this was only practice and should not count. Subsequent batches did not stain properly, as had often been the case, but *Nature*'s investigators considered these the true results. For these and many other scientific reasons, Benveniste objected to the investigator's determination that his team's findings were erroneous. However, the behavior of the investigative team drew the loudest criticism from Benveniste. The investigative team decided to single blind the results (to Benveniste's staff) and then, apparently to elicit fraud, the magician folded the code into tin foil and taped it to the laboratory ceiling while a video camera taped the procedure. At one point, Benveniste and Maddox reportedly asked Stewart to stop screaming. During one of the most delicate parts of the testing procedure, Randi (the magician) started to perform magic tricks, thereby distracting the laboratory staff. There is little wonder, then, at Benveniste's outrage or his question:

... are all these results "made up" as snapped at me by Stewart, the very referee who cleared the paper with raw data and statistics in hand? Why then accept a paper on 13 June to publish June 30th to destroy on 8 July data so easily spotted as wrong or made up? Is it a display to the world of the almighty anti-fraud and heterodoxy squad?[124]

When *Nature* printed a *post hoc* defense of the editor's decision to publish the original article, it carried the inflammatory title, "When To Publish Pseudoscience." The storm of controversy grew and grew. The matter was discussed in the *New York Times* and

several popular European newspapers. One article included accusations of fraud against Benveniste by a French Nobel laureate, against whom Benveniste later won a libel action.

Although the director-general of INSERM chastised Benveniste for his penchant for media attention, he protested the investigation to *Nature*. He commented on the "oddness of the investigative panel," the "unprecedented" decision to send such a team, the "offensive content" of the conclusions, and the "questionable ulterior justifications of the journal regarding its real motivations."[125]

Five years later, *Nature* published an unsuccessful replication of Benveniste's work by Hirst and associates, possibly closing off this line of inquiry.[126] This group of investigators criticized *Nature* both for initially publishing Benveniste's work and for then savaging it. Many commentators believed that the whole episode was essentially a publicity stunt by the editor of *Nature*, one with a chilling effect on rational scientific discourse of controversial subject matter.

Stewart continued to pursue scientific misconduct and was the center of other controversial allegations, including an accusation of plagiarism against historian Stephen Oates and an investigation of a 1986 paper, coauthored by Nobel laureate David Baltimore, published in *Cell*. These incidents drew attention and embarrassment to the NIH. Five years after the Benveniste incident, the NIH told Stewart to stop investigating scientific misconduct and reassigned him within the NIH.

Toxicology

The most commonly used model for investigating the biologic effects of homeopathic dilution is toxicologic research. Various investigators have conducted toxicologic studies over the past 45 years, beginning with experiments by Lapp, Wurrmser, and Ney with rats poisoned by arsenic.[127] The treatment group received homeopathic dilutions of arsenic 7C (1×10^{-14}). Lapp compared the rate of clearance of the poison in homeopathically treated rats with that of the untreated control group. Cazin and associates replicated this work.[128] Fisher and associates unsuccessfully attempted to extend the model to lead poisoning treated with a postavogadran dilution 200C (1×10^{-400}). His group found homeopathy inferior to a chelating agent and not significantly different from distilled water.[129]

A group led by Klaus Linde conducted a meta-analysis and critical review of published and unpublished research on this topic, published in 1994 by *Human and Experimental Toxicology*.[130] They found reports of 135 experiments, 76% of which were conducted by French researchers. Fewer than 10% were published in conventional medical journals.

Investigators obtained sufficient information for quality assessment in 116 of the experiments. The quality of the experiments was quite low, although it was improving in the more recent publications. Fewer than 2% of the experiments were randomized. Descriptions of the dilution process were common deficiencies, with fewer than 1% describing contamination precautions. Fewer than 8% of the experiments were blinded.

Of all the experiments, 40 used dilutions beyond the point of expected physiologic effects (12C or 24X, 1×10^{-24}) and had adequate quality to allow reevaluation. Of the 40, 27 had results favoring homeopathy, 26 of the better quality experiments were adequately similar to allow formal meta-analysis. Of these 26, 14 studied homeopathic treatment of mercury toxicity and 12 the treatment of arsenic poisoning.

The mercury set was a series of experiments with mice that received lethal doses of mercury. The mice in the nine experiments using daily injections of the 15C (1×10^{-30}) preparation had a 40% decreased mortality rate at 10 days (95% CI 21.8%-58.1%) compared with controls. The other five studies used a 5C (1×10^{-10}) preparation to reduce mortality by 7.2% (95% CI 10.1%-24.6%) over controls.

The other series used arsenic-poisoned rats and measured clearance of the poison from the bodies via urine and stool. The treatment was a 7C (1×10^{-14}) preparation of As_2O_3 administered in a variety of protocols. Compared with controls, treated rats increased their elimination of arsenic by 19.6% (95% CI 6.9%-32.4%) in urine and 25.5% (95% CI 8.9%-42.1%) in stool, thereby reducing blood levels by an average of 6.1% (95% CI 3.2%-9.2%) greater than controls.

Linde identified 34 better-quality trials of inorganic toxins, 28 of which had positive findings. Only 1 of the 22 experiments using organic compounds met minimal quality standards. That trial was positive. Of the 26 plant studies, six were of acceptable quality, only two of which had positive results. Six of the seven acceptable experiments using cell or embryo cultures reached positive conclusions. The quality of all seven studies of isolated organs was too poor to allow for assessment.

Linde and his colleagues pointed out that studies of postavogadran dilutions (12C or 24X, 1×10^{-24}) had the highest quality. More than 70% of those studies showed positive outcomes. They also commented that the principle of hormesis (the opposite physiologic effect at a low dose) has been studied for many years and could be important to the action of homeopathically diluted substances. In closing, they wrote, "While current research is not conclusive in this area, there is sufficient evidence to explore SAD [serial agitated dilution] preparations as a possible approach to protecting against intoxication."[130]

Miscellaneous Life Sciences

Silicea as a homeopathic remedy is known useful when patients experience recurrent infections characterized, in part, by sluggish immune response. Davenas and associates ran a series of experiments measuring the activity of mouse macrophages following homeopathic doses (1×10^{-11} and 1×10^{-19}) of silica.[131] The authors concluded, "These results demonstrate clear ex vivo cellular effect of high dilutions of silica, that cannot be explained in our present state of knowledge."[131] Oberbaum and associates conducted another trial of homeopathic silicea.[132] They found that homeopathically diluted silicea had a beneficial effect on wound healing in mice.

Experiments on the effects of homeopathic preparations on living systems have taken many shapes over many decades. In 1902, Jousset studied the effect of homeopathically diluted silver nitrate on the growth of *Aspergillus*.[133] Kolisko[134] and Roy[135] investigated the stimulatory and suppressive effects of homeopathic dilutions on barley and wheat growth. Boyd demonstrated effects of postavogadran dilutions of mercuric chloride on starch enzymes.[136]

Endler and associates conducted a series of experiments using postavogadran homeopathic dilutions of thyroxine to inhibit tadpole-to-frog metamorphosis.[137] These studies are intriguing for two reasons. First, they demonstrated a physiologic effect from a preparation that should not have contained any molecules of thyroxine. The second surprise is that thyroxine usually accelerates the metamorphic process. Here, diluted homeopathically, it exhibited suppressive effects. An interesting footnote to this series is the age of this line of investigation. As early as 1927, investigators began assessing the effects of homeopathic dilutions on developing tadpoles.[138]

There have been a large number of animal, organ, tissue, and cellular studies evaluating aspects of homeopathic principles published in scientific journals, far too many to examine here. To more fully explore these areas of homeopathic research, refer to books by Bellavite[139] and Endler and associates.[140]

Fundamental Science

Defining a mechanism of action would irrevocably alter the debate about homeopathy. The improbability of homeopathy is such a fundamental barrier that it stymies unbiased critical thought for many. Although some, like Eskinazi in *Archives of Internal Medicine,*[141] argue that conventional science and pharmacologic research already encompass the most unlikely homeopathic principles, most physicians are either unaware of these findings or believe that homeopathy needs additional explanation.

Similia

Since the 1990s, van Wijk and Wiegant have been researching the similia (like cures like) principle, the core concept of homeopathy.[142,143] Their experiments use cultured mammalian cells measuring the response to a stressor, recovery rate, and resistance to subsequent exposures to the stressor. Stressors they have examined include sodium arsenite, cadmium, and, broadening their approach, heat stress. They found that a limited exposure to any of these stressors was followed initially by increased sensitivity to the stressor but subsequently by increased resistance to the stressor. This response was mediated by an acceleration of self-repair mechanisms in the cells and occurred only when the cells were partially damaged by the initial stressor. The response was stressor specific; arsenite exposure, for example, was not protective for subsequent heat stress.

The medical literature is full of publications documenting the nearly ubiquitous tendency of conventional medications to create paradoxic drug effects. Although hundreds of articles have touched on this aspect of medicine, little systematic investigation of the general principle has been conducted. Some observers point to paradoxic effects as support of the homeopathic principle of like cures like. Homeopaths

may simply be focusing attention on the rare or delayed effects of medication.

Hormesis has a great deal of research support but an inversely proportional level of awareness among clinicians.[144] Its effects are well documented in radiation biology, where it has been called "the issue of the decade."[145] Recognition of the health benefits of low-level radiation is growing, as is awareness of the detrimental effects of high doses of radiation.[145-148] There is discussion of the role of hormesis in promoting longevity following caloric restriction, and of the health effects of low-level toxin exposure.[149-153] Hormesis is yet another phenomenon that suggests that every influence can have positive and negative repercussions. Many questions await answers.

Potentization

Although the ability of postavogadran dilutions to have biologic effects is not the most essential tenet of homeopathic medicine, it does appear to be the most scientifically unacceptable. As Schulte wrote, "Any fundamental research into homeopathy has to address the problem of apparent information transfer and information storage in aqueous solutions, as well as the subsequent mechanism of transfer to a physiologic system."[154] This single element, the one explanation essentially absent from Hahnemann's meticulously recorded development of theoretic and clinical homeopathy, is either the most intriguing or the most frustrating aspect of the study of homeopathy, depending on the viewer's perspective. The best starting point for readers who desire to consider fundamental research pertaining to homeopathic potentization is Schulte's paper.

Although Schulte's article is the best summary of recent scientific investigations, this most perplexing facet of homeopathic philosophy has been a popular topic in homeopathic literature for many decades. Stephenson and associates wrote several theoretic pieces published during the 1960s in the *Journal of the American Institute of Homeopathy.*[155-157] In these articles and others, he attempted to summarize scientific research on microdilutions and use principles of nuclear physics to explain homeopathic theory.[158,159] Stanford professor William Tiller also wrote a series of articles considering theoretic scientific models that could help explain the actions of homeopathic dilutions and the concept of similars.[160,161]

As early as the mid 1960s, investigators attempted to use nuclear magnetic resonance (NMR) imaging to assay homeopathic remedies.[162,163] These homeopathic experimenters found no effects when the homeopathic dilutions were prepared in plastic- or paraffin-lined glass containers. Since then we have learned that most forms of glass release paramagnetic ions into solutions that can lead to false changes in NMR readings. Papers on this topic continue to be published, but nearly all of them are difficult to interpret because of inadequate controls for contamination by dissolved gases and metal ions from glass.[164-167] In a recent issue of the *British Homeopathic Journal,* two of the foremost researchers in this field urged cautious interpretation of current data and called for high-quality systematic protocols to provide better data in the future.[168]

David Anick, MD, PhD, has proposed several methods by which materials might retain chemical if not biologic effects as homeopathic dilutions. One example is that of "water wires," which are a well-known biologic phenomenon that allows transmission of charged particles through water at a much faster rate than the process of dilution. Another possibility discussed by Anick was the idea that aberrations in the length of hydrogen bonds in water could allow marked and persistent differences between seemingly identical water-based solutions.[169]

Shui-Yin Lo has conducted a series of experiments in which aqueous dilutions apparently produced crystalline structures in the water.[170] Because concentrated solutions have a high degree of intermolecular interaction, these organized molecules appear to be significant only in very dilute solutions. These crystals are thus vulnerable to the types of environmental conditions (e.g., sunlight, heat, strong magnetic fields) that are traditionally thought to damage homeopathic remedies.

The investigation of homeopathic principles on the level of basic science is proceeding vigorously. Investigators have proposed a number of interesting possibilities. None of these, with the possible exception of hormesis, is firmly established. No single theory adequately accounts for both of the essential homeopathic principles, similia and potentization. We remain a long way away from understanding how these extreme dilutions can directly create clinical effects.

Creative Homeopathic Research

Research is a creative activity. Although many falsely believe that research is extremely straightforward and necessitates the most linear thinking in medicine, in actuality, any good researcher must think creatively to ask the right question and then design a protocol to answer that question. A number of creative homeopathic researchers have taken steps to stretch their research designs. Several investigators have designed trials incorporating homeopathic principles, such as using the traditional aggravation of symptoms as an outcome measure. One study tested the reliability of homeopathic proving methodology as a measure of the validity of homeopathy itself.[171]

Every well-trained homeopath recognizes that each homeopathic remedy encompasses a complex pattern of symptoms. Because certain remedies are more commonly linked to certain illness states, the first stage of a study by Davidson and associates was to survey a panel of homeopathic experts to determine the most common remedies for phobic anxiety disorders.[172] Then, they recruited patients meeting conventional criteria for this disorder. From the patients they collected additional information, such as the specific characteristics of their anxiety, food desires, and temperature tolerance. Finally, investigators applied a statistical technique (grade of membership analysis) to determine whether the patients' symptoms were clustered like the homeopathic remedies commonly prescribed for this group of patients. For example, a *Lycopodium clavatum* patient can experience symptoms of agoraphobia, but will also usually have indigestion (especially bloating after meals) and a craving for sweets, and tends to be groggy in the mornings. However, an *Arsenicum* patient will have different specific fears, greater restlessness with the anxiety, and, usually, great sensitivity to cold than a *Lycopodium* patient. The study showed that patients with phobic anxiety disorders tend to experience clusters of symptoms that often parallel the homeopathic classifications.

HOMEOPATHIC RESEARCH— WHERE DO WE GO FROM HERE?

When the Homeopathic Research Network was founded in 1993, the organizational objective was "to prove and improve homeopathy." Two different but overlapping research efforts were (and are) needed. One effort is to demonstrate that homeopathy has real effects, to "prove homeopathy," in other words.

When considering homeopathy as a clinical practice, the significance of those effects must be defined by patient benefit. For two centuries patients and clinicians have used homeopathy despite the absence of scientific recognition; this itself is a form of "proof" that it works. The community of clinical homeopaths has been arguing about the proper application of homeopathic methods for very nearly that entire time. Improving the clinical practice of homeopathy will benefit patients. Settling these disputes would certainly make homeopathic gatherings more peaceable, if less exciting.

Proving Homeopathy

To define a mechanism of action of high dilutions, researchers must do the following:
- Define a mechanism of action of high dilutions
- Continue basic sciences investigation of the similia principle
- Replicate trials
- Investigate patient benefit rather than placebo differentiation

Although the first two points are obviously important, the latter two bear further comment. A single, favorable trial, no matter how elegant, means little until independent investigators confirm the finding. Replication is absolutely essential. Understanding the degree of homeopathy's clinical effect is essential in determining its benefit to patients. In addition, the complexity of the placebo response and its variability by disease and patient characteristics conspire to limit the value of simple placebo-controlled trials. Placebo trials should not be abandoned, but rather examined carefully and used selectively.

Improving Homeopathy

Realistically, it is important to accept that regardless of the findings of scientific research, people will continue to use homeopathic medicine for the foreseeable future. One hundred highly publicized negative trials would not end a system of medicine so well established by tradition and familiar to hundreds of millions worldwide. Some homeopaths therefore argue that research has nothing to offer those who would continue to use homeopathy. However, research can still play a role in this independent-minded community.

There are many disagreements about the correct methods of homeopathic clinical practice, including disputes about dosing regimens (potency and frequency), the clinical effects of interactions between concurrently administered homeopathic medicines, antidotes, the diagnostic accuracy of electronic devices, adverse effects of homeopathy, and the relative benefit of differing styles of homeopathic prescribing (classical or otherwise). Research can be a powerful tool to settle these clinical disputes.

SUMMARY

Does homeopathy work? Is homeopathy effective for certain conditions? Research is the customary means we use to settle such questions. Unfortunately, it is not easy to conduct good research in homeopathy. Furthermore, it takes a substantial mass of excellent research to shift the weight of medical opinion on controversial topics such as homeopathy. Because we do not have such a strongly compelling body of research favoring homeopathy, research has yet to provide conclusive answers to these questions.

In some ways, research has made homeopathy more mysterious. A decade ago, very few physicians would have predicted that any good study would produce a result favorable to homeopathy. However, many good studies have done just that. At the same time, many good studies do not support homeopathy. That homeopathy has not simply shriveled up under the bright light of scientific examination is surprising and intriguing. Research has given us a sense of what needs to be done. We have much yet to learn.

References

1. Coulter H: *The origins of modern western medicine,* Berkeley, Calif., 1988, North Point Press.
2. Dimond E, Kittle C, Crockett J: Comparison of internal mammary artery ligation and sham operation for angina pectoris, *Am J Cardiol* 1960:483-486.
3. Wharton R, Lewith G: Complementary medicine and the general practitioner, *BMJ (Clin Res Ed)* 292(6534): 1498-1500, 1986.
4. Gonzales R, Steiner JF, Sande MA: Antibiotic prescribing for adults with colds, upper respiratory tract infections, and bronchitis by ambulatory care physicians, *JAMA* 278(11):901-904, 1997.

5. Pichichero ME: Understanding antibiotic overuse for respiratory tract infections in children, *Pediatrics* 104(6):1384-1388, 1999.

6. Watson RL, Dowell SF, Jayaraman M et al: Antimicrobial use for pediatric upper respiratory infections: reported practice, actual practice, and parent beliefs, *Pediatrics* 104(6):1251-1257, 1999.

7. Conly J: Controlling antibiotic resistance by quelling the epidemic of overuse and misuse of antibiotics, *Can Fam Physician* 44:1769-73, 80-84, 1998.

8. Lynoe N, Svensson T: Doctors' attitudes towards empirical data—a comparative study, *Scand J Soc Med* 25(3):210-216, 1997.

9. Greenhalgh T, Gill P: Pressure to prescribe, *BMJ* 315(7121):1482-1483, 1997.

10. Wears RL: What is necessary for proof? Is 95% sure unrealistic? *JAMA* 271(4):272, 1994.

11. Berman BM, Singh BB, Hartnoll SM, et al: Primary care physicians and complementary-alternative medicine: training, attitudes, and practice patterns, *J Am Board Fam Pract* 11(4):272-281, 1998.

12. Ernst E: Unconventional cancer therapies: what we need is rigorous research, not closed minds, *Chest* 117(2):307-308, 2000.

13. Ernst E, Resch KL: Reviewer bias against the unconventional? A randomized double-blind study of peer review, *Complement Ther Med* 7(1):19-23, 1999.

14. Jonas W: Alternative medicine and the conventional practitioner, *JAMA* 279(9):708-709, 1998.

15. Schwartz MP, Wagner PJ: Which medicines do our patients want from us? *J Fam Pract* 49:339-341, 2000.

16. Jonas WB: Alternative medicine—learning from the past, examining the present, advancing to the future (editorial), *JAMA* 280(18):1616-1618, 1998.

17. Crim C: Clinical practice guidelines vs actual clinical practice: the asthma paradigm, *Chest* 118 (suppl 2):62S-64S, 2000.

18. Ellrodt AG, Conner L, Erieding M et al: Measuring and improving physician compliance with clinical practice guidelines: a controlled interventional trial, *Ann Intern Med* 122(4):277-282, 1995.

19. Vinker S, Nakar S, Rosenberg E, et al: Attitudes of Israeli family physicians toward clinical guidelines, *Arch Fam Med* 9(9):835-840, 2000.

20. Lewis LM, Lasater LC, Ruoff BE: Failure of a chest pain clinical policy to modify physician evaluation and management, *Ann Emerg Med* 25(1):9-14, 1995.

21. Gonzales R, Barrett PH Jr, Crane LA, et al: Factors associated with antibiotic use for acute bronchitis, *J Gen Intern Med* 13:541-548, 1998.

22. Hueston WJ, Hopper JE, Dacus EN, et al: Why are antibiotics prescribed for patients with acute bronchitis? A postintervention analysis, *J Am Board Fam Pract* 13(6):398-402, 2000.

23. Worrall G, Freake D, Kelland J et al: Care of patients with type II diabetes: a study of family physicians' compliance with clinical practice guidelines, *J Fam Pract* 44(4):374-381, 1997.

24. Zerr DM, Del Beccaro MA, Cummings P: Predictors of physician compliance with a published guideline on management of febrile infants, *Pediatr Infect Dis J* 18(3):232-238, 1999.

25. Seto TB, Kwiat D, Taira DA et al: Physicians' recommendations to patients for use of antibiotic prophylaxis to prevent endocarditis, *JAMA* 284(1):68-71, 2000.

26. van Weel C, Knottnerus JA: Evidence-based interventions and comprehensive treatment, *Lancet* 353:916-918, 1999.

27. Holdaway IM, Evans MC, Frengley PA et al: Related Articles Investigation and treatment of renal calculi associated with hypercalciuria, *J Endocrinol Invest* 5:361-365, 1982.

28. Evans RA, Maher PO, Agostino M et al: Investigation and treatment of renal calculi, *Med J Aust* 143:278-281, 1985.

29. Borghi L, Schianchi T, Meschi T et al: Comparison of two diets for the prevention of recurrent stones in idiopathic hypercalciuria. *N Engl J Med* 46(2):77-84, 2002.

30. Martini LA, Wood RJ: Should dietary calcium and protein be restricted in patients with nephrolithiasis? *Nutr Rev* 58(4):111-117, 2000.

31. Acupuncture, *NIH Consens Statement* 15(5):1-34, 1997.

32. NIH Consensus Conference: Acupuncture, *JAMA* 280(17):1518-1524, 1998.

33. Bareta JC: Evidence presented to consensus panel on acupuncture's efficacy, *Altern Ther Health Med* 4(1):22-30, 102, 1998.

34. Wootton J: National Institutes of Health consensus development statement on acupuncture, *J Altern Complement Med* 3(4):419-420, 1997.

35. Brody H: The lie that heals: the ethics of giving placebos, *Ann Intern Med* 97(1):112-118, 1982.

36. Lynoe N: Is the effect of alternative medical treatment only a placebo effect? *Scand J Soc Med* 18(2):149-153, 1990.

37. Joyce CR: Placebo and complementary medicine, *Lancet* 344(8932):1279-1281, 1994.

38. Jonas WB (editorial): Magic and methodology: when paradigms clash, *J Altern Complement Med* 5(4):319-321, 1999.

39. Treuherz F: Correspondence and *Hecla lava*: the origins of Kent's homeopathy, *JAIH* 77:130-149, 1984.

40. Jacobs J, Jimenez LM, Gloyd SS et al: Treatment of acute childhood diarrhea with homeopathic medicine: a randomized clinical trial in Nicaragua, *Pediatrics* 93(5):719-725, 1994.

41. Johnson AG: Surgery as a placebo, *Lancet* 344(8930):1140-1142, 1994.

42. Harrington A: *The placebo effect,* Cambridge, Mass., 1997, Harvard University Press.

43. Gotzsche PC: Is there logic in the placebo? *Lancet* 344(8927):925-926, 1994.

44. Gotzsche PC: Placebo effects: concept of placebo should be discarded, *BMJ* 311(7020):1640-1641, 1995.

45. Benson H, McCallie DP Jr: Angina pectoris and the placebo effect, *N Engl J Med* 300(25):1424-1429, 1979.

46. Kleinman I, Brown P, Librach L: Placebo pain medication: ethical and practical considerations, *Arch Fam Med* 3:453-457, 1994.

47. Shapiro AK, Struening EL, Barten H et al: Correlates of placebo reaction in an outpatient population, *Psychol Med* 5(4):389-396, 1975.

48. Stagno SJ, Smith ML: The use of placebo in diagnosing psychogenic seizures: who is being deceived? *Semin Neurol* 17(3):213-218, 1997.

49. Hrobjartsson A, Gotzsche PC: Is the placebo powerless? An analysis of clinical trials comparing placebo with no treatment, *N Engl J Med* 344(21):1594-1602, 2001.

50. Levine JD, Gordon NC, Fields HL et al: The mechanism of placebo analgesia, *Lancet* 2(8091):654-657, 1978.

51. Olness K, Ader R: Conditioning as an adjunct in the pharmacotherapy of lupus erythematosus, *J Dev Behav Pediatr* 13(2):124-125, 1992.

52. Wolf S: Effects of suggestion and conditioning on the action of chemical agents in human subjects: the pharmacology of placebos, *J Clin Invest* 29:100-109, 1950.

53. Coronary Drug Project: Influence of adherence to treatment and response of cholesterol on mortality in the Coronary Drug Project, *N Engl J Med* 303:1038-1041, 1980.

54. Ader R, Cohen N: Behaviorally conditioned immunosuppression, *Psychosom Med* 37(4):333-340, 1975.

55. Rowbotham DJ (editorial): Endogenous opioids, placebo response, and pain, *Lancet* 357(9272):1901-1902, 2001.

56. Rochon PA, Binns MA, Litner JA et al: Are randomized control trial outcomes influenced by the inclusion of a placebo group?: a systematic review of nonsteroidal antiinflammatory drug trials for arthritis treatment, *J Clin Epidemiol* 52(2):113-122, 1999.

57. Kleijnen J, de Craen AJ, van Everdingen J et al: Placebo effect in double-blind clinical trials: a review of interactions with medications, *Lancet* 344(8933):1347-1349, 1994.

58. Skovlund E: Should we tell trial patients that they might receive placebo? (letter), *Lancet* 337(8748):1041, 1991.

59. Rothman KJ, Michels KB: The continuing unethical use of placebo controls [see comments], *N Engl J Med* 331(6):394-398, 1994.

60. Ware JE: Measuring patients' views: the optimum outcome measure, *BMJ* 306(6890):1429-1430, 1993.

61. Gotzsche PC: Sensitivity of effect variables in rheumatoid arthritis: a meta-analysis of 130 placebo controlled NSAID trials, *J Clin Epidemiol* 43(12):1313-1318, 1990.

62. Dean ME: A homeopathic origin for placebo controls: "an invaluable gift of God," *Altern Ther Health Med* 6(2):58-66, 2000.

63. Kaptchuk TJ: Intentional ignorance: a history of blind assessment and placebo controls in medicine, *Bull Hist Med* 72(3):389-433, 1998.

64. Lown B: Preface to *The lost art of healing,* Boston, 1996, Houghton Mifflin.

65. Gibson RG, Gibson SL, MacNeill AD et al: Homeopathic therapy in rheumatoid arthritis: evaluation by double-blind clinical therapeutic trial, *Br J Clin Pharmacol* 9:453-459, 1980.

66. Shipley M, Berry H, Broster G et al: Controlled trial of homeopathic treatment of osteoarthritis, *Lancet* 1(8316):97-98, 1983.

67. Homoeopathy, *Lancet* 1(8322):482, 1983.

68. Wiesenauer M, Gaus W: Double-blind trial comparing the effectiveness of the homeopathic preparation Galphimia potentiation D6, Galphimia dilution 10(-6) and placebo on pollinosis, *Arzneimittelforschung* 35(11):1745-1747, 1985.

69. Blackley CH: *Br Homeopath J* 29:238-286, 1871.

70. Blackley CH: *Br Homeopath J* 29:477-501, 1871.

71. Blackley CH: *Br Homeopath J* 29:713-736, 1871.

72. Blackley CH: *Br Homeopath J* 30:246-274, 1872.

73. Blackley CH: *Br Homeopath J* 30:417-449, 1872.

74. Blackley CH: *Br Homeopath J* 30:656-678, 1872.

75. Blackley CH: *Br Homeopath J* 31:77-103, 1873.

76. Milspaugh CF: *New, old and forgotten remedies,* Philadelphia, 1900, Boericke and Tafel.

77. Reilly DT. Taylor MA, McSharry C et al: Is homoeopathy a placebo response? Controlled trial of homoeopathic potency, with pollen in hayfever as model, *Lancet* 2(8512):881-886, 1986.

78. Editorial: Quadruple-blind, *Lancet* 1:914(8643), 1989.

79. Ferley JP, Zmirou D, D'Adhemar D et al: A controlled evaluation of a homoeopathic preparation in the treatment of influenza-like syndromes, *Br J Clin Pharmacol* 27(3):329-335, 1989.

80. Personal communication with Thierry Boiron, President and CEO of Boiron USA, 2000.

81. Fisher P, Greenwood A, Huskisson EC et al: Effect of homeopathic treatment on fibrositis (primary fibromyalgia), *BMJ* 299(6695):365-366, 1989.

82. Kleijnen J, Knipschild P, ter Riet G: Clinical trials of homeopathy, *BMJ* 302(6772):316-323, 1991 (published erratum appears in *BMJ* 302(6780):818, 1991).

83. Kleijnen J, Knipschild P: The comprehensiveness of Medline and Embase computer searches: searches for controlled trials of homoeopathy, ascorbic acid for common cold and ginkgo biloba for cerebral

insufficiency and intermittent claudication, *Pharm Week Bl Sci* 14(5):316-320, 1992.

84. Andrade LE, Ferraz MB, Atra E et al: A randomized controlled trial to evaluate the effectiveness of homeopathy in rheumatoid arthritis, *Scand J Rheumatol* 20(3):204-208, 1991.

85. Jacobs J, Jimenez M, Gloyd S et al: Homeopathic treatment of acute childhood diarrhea, *Br Homeopath J* 82(5):83-86, 1993.

86. Carlston M: Homeopathic diarrhea trial, *Pediatrics* 95(1):159 (discussion 160), 1995.

87. Jacobs J, Jimenez M, Malthouse S et al: Homeopathic treatment of acute childhood diarrhea: results from a clinical trial in Nepal, *J Altern Complement Med* 6(2):131-139, 2000.

88. de Lange de Klerk ES, Blommers J, Kuik DJ et al: Effect of homoeopathic medicines on daily burden of symptoms in children with recurrent upper respiratory tract infections, *BMJ* 309(6965):1329-1332, 1994.

89. Reilly D, Taylor MA, Beattie NG et al: Is evidence for homoeopathy reproducible? *Lancet* 344(8937):1601-1606, 1994.

90. Lokken P, Straumsheim PA, Tveiten D et al: Effect of homoeopathy on pain and other events after acute trauma: placebo controlled trial with bilateral oral surgery, *BMJ* 310(6992):1439-1442, 1995.

91. Campbell A: Two pilot controlled trials of arnica montana, *Br Homeopath J* 65:154-158, 1976.

92. Hart O, Mullee MA, Lewith G et al: Double-blind, placebo-controlled, randomized clinical trial of homoeopathic arnica C30 for pain and infection after total abdominal hysterectomy, *J R Soc Med* 90(2):73-78, 1997.

93. Vickers AJ: Can acupuncture have specific effects on health? A systematic review of acupuncture antiemesis trials, *J R Soc Med* 89(6):303-311, 1996.

94. Tveiten D, Bruseth S, Borchgrevink CF et al: Effect of arnica D 30 during hard physical exertion. A double-blind randomized trial during the Oslo marathon 1990, *Tidsskr Nor Laegeforen* 111(30):3630-3631, 1991.

95. Tveiten D, Bruseth S, Borchgrevink CF et al: Effects of the homeopathic remedy arnica D 30 on marathon runners: a randomized double-blind study during the 1995 Oslo marathon, *Complement Ther Med* 6:71-74, 1998.

96. Vickers AJ, Fisher P, Smith C et al: Homeopathic arnica 30x is ineffective for muscle soreness after long-distance running: a randomized, double-blind, placebo-controlled trial, *Clin J Pain* 14(3):227-231, 1998.

97. Ludtke R, Wiesenauer M: A meta-analysis of homeopathic treatment of pollinosis with Galphimia glauca, *Wien Med Wochenschr* 147(14):323-327, 1997.

98. Linde K, Clausius N, Ramirez G et al: Are the clinical effects of homeopathy placebo effects? a meta-analysis of placebo-controlled trials, *Lancet* 350(9081):834-843, 1997 (published erratum appears in *Lancet* 351[9097]:220, 1998).

99. Weiser M, Strosser W, Klein P: Homeopathic vs conventional treatment of vertigo: a randomized double-blind controlled clinical study, *Arch Otolaryngol Head Neck Surg* 124(8):879-885, 1998.

100. Brigo B: Homeopathic treatment of migraine: a sixty case, double blind, controlled study (homeopathic remedy versus placebo). Paper presented at the proceedings of the 42nd LMHI (Liga Medicorum Homoeopathica Internationalis) Congress, Arlington, Va., 1987. (http://www.lmhi.net/)

101. Walach H, Haeusler W, Lowes T et al: Classical homeopathic treatment of chronic headaches, discussion 01, *Cephalalgia* 17(2):119-126, 1997.

102. Whitmarsh TE, Coleston-Shields DM, Steiner TJ: Double-blind randomized placebo-controlled study of homoeopathic prophylaxis of migraine, *Cephalalgia* 17(5):600-604, 1997.

103. Consensus statement: The Commonweal Conference on Homeopathy in Human and Veterinary Medicine, *Hom Int* (2):24-25, 1998.

104. Linde K, Melchart D: Randomized controlled trials of individualized homeopathy: a state-of-the-art review, *J Altern Complement Med* 4(4):371-388, 1998.

105. Chapman EH, Weintraub RJ, Milburn MA et al: Homeopathic treatment of mild traumatic brain injury: a randomized, double-blind, placebo-controlled clinical trial, *J Head Trauma Rehabil* 14(6):521-542, 1999.

106. Linde K, Scholz M, Ramirez G et al: Impact of study quality on outcome in placebo-controlled trials of homeopathy, *J Clin Epidemiol* 52(7):631-636, 1999.

107. Taylor MA, Reilly D, Llewellyn-Jones RH et al: Randomised controlled trial of homeopathy versus placebo in perennial allergic rhinitis with overview of four trial series, *BMJ* 321:471-476, 2000.

108. Jacobs J, Chapman EH, Crothers D: Patient characteristics and practice patterns of physicians using homeopathy, *Arch Fam Med* 7(6):537-540, 1998.

109. Jacobs J, Springer DA, Crothers D: Homeopathic treatment of acute otitis media in children: a preliminary randomized placebo-controlled trial, *Pediatr Infect Dis J* 20(2):177-183, 2001.

110. Williams RL, Chalmers TC, Stange KC et al: Use of antibiotics in preventing recurrent otitis media and in treating otitis media with effusion: a meta-analytic attempt to resolve the brouhaha, *JAMA* 270:1344-1351, 1993.

111. Culpepper L, Froom J: Routine antimicrobial treatment of acute otitis media: is it necessary? *JAMA* 278:1643-1645, 1997.

112. Rosenfeld RM: An evidence-based approach to treating otitis media, *Pediatr Clin North Am* 43:1165-1181, 1996.

113. Bollag U: Cause of otitis media, *Lancet* 357:311, 2001.

114. Droste JH, Wieringa MH, Weyler JJ et al: Does the use of antibiotics in early childhood increase the risk of asthma and allergic disease? *Clin Exp Allergy* 30(11):1547-1553, 2000.

115. Wickens K, Pearce N, Crane J et al: Antibiotic use in early childhood and the development of asthma, *Clin Exp Allergy* 29(6):766-771, 1999.

116. von Hertzen LC: Puzzling associations between childhood infections and the later occurrence of asthma and atopy, *Ann Med* 32(6):397-400, 2000.

117. Davenas E, Beauvais F, Amara J et al: Human basophil degranulation triggered by very dilute antiserum against IgE, *Nature* 333(6176):816-818, 1988.

118. Strachan DP: Family size, infection and atopy: the first decade of the "hygiene hypothesis, *Thorax* 55(suppl 1):S2-10, 2000.

119. Poitevin B, Aubin M, Benveniste J: Approach to the quantitative analysis of the effect of Apis mellifica on the in vitro human basophil degranulation, *J Innov Tech Biol Med* 7:64-68, 1986.

120. When to believe the unbelievable (editorial), *Nature* 333:787, 1988.

121. Anderson C: Robocops: Stewart and Feder's mechanized misconduct search, *Nature* 350(6318):454-455, 1991.

122. Maddox J, Randi J, Stewart WW: High-dilution experiments a delusion, *Nature* 334(6180):287-290, 1988.

123. Maddox, J: (letter) *Nature* 333:795, 1988.

124. Benveniste J: Dr. Jacques Benveniste replies, *Nature* 334(6180):291, 1988.

125. Coles P: Benveniste controversy. INSERM closes the file, *Nature* 340(6230):178, 1989.

126. Hirst SJ, Hayes NA, Burridge J et al: Human basophil degranulation is not triggered by very dilute antiserum against human IgE, *Nature* 366(6455):525-527, 1993.

127. Lapp C, Wurrmser L, Ney J: Mobilisation de l'arsenic fixe chez le cobaye sons l'influence des doses infinitesimal d'arseniate, *Therapy* 13:46-55, 1958.

128. Cazin JC, Cazin M, Gaborit JL et al: A study of the effect of decimal and centesimal dilutions of arsenic on the retention and mobilization of arsenic in the rat, *Hum Toxicol* 6(4):315-320, 1987.

129. Fisher P, House I, Belon P et al: The influence of the homoeopathic remedy plumbum metallicum on the excretion kinetics of lead in rats, *Hum Toxicol* 6(4):321-324, 1987.

130. Linde K, Jonas WB, Melchart D et al: Critical review and meta-analysis of serial agitated dilutions in experimental toxicology, *Hum Exp Toxicol* 13:481-492, 1994.

131. Davenas E, Poitevin B, Benveniste J et al: Effect on mouse peritoneal macrophages of orally administered very high dilutions of silica, *Eur J Pharmacol* 135(3):313-319, 1987.

132. Oberbaum M, Markovits R, Weisman Z et al: Wound healing by homeopathic silica dilutions in mice, *Harefuah* 123(3-4):79-82, 156, 1992.

133. Bertrand G: The extraordinary sensitiveness of aspergillus niger to manganese, *Comptes Rendus Académie des Science* 154:616, 1912.

134. Kolisko L: Physical and physiological demonstration of the effect of the smallest entities, *Der Kommende Tag* 1-10, 1923.

135. Roy J: The experimental justification of the homeopathic dilution, *Le Bulletin Médical* 46:528-531, 1932.

136. Boyd WE: The action of microdoses of mercuric chloride on diastase, *Br Homeopath J* 31(5):106-111, 1941.

137. Endler PC, Pongratz W, Van Wijk R et al: Effects of highly diluted succussed thyroxine on metamorphosis of highland frogs, *Ber J Res Hom* 1(3):151-160, 1991.

138. Konig K: On the effect of extremely diluted ("homeopathic") metal salt solutions on the development and growth of tadpoles, *Zeitschrift für die Gesamte Experimentelle Medizin* 56:581-593, 1927.

139. Bellavite P, Signorini A (contributor): *Homeopathy: a frontier in medical science*, Berkeley, Calif., 1995, North Atlantic Books.

140. Endler PC, Schulte J: *Ultra high dilution, physiology and physics*, Dondrecht, The Netherlands, 1994, Kluwer Academic.

141. Eskinazi D: Homeopathy re-revisited: is homeopathy compatible with biomedical observations? *Arch Intern Med* 159(17):1981-1987, 1999.

142. Van Wijk R, Wiegant FA: *Cultured mammalian cells in homeopathy research: the similia principle in self-recovery*, Utrecht, Netherlands, 1994, Utrecht University.

143. Van Wijk R, Wiegant FA: The similia principle as a therapeutic strategy: a research program on stimulation of self-defense in disordered mammalian cells, *Altern Ther Health Med* 3(2):33-38, 1997.

144. Calabrese EJ, Baldwin LA: The marginalization of hormesis, *Hum Exp Toxicol* 19(1):32-40, 2000.

145. Pollycove M: The issue of the decade: hormesis, *Eur J Nucl Med* 22(5):399-401, 1995.

146. Sheppard SC, Guthrie JE, Thibault DH: Germination of seeds from an irradiated forest: implications for waste disposal, *Ecotoxicol Environ Saf* 23(3):320-327, 1992.

147. Rattan SI: Repeated mild heat shock delays ageing in cultured human skin fibroblasts, *Biochem Mol Biol Int* 45(4):753-759, 1998.

148. Calabrese EJ, Baldwin LA: U-shaped dose-responses in biology, toxicology, and public health, *Annu Rev Public Health* 22:15-33, 2001.

149. Neafsey PJ: Longevity hormesis: a review, *Mech Ageing Dev* 51(1):1-31, 1990.

150. Turturro A, Hass BS, Hart RW: Does caloric restriction induce hormesis? *Hum Exp Toxicol* 19(6):320-329, 2000.

151. Masoro EJ: Caloric restriction and aging: an update, *Exp Gerontol* 35(3):299-305, 2000.

152. Kmecl P, Jerman I: Biological effects of low-level environmental agents, *Med Hypotheses* 54(5):685-688, 2000.

153. Calabrese EJ, Baldwin LA, Holland CD: Hormesis: a highly generalizable and reproducible phenomenon with important implications for risk assessment, *Risk Anal* 19(2):261-281, 1999.

154. Schulte J: Effects of potentization in aqueous solutions, *Br Homeopath J* 88(4):155-160, 1999.

155. Stephenson JH: On possible field effects of the solvent phase of succussed high dilutions, *JAIH* 57:259-261, 1966.

156. Barnard GP, Stephenson JH: Microdose paradox: a new biophysical concept, *JAIH* 277-286, 1967.

157. Barnard GP, Stephenson JH: Fresh evidence for a biophysical field, *JAIH* 62:73-85, 1969.

158. Stephenson JH: A review of investigations into the action of substances in dilutions greater than 1×10^{-24} (microdilutions), *JAIH* 48:327-355, 1955.

159. Stephenson JH: Homeopathic philosophy in the light of twentieth century physics, *JAIH* 66-69, 1960.

160. Tiller W: A rationale for the homeopathic "Law of Similars" *Journal of Homeopathic Practice* 2(1):48-52, 1979.

161. Tiller W: A rationale for the potentizing process in homeopathic remedies, *Journal of Homeopathic Practice* 2(1):53-59, 1979.

162. Smith RB, Boericke GW: Modern instrumentation for the evaluation of homeopathic drug structure, *JAIH* 59:263-280, 1966.

163. Smith RB, Boericke GW: Changes caused by succussion on NMR patterns and bioassays of BKTA succussions and dilutions, *JAIH* 61:197-212, 1968.

164. Sukul A, Sarkar P, Sinnababu SP et al: Altered solution structure of alcoholic medium of potentized Nux vomica underlies its antialcoholic effect, *Br Homeopath J* 89(2):73-77, 2000.

165. Poitevin B, Demangeat JL: Effects of potentization, *Br Homeopath J* 89(3):155-256, 2000.

166. Milgrom LR, King KR, Lee J et al: On the investigation of homeopathic potencies using low resolution NMR T2 relaxation times: an experimental and critical survey of the work of Roland Conte, *Br Homeopath J* 90:5-13, 2001.

167. Aabel S, Fossheim S, Rise F: Nuclear magnetic resonance (NMR) studies of homeopathic solutions, *Br Homeopath J* 90(1):14-20, 2001.

168. Demangeat JL, Poitevin B: Nuclear magnetic resonance: let's consolidate the ground before getting excited! *Br Homeopath J* 90(3):2-4, 2001.

169. Anick D: *Complexes of short hydrogen bonds: the active ingredient in homeopathy?* Homeopathic Research Network Fourth Scientific Symposium, Washington, DC, 1998, Homeopathic Research Network.

170. Lo S-Y: *IE crystals and homeopathy*, Homeopathic Research Network Third Scientific Symposium, San Francisco, 1995, Homeopathic Research Network.

171. Walach H: Does a highly diluted homoeopathic drug act as a placebo in healthy volunteers? Experimental study of belladonna 30C in double-blind crossover design—a pilot study, *J Psychosom Res* 37(8):851-860, 1993.

172. Davidson J, Woalbury M, Morrison R: Multivariate analysis of five homoeopathic medicines in a psychiatric population, *Br Homeopath J* 84:195-202, 1995.

Suggested Readings

Bellavite P, Signorini A. *Homeopathy: a frontier in medical science*, Berkeley, 1995, North Atlantic Books.

Endler PC, Schulte J: *Ultra high dilution, physiology and physics*, Dondrecht, 1994, Kluwer Academic.

Ernst E, Hahn EG (editors): *Homeopathy. a critical appraisal*, Oxford, 1998, Butterworth-Heinemann.

Harrington A: *The placebo effect*, Cambridge, Mass., 1997, Harvard University Press.

Lown B: *The lost art of healing*, Boston, 1996, Houghton Mifflin.

Shapiro A, Shapiro E: *The powerful placebo*, Baltimore, 1997, Johns Hopkins University Press.

Spiro H: *The power of hope: a doctor's perspective*, New Haven, Conn., 1998, Yale University Press.

Van Wijk R, Wiegant FA: *The similia principle in surviving stress: mammalian cells in homeopathy research*, Utrecht, The Netherlands, 1997, Utrecht University.

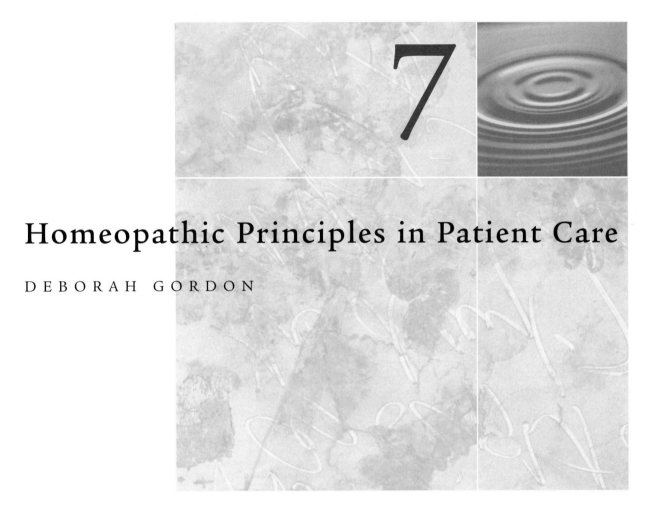

Homeopathic Principles in Patient Care

DEBORAH GORDON

This chapter describes the process of patient care in a clinical setting, summarizing and explaining the steps taken by the homeopath.

THE HOMEOPATHIC APPROACH TO THE PATIENT

The homeopathic approach to the patient is derived from the goal of the homeopathic consultation, to understand the state of the patient well enough to select the appropriate homeopathic treatment. Understanding a patient begins with the medical diagnosis and expands to include the particular aspects of the patient's illness, history, and personality. The homeopath is interested in understanding the uniqueness of the illness and the person who has the illness. What makes this person's illness

peculiar to him or her? What makes this person tick? What are the patient's unique habits and attitudes? The homeopath will rely on observation and examination, oral communication, and written records to make a comprehensive homeopathic evaluation.

Initial Contact

Observation begins with the first contact between homeopath and patient. In small practices, some homeopaths schedule appointments personally, whereas in larger practices the task is delegated. Unusual patient attitudes, varying from extreme shyness to urgent demands for prompt appointments, are noted. It is not unusual for a homeopath with a full practice to have a waiting time of several months for scheduling new patients, and this is quite disconcerting to some patients.

Although homeopaths vary in their routines for scheduling patients and obtaining medical histories, it is a common convention of practice that the homeopath goes to the waiting room to greet the patient and lead the way to the consultation room. While approaching the waiting patient, the homeopath seeks useful observations that express something of the nature of the patient, including posture, level and choice of activity, interaction with other waiting patients, general appearance, and whether the patient has come to the consultation alone or with others. Although no conclusions can be drawn at this time, it may prove useful in the final understanding to remember whether the patient was humming and staring out the window, arguing with the front desk, or quietly reading.

Most homeopaths request that the patient complete a history form before the appointment. Forms vary from single pages that contain typical medical information (e.g., previous illnesses, surgeries, family history, and allergies) to lengthy forms that introduce the patient to the homeopathic line of questioning (e.g., content of dreams, sleep patterns, details of the emotional aspects of the patient's history).

Medical records from other practitioners, conventional and complementary, are important parts of the full evaluation of the patient.

The Homeopathic Consultation

The consultation ideally occurs in a quiet room, comfortably furnished with chairs for all, a writing desk for the homeopath, and reference books or a computer. Homeopaths who see children usually provide toys or drawing materials so the children may have some freedom of movement or play. An examination table and equipment may be in a corner of the room or may be located elsewhere. The interview may be videotaped for purposes of case analysis and teaching. Informed consent is required for videotaping.

Style of Interview

Throughout the interview, each line of questioning is initiated with an open-ended approach, which allows the patient to express fully everything that he or she has intended to tell the homeopath, in his or her own words and manner. The patient may begin speaking without any prompting from the homeopath, or may sit quietly and wait for a question. Some homeopaths spend a minute or two looking through the patient's forms to allow the patient time to adapt to the room and inspect diplomas or photographs if he or she so desires.

The homeopath will begin the interview with a simple question, "What may I do for you?" or "What brings you here today?" The question may be joined to a brief statement about the purpose of the interview: "I am interested in learning as much as possible about your medical problems and about you personally. Please start wherever you like and tell me about yourself." The homeopath listens to everything the patient says without interruption, unless the patient is drifting seriously off course. To minimize any possible influence on what the patient is saying, the practitioner's nonverbal responses are neutral or gently supportive and encouraging.

Content of the Examination

A homeopathic interview covers three types of information:

1. Chief and secondary complaints
2. Review of systems
3. The nature of the person

The order in which information is gathered varies among practitioners and according to the way in which the patient reveals the information. Observations regarding the patient's nature are made throughout the interaction.

The chief complaint is usually the patient's starting point. The homeopath asks patients to tell the story of the problem in their own words. The homeopath is first interested in the patient's perceptions—how the illness is experienced and how it affects the life of the patient.

The patient's answer is *always* helpful, even if it is not what the homeopath has asked for. If the patient chooses to describe his or her illness by listing the doctors consulted and what those doctors tested, diagnosed, and treated, the homeopath regards that orientation as valuable information; for some reason, as yet unknown, the patient has chosen to talk about what medical specialists have said rather than about his or her own experience. That observation is filed away and will be considered in the analysis, but important information is still needed regarding the complaint.

The homeopath must understand the nature of the complaint with great clarity to make an accurate homeopathic analysis. Beginning with open-ended questions and eventually becoming as specific as necessary, the homeopath wants to learn about the onset of the condition, the nature of the patient's symptoms, and the management of the problem.

The homeopathic consideration of possible causation expands on the conventional view. A homeopath will want to know about risk factors and specific events in the patient's history that may, from a homeopathic perspective, be associated with the problem. For patients who lack typical risk factors, homeopaths will often discover contributing or inciting events that are not typically considered a "cause" of the problem. Box 7-1 provides examples of typical questions asked in homeopathic analysis.

For example, if an elderly, lifelong smoker develops severe asthma, both traditional and homeopathic analysis may attribute the cause to smoking. However, a similarly afflicted young nonsmoker, with no personal or family history associated with risk of asthma, may reveal that the asthma began after a significant life event. Understanding the nature of this life event may provide the clue to the homeopathic analysis and successful treatment.

To understand the nature of the symptoms in terms that will be useful for homeopathic analysis, the homeopath may simply pay close attention to the spontaneous telling of a related story, or may have to resort to a series of questions. Questions always be as open-ended as possible at first, and become increasingly specific as key pieces of the puzzle are sought. The specific characteristics that ameliorate or intensify the symptoms are called *modalities* and are very helpful to the homeopath during the process of sorting out what is distinctive about this particular patient (Box 7-2).

All medical practitioners are interested in what the patient is and has been doing for the problem. Securing information about previous and current medications and their benefits and adverse effects is standard practice in conventional and homeopathic medical consultations. In some instances the information will prove particularly useful in a homeopathic analysis. Differential diagnosis to select the appropriate homeopathic remedy may hinge on prior

---

BOX 7-1

Typical Questions Asked in Homeopathic Analysis

When did the problem start?

How exactly did it start?

What else was happening in your life at that time or in the preceding few months or even years?

That is, did you have any preceding medical problems or medical treatments, even if they seem unrelated?

Were there any significant changes or events in your personal life?

What was your stress level at the time the problem started?

How did that stress feel in your own experience?

What did you think was happening before you went to the doctor for a diagnosis?

BOX 7-2

Questions a Homeopath Asks to Understand the Nature of the Patient's Symptoms

Please describe the sensations of your problem as clearly as you can.

What is the location, nature, and timing of the pain, and what makes it better or worse? (The homeopath will investigate carefully this concept of modalities. Many patients, at first consideration, will simply reply that some medication takes away the pain. However, with a little patience, and a little patient education, many patients actually reveal some amazing and homeopathically useful modalities for their chief complaint. Homeopaths are looking for unusual and individualized modalities, such as those illustrated by the following statements: "My period stops if I get my feet wet," or "My throat feels burning hot, but the only thing I want to drink is tea, which makes it feel better." These are very unusual, and therefore useful, modalities.)

Considering the modalities, is there any position, activity, rest, weather, season, or direct application that affects the symptoms?

Does the pain extend to other parts of your body?

Are any other symptoms associated with the main symptoms?

How is your mental and emotional state associated with this condition?

How does this condition affect your life?

What is the hardest thing for you about this problem?

medical treatment. For example, exertional asthma following cortisone prescribed as treatment for poison oak may be treated differently from exertional asthma that followed a hysterectomy. Although the impact of the medical problem on the patient's life is an area of interest to conventional and homeopathic practitioners, homeopaths may probe further to find out more about the person and how he or she handles the stress of illness (Box 7-3).

The attention paid to the characteristics of the chief complaint is quite time consuming. However, to fully understand the patient, the homeopath must learn of all aspects of the patient's health. Therefore the same degree of attention must be paid to any other symptoms the patient experiences. Generally speaking, most of these symptoms come up during the investigation into the chief complaint. A formal review of systems to uncover any omissions is still a good idea.

The homeopath makes an assessment of the nature of the patient as a person, including personality, familial and other relationships, social situation, coping mechanisms, and other areas of interest as indicated in each interview. Clearly, understanding the nature of the person is challenging, as is eliciting information that will lead to such an understanding and evaluating it without prejudice. The homeopath must approach the interview with an open mind, free from preconceptions about the patient and his or her illness, and free from distraction with personal matters. In the midst of a busy schedule, it can be difficult to listen attentively and to refrain from making undue associations or presumptions regarding the patient's story.

BOX 7-3

Typical Questions a Homeopath May Ask to Ascertain the Effect of an Illness

What have you done for this problem and what was the effect of that treatment?

What are you still doing for the problem? Are you taking medications? Are you receiving other therapies, either conventional or alternative?

What treatments have you pursued or are you pursuing for other conditions?

What is the hardest part of this illness in your experience?

What do you miss the most in your life, and what is your feeling about that?

The personal nature of the interview can surprise patients who may arrive with a list of medications, previous test results, and a series of diagnoses. Patients new to homeopathy may experience an initial unease when asked to talk about themselves. After the initial surprise, most patients are gratified to learn that less importance is placed on the diagnosis and more emphasis on the person who has the illness. Patients find a way to tell the story that reveals who they are. The open-minded homeopath will sit back with confidence and curiosity, gleaning much that contributes to his or her understanding.

Every patient will reveal nonverbal information. Babies clutch a parent's arm (fearfully? mischievously? angrily? jealously?) or upset the entire toy basket; children sit forward with eager involvement or absentmindedly handle books on a low shelf; adults sit back with arms folded or lay out neatly typed lists of previous medical consultations. Nervous laughter, unconscious gestures, even the nature of clothing selected—all contain information that may be helpful.

Information may be solicited with a simple request that the patient talk about himself or herself, such as, "I think I understand quite a lot about your physical complaints. Now, to select the right treatment for you, I would like to know as much as possible about the rest of you. Who are you, and how would you describe your temperament?" For most patients, this is indeed a challenging task that unfolds with the combined efforts of patient and homeopath.

Each homeopath develops a personal interviewing style, which may appear similar to the style of psychotherapeutic assessment. The following are some of the interview techniques used by homeopaths.

Practicing active silence: Watching and waiting can be a valuable tool, allowing the homeopath to observe and the patient to decide what he or she would like to talk about.

Eliciting a story: The homeopath may try to elicit a story (What happened at recess today? Tell me about the last time you were really upset.) or an unconscious theme (Have you ever had any frightening or recurring dreams? Do you have any fears or phobias?) It is not unusual to hear stories, perhaps previously unshared, that have troubled a patient, or to follow the patient as he or she recognizes a recurring theme in the chain of events described.

Asking for reports from others: What important friends or relatives say about the patient, or what the patient believes they may say, can be revealing. (What would your wife say is your best quality? Your worst?) Reports from others must always be considered in context, keeping in mind the primary goal of the interview, which is to learn the patient's experience in his or her own words. Observations of others regarding the patient's behavior are of secondary, although sometimes quite useful, importance.

Noticing dropped clues: Inadvertent communications may influence the therapist's thinking about the patient. If a patient makes an offhand remark, expresses an inappropriate emotion, speaks to himself or herself as an aside, or substitutes one word for another, the homeopath is entitled to consider whether the "mistake" may be interpreted as significant. For example, if a patient mistakenly refers to her husband as "my father," it is reasonable to learn more about her relationship with her father and to assess whether any unresolved themes from that relationship are exerting an influence in her current life.

The standard of practice is to start with a simple sentence or question and listen without interruption to the patient's answer. If more information is needed, questioning proceeds with simple or open-ended inquiry and becomes specific only to clarify information.

An important part of every medical evaluation is the physical examination, and this is true in homeopathy as well. Important information can be obtained about the patient's general level of health and fitness, the accuracy of the patient's description of his or her condition, and possibly about health concerns that the patient is unaware of.

In addition, the homeopath may gather particularly useful information from items of little interest in a conventional evaluation. For example, imagine the physician is examining two children with chronic respiratory infections, considering which remedy might be appropriate for each. One child has a bluish tint to her sclera, an indication to consider the remedy *Carcinosin*. The other child has a streak of hair growing down the midline of the back, overlying the spine, an indication for the remedy *Tuberculinum*. The final choice of remedy will be based on the totality of factors, but in these cases, the physical examination has added distinguishing clues.

Certain details of the patient's nature are of peculiar interest to homeopaths because they correspond to indications for specific remedies. The homeopath must inquire about that body of information referred to as *generals*, meaning details that describe the patient's general tendencies. Generals fall roughly into two categories: preferences and modalities.

Regarding preferences, the homeopath wants to know about food cravings and aversions, sleep position and patterns, and whether the patient is more on the warm side or the chilly side.

Food cravings and aversions are helpful when they reflect true choices on the part of the patient. The foods that a patient strongly likes or dislikes may be quite different from the foods chosen or avoided at mealtime, because those choices may be made for health reasons or, for children particularly, made by other people. In addition to specific food desires and aversions, the patient is questioned regarding specific tastes: sweet, sour, salty, spicy, or smoked. The nature and intensity of the patient's general thirst is also important.

Sleep patterns involve the patient's physical position during sleep and the length and quality of sleep. Again, the question is of preference, not of selection. A patient may sleep on his back with a pillow under his knees on the advice of his physician, but, given the choice or an unusual bed, he or she may find himself on his abdomen. Other significant information may include the patient's natural patterns of sleep and waking, and whether he or she feels refreshed on waking. Napping may be soothing or only aggravate an afternoon sense of fatigue.

A simple piece of information that is sometimes difficult to elicit is the patient's sense of temperature, quite separate from both emotional temperament and degree of fever or chill as measured by a thermometer. Some homeopathic remedies are specifically indicated for people who tend to feel chillier than others, whereas other remedies are for people who are on the warm side. Most people have not reflected on this characteristic, so a bit of questioning is needed to find out, "Are you usually warmer or cooler than those around you? Do you turn the thermostat up or down more often? Do you wear shorts in the winter or a sweater in the summer?"

Once the homeopath acquires information about the modalities of the chief complaint and other physical complaints, it is important to know whether any general modalities apply to the patient as a whole. Sample modalities of a general nature include seasons, locations (e.g., the seashore or the mountains), weather conditions, time of day, particular activities (e.g., ascending stairs, reading, playing the piano), and bodily functions (e.g., diarrhea, menses, sleep). Rather than question the patient specifically regarding an infinite list of possible modalities, the homeopath instead strives to notice information revealed about these modalities during the general interview, and questions further as needed.

For example, it is not uncommon for a patient with headaches to relate the timing of the headaches to changing weather patterns. However, if a patient says that not only the headaches, but his or her allergies and general energy level become problematic when the weather changes, the homeopath will want to know specifically what sort of a change and when does the aggravation come relative to that change. "Oh, I'm worse when it's threatening rain, and once it starts to rain, I feel actually a bit better." This statement provides two items of information, namely that the patient is worse before a storm and better during rainy or wet weather.

The homeopath is of course interested in what is relevant in conventional medical evaluations, including a review of systems and personal and family medical histories. Areas of particular interest regarding the personal medical history include problems and treatments that preceded the onset of the chief complaint, as well as the history of vaccinations, injuries, and surgeries. Some remedies are particularly indicated for postoperative complaints, whereas others are more appropriate for complaints associated with a recent vaccination. The family history is often contributory, because certain hereditary tendencies considered in homeopathic analysis not usually considered in conventional medicine. Areas of particular interest include history of cancer, tuberculosis, syphilis, gonorrhea, and epilepsy. Also of interest are instances of heart disease and diabetes, particularly when such instances have an early age of onset. Homeopaths practicing in certain locales would also be interested in history of leprosy, typhoid, and other epidemic and endemic diseases.

CASE ANALYSIS AND REMEDY SELECTION

Having gathered necessary information about the patient, the homeopath is faced with the task of synthesizing the information in such a way that the correct homeopathic remedy may be selected. Case analysis is directed at developing an organized homeopathic picture of the patient that corresponds to a similarly organized picture of a homeopathic remedy.

Case Analysis

The patient's story is organized into the homeopathic picture, which always includes and expands upon a conventional understanding of the patient. The physician seeks to identify all distinctive qualities of illness and temperament that characterize the patient, to understand what is particular about the expression of illness in the patient. The physician considers all information gathered and must make a sensible analysis by answering a series of questions.

What Is the Central Feature of the Case?

The most important part of the analysis is to identify the central feature or disturbance, which may or may not be the same as the patient's chief complaint. The central disturbance may be on one or more of three important levels—physical, emotional, or mental. The homeopath must identify and understand the central feature as the basis for selecting the appropriate remedy.

Samuel Hahnemann, in the *Organon of Medicine*, summarized this mandate as follows:

A physician must . . . clearly realize what is to be cured in diseases, that is, in each single case of disease. . . . It will help the physician to bring about a cure if he can find out the data of the most probable cause of an acute disease, and the most significant factors in the entire history of a protracted wasting sickness, enabling him to find out its fundamental cause.[1]

Hahnemann continues over many paragraphs to describe different aspects of what is referred to here as the *central feature*. The concept of a central feature is important, and is peculiar to homeopathic analysis. Although there are distinguishing characteristics among individual homeopaths at an advanced level of analysis, as a group homeopaths share an understanding about health and disease that varies somewhat from conventional medical understanding.

The totality of symptoms must be considered in every case. It is important to remember that, unlike conventional medicine, the pathologic diagnosis is only a possible starting point for the homeopathic diagnosis. The homeopath seeks the distinguishing aspects of the complaint and the person who has the complaint, so that the Law of Similars may be applied and a homeopathic remedy chosen—one that has been shown to cause or cure the particular complaints of the patient. *Totality* does not necessarily imply a complete and exhaustive review of systems, but rather the importance of the whole picture. In an acutely ill patient, it may be the intensity of symptoms and the level of the energy or malaise that represents the totality of the illness picture. However, in a case of chronic rheumatoid arthritis, much more information (a complete review of systems, as well as an understanding of the patient's nature or personality) is needed, because the patient's disease response is all encompassing.

In chronic cases, the overview is usually quite broad. Many aspects of the patient's life will be considered in search of emotional themes, limitations on any level, and distinguishing details that may not be pathologic but are nonetheless characteristic, such as food preferences and sleep habits.

The consideration of acute cases is more clearly focused for several reasons. First and foremost, it is usually the case that when an individual is sufficiently ill to merit attention, the defining aspects of the case are often quite clear. The physician is less interested in a global picture of the patient and more interested in a snapshot that answers the question, "How are you different from your normal state?" Answers to this question include acute physical symptoms and important general or emotional features. For example, a patient with an acute sore throat will usually be very clear about the nature of the pain and the accompanying modalities, as well as his or her general level of heat or chilliness, thirst, appetite, and mood. "I don't have time for these questions, just get me well . . . now!" provides sufficient information about the patient's emotional state, as does, "I really don't know. I don't care. Leave me alone, I want to go home."

The totality of symptoms is organized according to a functional hierarchy of symptoms, from most to least severe. In a general sense, any disturbance on a mental level (e.g., dementia, thought disorder) is usually the most severe and disabling, followed by emotional disturbance (e.g., depression, anxiety) and finally by disease of the physical body. At each level, an appropriate internal hierarchy is structured based on the degree to which the problem compromises health, so that within the level of physical symptoms,

heart disease is more serious than skin disease. The hierarchy is flexible and based on logic, such that for every patient the totality of symptoms must be analyzed, with due regard to severity of each symptom, in the context of the life of the patient. Where is the patient most restricted or disabled? What level of dysfunction or suffering is most acute? What improvement would most benefit the patient?

Considering a totality of symptoms in each patient, the most crucial area or level of disturbance becomes the central feature of the case and the key to a successful prescription. Two examples illustrate this point.

First, although skin disease (physical) is almost always less disabling than mental or emotional symptoms, a severe dermatitis, with intolerable itching, swelling, and even bleeding, is more disabling than a mild case of situational anxiety, even though anxiety resides on the deeper (emotional) level.

Second, a patient's primary complaint is chronic eczema, but further questioning reveals that he or she struggles chronically with depression. A thorough exploration and analysis of the depression reveals an unresolved grief in the patient's childhood. The homeopath understands that the depression reveals a disturbance on a level more central than the skin, and so selects the remedy based primarily upon the understanding of the depression. A remedy selected with this understanding is most likely to address both the depression and the eczema and lead to a successful outcome.

What Are the Strange, Rare, and Peculiar Aspects to the Case?

It is essential that the physician have an understanding of both medical pathology and human nature upon which to base his or her evaluation. Crucial to a correct homeopathic prescription is the identification of aspects of the case that are unexpected, distinguishing symptoms that are thus considered strange, rare, and peculiar.

Symptoms may be considered strange, rare, and peculiar by several different criteria. A symptom may be quite unusual and striking by its very nature, or by its intensity or frequency, or it may be unusual only in the context of the particular patient and his or her illness or personality.

For example, a patient with a severe sore throat states that the pain is eased only by eating solid food and is made worse by swallowing liquids. This unusual modality becomes a central feature in understanding the patient and making the correct prescription.

In another case, a patient with migraines since a business failure is presumed to be suffering financial worries. The patient reports that he or she worries constantly about money and making ends meet. Further inquiry reveals that because of a generous inheritance the patient has no real basis for financial concern.

Finally, a patient with allergic rhinitis sneezes for several hours each morning on waking, or hiccups after each sneeze. Patients with allergic rhinitis are *expected* to sneeze most when they are most exposed to allergens. However, patients whose sneezing becomes strongest according to the time of day, or who follow an allergic sneeze with a hiccup, are revealing individual symptoms uncommon in this condition.

Is There Clear Causation?

The homeopathic physician will inquire carefully into the circumstances surrounding the beginning of an illness, looking for an event or a condition that may have precipitated the lapse in health. An essential assumption in homeopathic perspective is that a healthy body operates to preserve homeostasis; confronted with stress of any sort, the organism will seek to maintain a healthy state. When the homeostatic mechanism fails, illness ensues as a result of a particular stressor affecting a particular weakness of the organism.

To evaluate stress or causation, the homeopath examines factors that are usually considered, such as habits, lifestyle, and infectious disease, but expands the analysis to identify specific stressors. Selection of the appropriate homeopathic remedy will vary, depending on whether the stress is the grief of an emotional loss, the shock of a near-accident, or overwork associated with final examinations for a college student. The specific nature of the stress and the patient's reaction to it are important factors to understand.

Is the Case Acute or Chronic?

In most cases the answer to this question is not difficult, yet it must still be carefully considered. The important point is to question when the patient was last in good health, which necessitates understanding what good health is for that patient. The patient's sense of well being is one possible guideline, the report of family members is another.

In the case of recurring acute illness, such as repeated otitis media in children, the homeopath will consider whether the tendency to such problems is chronic, or whether the child is generally healthy but has been unable to successfully heal an acute illness. If the condition is the result of a chronic weakness, consideration of the complete history may lead to a treatment that eradicates the tendency to ear infections. In the second circumstance, treating it with a homeopathic remedy as opposed to using the suppressive antibiotic may enable the child's immune system to eradicate the infection, which then does not reappear.

What Other Features Are Important to the Case?

While evaluating the totality of symptoms and the patient as a whole, a great deal of information may be acquired that does not seem central to the case at hand. Considering a wide variety of information offers the homeopath the opportunity to develop a greater sense of patience, to resist the urge to discard what seems irrelevant. At times what seems most irrelevant will in fact be important to understanding the patient or may provide an essential clue in the search for the correct remedy.

As the physician gains clinical experience and increased familiarity with homeopathic medications, the process of sorting valuable information from the merely extraneous becomes more efficient. The skill of effective analysis at this level is best acquired in a clinical situation, working with the guidance of an experienced homeopath.

What Features of the Patient's Life or Lifestyle Contribute to the Disease Process?

In general, the answers to this question overlap broadly with conventional understanding of how lifestyle affects health. Lifestyle choices clearly have an influence on certain states of health or illness, and each physician develops a personal style for advising patients regarding those choices. Homeopaths are usually very successful at helping patients change unhealthy lifestyle habits.

Consider the example of a heavy coffee drinker who has problems with insomnia. Obviously, any physician would consider counseling the patient about the relationship between coffee and sleeplessness.

However, the homeopath will also consider the patient's craving for coffee as a symptom, and if the remedy selected has been observed to decrease a coffee craving, the homeopath may choose to sit in silence while waiting to see whether the patient's craving changes without counseling.

Many other choices are not so clear cut—many are controversial—and the decisions made by homeopaths regarding the importance and effectiveness of lifestyle counseling are as personal as the choices made by conventional physicians.

Selecting the Remedy: Resource Texts

Once the patient's information is organized into a homeopathic picture, the physician will search for a corresponding homeopathic medicine. A homeopathic medicine will be sought based on its predictable effectiveness in treating the picture of the patient arranged in the case analysis. The physician has three types of sources in which to search for information about the homeopathic remedies.

Homeopathic Provings

Homeopathic medicines develop indications for clinical usefulness depending on their performance in clinical trials, which in homeopathic practice are called *provings*. The nature of provings has evolved somewhat over the 200-plus years of homeopathic practice, but the process of information gathering remains the same. In modern clinical provings, carefully controlled and supervised groups of individuals ingest one or more doses of an unidentified homeopathic remedy and carefully record all symptoms or changes in their normal state. Symptoms will range from the content of dreams, changes in emotional state, and physical sensations to actual physical changes. Symptoms are reviewed for accuracy and collated among different provers to provide a comprehensive list of symptoms caused by that particular remedy, arranged in groupings of body parts affected. Symptoms in the categories of *mind* and *generalities* may predominate for some remedies, or other specific areas, such as *head, stomach,* or *sleep,* may be affected, depending on the scope of action of the particular remedy.

Information has been retained from provings that have varied widely in their clinical design over the last two centuries, ranging from single provers to large groups, from seemingly innocuous inactive substances to quite potent and drastically acting ones. Information has been added in a similar fashion when poisonings have occurred, although poisoning symptoms are generally less reliable for clinical applications than proving ones. For example, the homeopathic remedy made from mercury is not toxic as a remedy (referred to as *Mercurius vivus* or *Mercurius solubilis*), but elicits symptoms if administered in a proving. Symptoms observed during historical episodes of poisoning from mercury (environmental or iatrogenic) are striking but are less useful in clinical practice. Poisoning symptoms are retained in the clinical texts for the sake of completeness, interest, and possible application.

The most comprehensive record of provings is a 12-volume set collected by T.F. Allen, MD, which lists proving substances in alphabetical order.[2] This reference provides a comprehensive list of the symptoms associated with substances at that time. For example, the listing for the homeopathic remedy made from mercury (formal name is *Mercurius solubilis* or *Mercurius vivus*) is fairly long, running for 28 pages in a typical edition. Provings completed since Allen's work was published are published individually, in collections, or in homeopathic journals.

The following are excerpts from the symptom list for *Mercurius vivus*. The first information provided is about the substance itself.

> Hydrargyrum, an elementary body. (Mercurius vivus, Quicksilver.)
> Preparation for use, Triturations.
> Mercurius solubilis, Hahnemanni.
> Hydrargyrum oxydulatum nigrum (Ammonionitricum) $N_2O_{53}Hg_{2O} + 2NH_3$.
> Precipitated black oxide of Mercury, with varying (according to temperature) amounts of Nitric acid and Ammonia.
> Preparation for use: Triturations.[2]

General symptoms often appear in narrative form.

After he had taken the fourth powder I was summoned to see him, when he informed me that catarrhal symptoms were much improved, but he was then having a most violent facial neuralgia on the right side, originating in the dental nerve, and radiating upwards over the side of the face.

This he first felt after taking the second dose, and immediately after each of the two last the aggravation was marked and intense, so much so, that he felt that he could not take another dose.

I discontinued the remedy and the difficulty soon subsided.

His teeth, which are carious, are becoming loose; there is a white line, from undue epithelial secretions, at the margin of the gums; there are great tremors, approaching to paralysis, and an indecision in speaking, resembling stammering.

He has lost two stone weight during the last two years.

The tongue is wavy from nervous debility, and he suffers from nocturnal perspirations; memory is rather failing, and appetite is bad.

Pale, weak, and anxious-looking, with a slow but regular pulse; tongue furred; teeth mostly greenish black and carious; skin generally dry and cold.

Teeth, lower incisors, pegged, flattened at the top, the center brown, the enamel everywhere deficient.

All of them chipped and decayed.[2]

A section on *generalities* lists conditions affecting the whole person, as taken from various provings, poisonings, and clinical experience.

Emaciation.
He was emaciated and cachectic, and looked prematurely old.

It is certain that the children of the workers are affected with the mercurial poisoning; although it may be from the poison carried by the clothing.

A daughter, born during her mercurialism, was very small, only learned to walk when three years old, and never grew to be more than four feet in height; there was kyphoscoliotic curvature of the spine, the head was drawn to the chest and somewhat to the left side; there was very imperfect development of the muscle and bone.[2]

Symptoms of emotions, mental function, and dizziness are combined in a section of symptoms of the mind.

Emotional.
Mind, easily agitated.
Occasionally his mind seemed to wander.
Frightful images at night.
Hallucinations day and night.
Hallucination of mind, especially at night, with desire to escape.
Delirium; his speech was disconnected, and he would not answer questions; this delirium increased to a violent rage, so that the patient was obliged to be confined in a strait-jacket, with rolling of the eyeballs, clonic spasms, discharge of yellow, frothy liquid from the mouth and nose, and rattling in the trachea, followed by trismus and tetanus.
Delirium.
Constant weeping (elder).
Sadness.
Low-spirited.[2]

The final excerpt is take from a section that is highly characteristic for this remedy, a section referring to symptoms of the mouth.

Teeth.
Teeth black, loose.
Teeth turn yellow and become loose.
Thick gray coating on the teeth (after working fourteen days).
Teeth dirty-gray, loose.
Teeth foul.
Teeth thickly covered with tartar.
Carious teeth.
Decay of the teeth; they become loose in succession, and at the age of thirty she had lost six; they fell out at the slightest shock (after six years); most of the teeth, especially the molars, were gone; those that remained were blackened, laid bare, loose and carious (after thirty-eight years).
After a time, the teeth decay, become loose, of a grayish color, and fall out.
Since going into the works, he has been obliged to have several teeth removed.
All the teeth were loose.
Teeth loose, discolored
Teeth loose; at last drop out.[2]

Materia Medica and Keynotes

Although it is valuable for its completeness, the quoted reference for *Mercurius vivus* is incredibly cumbersome to use in an individual case. Over the last two centuries, various homeopathic physicians endeavored to create a simplified organization of the material in which they combined the most valuable symptoms gleaned from the provings and from the clinical experience of many homeopaths. The material is arranged alphabetically by substance and often serves as the confirming reference for practitioners.

The length and usefulness of different Materia Medica texts varies widely and becomes a choice guided by educational and clinical experience. The most widely accepted and revered text is generally thought to be the *Lectures on Homeopathic Materia Medica*, written by James Tyler Kent, MD, which was first published in 1904 and is still completely applicable in modern practice.

The following excerpts from Kent's chapter on the remedy *Mercurius* demonstrate the ease of use of Kent's presentation in a clinical setting as compared with the cumulative information presented in Allen's work. The text begins with a discussion of the substance and general features of its effects.

The pathogenesis of Mercury is found in the provings of Merc. viv. and Merc. sol., two slightly different preparations, but not different enough to make any distinction in practice.

Mercury is used in testing the temperature, and a Merc. constitution is just as changeable and sensitive to heat and cold. The patient is worse from the extremes of temperature, worse from both heat and cold. Both the symptoms and the patient are worse in a warm atmosphere, worse in the open air, and worse in the cold. The complaints of Mercury when sufficiently acute to send him to bed are worse from the warmth of the bed so that he is forced to uncover; but after he uncovers and cools off he gets worse again, so that he has difficulty in keeping comfortable. This applies to the pains, the fever, ulcers and eruptions and the patient himself.

He is an offensive patient. We speak of mercurial odors. The breath especially is very fetid, and it can be detected on entering the room; it permeates the whole room. The perspiration is offensive; it has a strong, sweetish, penetrating odor. Offensiveness runs all through; offensive urine, stool and sweat; the odors from the nose and mouth are offensive.

He is worse at night. The bone pains, joint affections and inflammatory conditions are all worse at night and somewhat relieved during the day. Bone pains are universal, but especially where the flesh is thin over the bones. Periosteal pains, boring pains, worse at night and from warmth of the bed. Mental symptoms: The mental symptoms, which still more deeply show the nature of the medicine, are rich. A marked feature running all through is hastiness; a hurried, restless, anxious, impulsive disposition. Coming in spells, in cold, cloudy weather, or damp weather, the mind will not work, it is slow and sluggish and he is forgetful. This is noticed in persons who are tending toward imbecility. He cannot answer questions right off, looks and thinks, and finally grasps it. Imbecility and softening of the brain are strong features. He becomes foolish. Delirium in acute complaints. From his feelings he thinks he must be losing his reason. Desire to kill persons contradicting her. Impulse to kill or commit suicide, sudden anger with impulse to do violence. She has the impulse to commit suicide or violent things, and she is fearful that she will lose her reason and carry the impulses out. Impulsive insanity, then, is a feature,

but imbecility is more common than insanity. These impulses are leading features. The patient will not tell you about his impulses, but they relate to deep evils of the will, they fairly drive him to do something. Given a Merc. patient, and he has impulses that he tries to control, no matter what, Merc. will do something for him. During menses, great anxiety, great sadness. Anxious and restless as if some evil impended, worse at night, with sweat. All these symptoms are common in old syphilitics, broken down after mercurial treatment and sulphur baths at the springs, with their bone pains, glandular troubles, sweating, catarrhs and ulcerations everywhere.[3]

The following, for comparison with Allen, are symptoms of the mouth.

Scorbutic gums in those who have been salivated [Editors note: When conventional physicians gave mercury to treat syphilis, they used the toxic effect of salivation as an indication that an adequate dosage had been administered to the patient. Thus "those who have been salivated."]. Rigg's disease; purulent discharge from around the teeth. Toothache; every tooth aches, especially in old gouty and mercurialized patients. Looseness of the teeth. Red, soft gums. Teeth black and dirty. Black teeth and early decay of the teeth in syphilitic children, like *Staph*. Copious salivation. Gums painful to touch. Pulsation in the gums and roots. Gums have a blue red margin, or purple color, and are spongy and bleed easily. Gums settle away, and the teeth feel long, and are elongated. Teeth sore and painful so that he cannot masticate. Abscesses of the gums and roots of the teeth. The taste, tongue and mouth furnish important and distinctive symptoms. As the tongue is projected it is seen to be flabby, has a mealy surface, and is often pale. The imprint of the teeth is observed all round the edge of the tongue. The tongue is swollen as if spongy, and presses in around the teeth and thus gets the imprint of the teeth. Inflammation, ulceration and swelling of the tongue are strong features. Old gouty constitutions have swollen tongue; the tongue will swell in the night and he will waken up with a mouthful. The taste is perverted, nothing tastes right. The tongue is coated yellow or white as chalk in a layer.[3]

More concise summaries of information regarding each remedy are compiled in collections of *keynotes*, in which data for each remedy may be limited to one or two pages. Texts of compiled materia medica and keynotes are very useful for confirming which information is relevant to a particular patient and for comparing the patient's symptom picture with the specifics of a particular remedy. Some homeopaths prescribe primarily based on a thorough understanding and grasp of the materia medica. This approach to prescribing requires tremendous strength of memory, given the size of the homeopathic pharmacopoeia and the truism that *any* remedy may be indicated in a particular case, regardless of the chief complaint.

The process of scanning all existing materia medica to find the material appropriate to a given patient has been simplified by computer programs that quickly access information matching search terms entered by the physician. However, because not all homeopaths have access to or choose to use computers, a written tool that evolved well before computers has made the work of homeopathy a little easier: the repertory.

Repertory

A later development in homeopathic literature that has proven immensely valuable to the practicing homeopath is a book (or computer program) referred to as a *repertory*. The repertories most commonly in use are modeled on a schema developed (in the original repertory) by James Tyler Kent. The most comprehensive modern version derived from the Kentian tradition is *The Complete Repertory*, by Roger van Zandvoort.

A Kent-based repertory is arranged in chapters covering symptoms of particular body parts (ranging from Mind to Extremities) and chapters referring to states of the entire body (i.e., Fever, Chill, Sleep, Skin, and Generalities). Within each chapter, symptoms are arranged alphabetically with extreme precision, elaborated on with extensive subrubrics, and, in the most modern repertories, elegantly cross-referenced to facilitate symptom location. For each symptom, there is a corresponding list of remedies that have either caused that symptom in a proving or poisoning or cured that symptom in clinical setting. Remedies are listed alphabetically for each symptom, and emphasis is given according to the strength of the association between the remedy and the symptom.

Following are rubrics representative of the materia medica and proving information for the remedy *Mercurius* cited previously. These rubrics are from the computerized version of *The Complete Repertory*, by Roger van Zandvoort.[4]

From the chapter on teeth, we find such rubrics as "TEETH; DIRTY look," with the remedies (abbreviated) "all-c., aur-m-n., caps., merc., pyrog." The fourth remedy in that series is "merc.," the abbreviation for *Mercurius*. This rubric would be considered any time the patient stated or the physician noted that even cleaned teeth appeared to be dirty.

Another rubric, "TEETH; LOOSENESS of" lists 97 remedies in various type styles to indicate different emphases. The remedy *Mercurius* is listed in bold type, indicating that the symptom has been repeatedly observed in provings or poisonings and that it has been cured in cases treated with *Mercurius*. (This rubric would be consulted for teeth which are indeed loose or for a strong sensation of looseness, regardless of the actual state of the teeth). The full list of remedies for this rubric is as follows:

acon., *alumn.*, *am-c.*, arg-n., arn., *ars.*, *aur.*, aur-ar., aur-m., *aur-m-n.*, aur-s., bar-c., bar-i., bar-m., bism., bor., *bry.*, *bufo*, calc., calc-f., calc-sil., camph., **Carb-an.**, **Carb-v.**, carbn-s., **Caust.**, cham., chel., *chin.*, cist., cocc., colch., com., *con.*, crot-h., dros., elaps, gels., gran., graph., hep., **Hyos.**, ign., iod., *kali-bi.*, *kali-c.*, kali-m., kali-n., kali-p., lac-c., lach., *lyc.*, *mag-c.*, mag-s., **Merc.**, **Merc-c.**, *mur-ac.*, naja, nat-ar., nat-c., nat-h., *nat-m.*, nat-p., nat-s., **Nit-ac.**, nux-m., *nux-v.*, olnd., op., *ph-ac.*, phos., phyt., plan., plat., *plb.*, psor., puls., rat., rheum, *rhod.*, *rhus-t.*, sang., scroph-n., *sec.*, *sep.*, **Sil.**, spong., stann., *staph.*, *sulph.*, syph., *tarent.*, thuj., tub., verat., **Zinc.**, zinc-p.[4]

To select a mental symptom for comparison, we can take a phrase from the paragraph on mental symptoms in Kent's *Materia Medica* on *Mercurius*: "Impulse to kill or commit suicide, sudden anger with impulse to do violence."[3] With a little experience we learn that the key word that guides the repertory search is *kill*, rather than *impulse*. Searching under the rubric *kill* for symptoms associated with *Mercurius*, the findings are abundant:

MIND; KILL, desire to: Many remedies, among them: merc

MIND; KILL, desire to; child, her own: androc., merc., plat.

MIND; KILL, desire to; hysterical melancholia, with: merc. alone, no other remedies.

MIND; KILL, desire to; knife, with a: . . . merc., . . .

MIND; KILL, desire to; person that contradicts her: Only merc.

MIND; KILL, desire to; sudden impulse to: . . .merc. . . .

MIND; KILL, desire to; sudden impulse to; herself (See also Fear; kill herself, that she might and Suicidal disposition): . . .merc., . . .

MIND; KILL, desire to; sudden impulse to; husband, her beloved: . . .merc. . . .

MIND; KILL, desire to; sudden impulse to; husband, her beloved; menses, particularly during, implores him to hide his razor: only merc.[4]

Familiarity with the repertory becomes one of the key features of most homeopathic physicians' prescriptive skills. The most comprehensive repertory text, the computer version of which has been used for these examples, runs a full 2830 pages in book form, and is well beyond the scope of fallible human memory.[4] Rubrics may contain one or hundreds of remedies. Careful use of the repertory by a conscientious practitioner reveals previously unnoticed rubrics almost daily.

The practitioner begins with the case analysis and the exact words of the patient, and translates that information into rubrics selected from the repertory. A comparison or cross-analysis of the rubrics, done by hand or through a computer program, will yield one or more remedies listed in most or all of the rubrics selected.

For example, a patient may offer the following as a chief or secondary complaint: "I'm having terrible trouble with my teeth and gums, so my dentist thought maybe homeopathy could help me. They're not actually falling out, but they seem loose to me and the dentist says that's not far from the truth. I really do brush them, but they look dirty, no matter what I do." Thus the rubrics are "TEETH, LOOSENESS of" and "TEETH; DIRTY look." The two rubrics are compared and only two remedies are listed in both rubrics: Aur-m-n *(Aurum muriaticum natronatum)* and Merc *(Mercurius,* as discussed).

Of course, during the interview a great deal more is learned about the patient, and the homeopath is particularly interested in any symptoms relating to emotions, personality, and mental state. Mental characteristics or symptoms are often the most significant and distinguishing aspects of the case.

For example, if the patient with the dental problem is encouraged to talk freely about himself, his relationships, and his personality, the homeopath listens patiently and with an open mind, confident that close attention will yield an answer. A statement such as, "You know, I don't really know why we're bothering with this. I don't care much about anything anymore and I couldn't care less whether my teeth fall out or not," would indeed be strange, rare, and peculiar, and may be translated into the mental rubric, "MIND; INDIFFERENCE, apathy; recovery, about his," for which three remedies are listed: ars., aur-m-n., calc. The homeopath would exercise clinical judgment, deciding whether this revelation is important to understanding the character of the patient. If so, the prescription is for the remedy aur-m-n.

On the other hand, the patient may mutter and spurt through an agitated depression, sorting through different life aspects. "My marriage? Oh, it's great, I guess, wait, that's not always true. Why just last night we had a HUGE fight, wow, I nearly forgot. When that happens I get so mad, I have to watch myself. I want to just run into the kitchen and grab a knife. I mean I would never kill her or anything, but the thought crosses my mind and it's almost as if I have to struggle against it."

Our previous example of rubrics for *Mercurius* included the rubric, "MIND; KILL, desire to; sudden impulse to; offense, for a slight: hep., merc., nux-v." If the physician believes that this rubric describes a significant aspect of the patient's character, he or she would select *Mercurius* as the appropriate remedy.

After scanning the repertory to compile a comprehensive list of remedies that may be useful in a particular case, the practitioner returns to the materia medica or provings for a fuller description of the remedy. Scores of authors have written in different languages over the last 200 years, adding to the wealth of information about homeopathic remedies. Clinical experience and training will enable the practitioner to develop techniques for selecting reliable texts and using keynotes, materia medica, and provings to compare what is known about a given remedy with what he or she has learned from the interview and case analysis.

Potency

After selecting the appropriate remedy, the homeopath makes a decision about the potency of the remedy. Homeopathic remedies in the United States are formulated in D (or X), C, and LM potencies, each letter the Roman numeral for a particular dilution. Thus a liquid form of the prepared medicine is diluted in 1:10 (X potency), 1:100 (C potency) or 1:50,000 (LM potency) solution of alcohol and water. With each dilution the remedy is succussed. The number of dilutions is matched with the appropriate Roman numeral to describe the potency. Common potencies include the following:

1. 6X, 12X and 30X are most commonly available in over-the-counter situations, and are safe for self-prescribing or beginning prescriptions.
2. 6C, 12C, 30C, 200C are commonly used by physician prescribers and describe a range of

low (6C, 12C), medium (30C), and high (200C) potencies.

3. A variation in nomenclature occurs in centesimal dilutions (1:100) beginning at 1000 centesimal dilutions; a shorthand is employed in which 1000C is written simply as 1M. Dilutions of higher potency continue in the shortened nomenclature; thus 10M, 50M, and CM (100M).

4. LM potencies are prepared at each sequential level, thus LM1, LM2, LM3, and so on, usually up to LM30. These potencies are usually prepared for the patient in a very dilute solution of alcohol in water, and administered in drops daily.

Unfortunately for the beginning practitioner, there are myriad systems to explain and advise on the selection of the correct potency. Clinical and educational experience weigh strongly on the beginning practitioner's first choices of potency. Fortunately, it is usually true that a correctly chosen remedy will act and be helpful in any potency; often the different potencies affect only the duration of action.

A simplified prescription schema limited to C and LM potencies is as follows: in acute illness, consider using the C potencies. Decide whether the key indicating symptoms (mental, physical, or emotional) are mild or intense. If the prescribing symptoms are intense, particularly if the mental or emotional symptoms are intense, you may use a high potency: 200C, 1M, or even 10M. A single dose of the remedy may suffice, or it may need to be repeated. Any need for repetition is determined by the response to the first dose; a favorable response followed by a return of some or all symptoms indicates a repetition of the remedy. It is more likely that repetition will be needed in the presence of fever.

If the prescribing symptoms are mild, you will do better with a lower potency, such as 6C, 12C, and perhaps 30C. With milder symptoms and lower potencies, the response to the remedy is often more gradual. When repetition is needed, the patient will start with a single dose and repeat that dose once or twice daily. It is very important in these situations in which patients with milder symptoms use lower potencies to tell the patient to stop taking the medicine when he or she starts to notice improvement. The remedy may be repeated later if the patient ceases to improve, but continued dosing may disrupt the improvement to a serious degree.

In chronic illness, proper potency may be determined along similar lines. Thus patients who are chronically ill, with one or a few clear symptoms that are clear, intense, or start from a single point in time, may be easily treated with a single dose of high-potency centesimal remedies, such as 200C or higher.

Chronic illness of an insidious, slowly evolving nature or with daily exacerbation may best be treated with daily homeopathic medicines. This may be accomplished by initiating treatment with a single dose of a high centesimal potency, and following that dose with daily low-potency dosing, such as 6C or 12C, or by using the LM potencies, which are most often used daily. Chronic patients who are also taking conventional or herbal medicines are often treated most effectively with LM potencies, so that the homeopathic remedy may easily and safely be taken daily.

Other Instructions

A controversial area of homeopathy among practicing homeopaths is the question of antidotes; that is, whether certain other substances can interfere with the curative action of the homeopathic remedy. Conventional (allopathic) medicines in some instances interfere with the action of the remedy. Decisions about concomitant medications are made on an individual basis, balancing two concerns. The prime concern, of course, is the patient's safety; many medications are taken because they are essential for the patient's health and well being. Such medications may be discontinued only if they are no longer considered essential. The second concern is the patient's health: dependence on medication for symptom relief can interfere with the body's ability to find its own reservoirs of healing in response to a correct homeopathic remedy. The patient and physician will discuss the interaction of medications and the homeopathic remedy.

For many years, practitioners in the United States have believed and observed that coffee, decaffeinated or regular, is an antidote for homeopathic remedies. At the same time, many practitioners in Europe and India (and many patients in the United States) have disregarded this caution without affecting remedy effectiveness. These two seemingly contradictory experiences are perhaps both true.

One possible explanation is that the nature of illness varies in different countries, and that illnesses in the United States, such as digestive complaints, stress-related illness, and nervous conditions, are in general more aggravated by coffee.

Another possible (or perhaps probable) explanation has to do with the degree of accuracy of the remedy. In a given case, acute or chronic, there may be one remedy that will act perfectly, yielding a gentle, rapid, and lasting cure. This remedy is considered the *simillimum*, and is sometimes elusive, particularly in chronic cases. In addition to the simillimum, there are likely many similar remedies that fall short of perfection but will act in a helpful way nonetheless. The simillimum may be less influenced by antidotes than are the similar but less-effective remedies. Thus it is more important for a beginning homeopath to caution patients about the use of antidotes, and less important for a more experienced homeopath.

Substances commonly considered antidotes are coffee, camphor (applied topically), menthol, and some conventional and herbal medicines. Certain medical practices are also considered antidotes, including dental procedures and certain kinds of hands-on medical treatment such as acupuncture or chiropractic. Beliefs and practices regarding these potential antidotes vary widely among different practitioners and are a continuing area of discussion and investigation.

In the *Organon of Medicine*, Samuel Hahnemann offered specific advice about the components of a healthy lifestyle that contribute to prompt healing in response to the remedy. Hahnemann distinguishes between diseases improperly called *chronic*, which respond to lifestyle adjustments, and those diseases that are truly chronic, which necessitate medical treatment. For patients entering medical treatment, Hahnemann offers a list of prohibitions that are nearly impossible to follow:

Patients with chronic diseases should avoid the following: coffee, fine Chinese tea and other herb teas, beers adulterated with medicinal vegetable substances, spiced chocolate, highly seasoned foods and sauces, vegetable dishes with herbs; chronically ill patients should also avoid every excess, even that of sugar and salt, alcoholic drinks not diluted with water, heated rooms, a sedentary lifestyle, excessive breast-feeding, long afternoon naps, etc.[1]

It is a rare practitioner who expects such rigid lifestyle standards of patients at this time. Homeopathic practitioners advise patients regarding lifestyle issues to varying degrees, according to the totality of their medical belief system. Thus physicians may advise their patients regarding alcoholic beverages, use of vaccinations, amount of exercise, and routine physical examinations, but the nature of such advice has no predictable common thread among homeopathic physicians.

Prognosis

Part of homeopathic prognosis is the immediate and long-term anticipated response to the remedy. The initial response to a correctly prescribed homeopathic remedy will follow one of three courses.

First, there may be no initial reaction; the response to the remedy is slow in onset and gradual in pace. This is the most likely response in chronic conditions that have not been treated with conventional, allopathic medication and that have evolved at a steady pace over the course of the illness. Chronic arthritis of a moderate degree, fatigue, and irritable bowel are conditions that may have been self-managed and slowly evolving, and may be slow to respond to a homeopathic remedy.

The second response is prompt and clear amelioration. A perfectly selected remedy given to a generally healthy patient with, at most, a few specific complaints is most likely to show this response pattern.

The third response is initial aggravation (worsening of symptoms in a pattern atypical for that patient). This aggravation may be brief or may introduce a gradual retracing of the chronic illness. An aggravation may apply to specific symptoms (e.g., headache, joint pain, sneezing) or to the patient's more general state (e.g., sleep patterns, energy levels). Patients with less vitality, multiple illnesses, or a history of medication for the symptoms are more likely to experience significant aggravation after the remedy. Healthy patients may also run through periods of aggravation, although these are usually short lived. A clear aggravation or a transient return of symptoms from the past are excellent prognostic signs for the future course of the illness.

Adverse responses or effects from the remedy are rare, but they do happen and must be distinguished from aggravations. Only a return of a previously experienced symptom, identical or slightly altered, may be considered an aggravation. A symptom completely new to the patient is considered an adverse response. A persistent aggravation or a serious adverse response are each an indication that the prescription was incorrect—either the remedy itself or its potency.

Long-term prognosis is an extremely complicated area in which clinical experience is a crucial factor. Patients new to homeopathy often inquire whether homeopathy can help with their specific diagnosis, a question that is almost impossible to answer reliably. Homeopathy can help with any condition, from the common cold to terminal illness. On the other hand, an incorrectly selected remedy will not help either a terminal illness or a common cold. If concern is limited to a select correctly prescribed remedy, which is a significant assumption, prognosis is more favorable in vital patients with clearly defined symptoms who have not been treated with numerous allopathic prescriptions, particularly immune-suppressing medications (e.g., corticosteroids, methotrexate). The prognosis is less favorable in more debilitated patients with vague and generalized symptoms and a history of using many medications.

The time course of response to a remedy varies as well, but one rule of thumb is that a chronic illness will resolve over a period of months loosely equal to the number of years the illness has been present. That number, already an approximation, may be doubled for patients middle-aged and older. However, even an illness predicted to resolve in 5 years is expected to show improvement, possibly significant improvement, in just the first few weeks of treatment.

CASE MANAGEMENT

Follow-up Evaluations

Patients with acute conditions are seen for follow-up examinations on a schedule similar to that in conventional medical practice. Any potentially serious condition is followed quite closely; illnesses expected to resolve without complication are treated and seen again only if the condition worsens.

Chronic illnesses are expected to take quite a different course under homeopathic treatment, and thus the follow-ups, at least initially, proceed at a different schedule. In chronic cases, some improvement is expected within the first few weeks; thus patients are typically seen for follow-up between 3 and 6 weeks.

Follow-up examinations are scheduled for 15 to 45 minutes, and are intended to evaluate the patient's response to the remedy in all areas disclosed in the initial interview. The chief complaint and other medical conditions or complaints are inquired after, as well as the patient's general state (e.g., energy, sleep, appetite) and specifics relevant to that patient. If a patient with a physical complaint is also found to have a lesser emotional problem, such as irritability or procrastination, it is important to ask in an open-ended way about these areas as well.

If the prescription is accurate, the patient is expected to move toward cure in a predictable fashion. Illness resolves in a logical fashion as the organism systematically seeks a homeostasis at a level of greater health. As observed and repeatedly confirmed in clinical experience, a patient's lifetime of complaints will resolve themselves in a sequence proceeding as follows: from those arising most recently to those from the distant past; from mental to emotional to physical complaints; from cephalad proceeding downward; and from internal, life-threatening conditions to superficial conditions. (A caveat that is not always confirmed is the expectation that the patient is not cured until the disease actually manifests on the superficial (epidermal) layer and presents as a rash.) In the mid-nineteenth century, Constantine Hering systematized these observations as the "Laws of Cure." This intellectual framework can be applied to evaluate the response to any therapeutic intervention.

The crucial determination the homeopath makes in the follow-up evaluation is whether the patient's overall level of health is moving in a direction of greater health toward cure. If the complaints have merely shifted around or (even worse) if the patients initial complaint has resolved while a more serious one has arisen (a process of suppression), the homeopath is not pleased with the results of treatment. Quite different from conventional practice, in homeopathy the overall picture must improve whether the chief complaint improves.

For example, consider a patient with chronic headaches who returns to say that he or she is delighted, the headaches are much better, but the patient had to see a psychiatrist because of the onset of a deep depression and is now on antidepressant medication. A conventional evaluation may not link the two complaints. The homeopath will consider that the prescription was wrong, and that the headaches have been suppressed into a more life-threatening condition, depression.

For another example, consider a patient with chronic headaches who reports that the headaches seem just as bad, but sleep and energy are so much better that he or she goes through the day joyfully and seems to handle the headaches much better than before. Although a conventional evaluation would be equivocal, the homeopath will be pleased, and will anticipate further improvement.

Further Prescribing

The second prescription is perhaps more problematic than the first. If the first remedy proves inaccurate and no healing response is seen, the case is considered as if new, and a new "first" prescription is made. Once a remedy is seen to have a curative effect, the question of "second prescription" arises and involves questions of when to repeat the remedy and when to change to a different remedy.

Duration of action of the initial prescription varies widely, and can be assessed only on individual clinical grounds. For example, a remedy taken for hay fever may prove curative, permanently, in one dose, or may need to be repeated twice daily at the height of the season and renewed annually. Given the wide variation, it is evident that communication between the homeopath and patient is required for appropriate guidance.

SUMMARY

It is undoubtedly evident from the previous discussion that many variables and variations are possible among different homeopathic practices. The physician who successfully practices homeopathy is similar to archetypes of physicians from the past, which may be thought incompatible in a world of modern medicine, managed care, and technologic sophistication. It is true that the homeopath spends more time with each patient than would be allowed by typical modern schedules, relies less on technologic diagnosis and newly patented prescription medication, and has idiosyncratic notions about the relationship between physical and emotional symptoms and the ability of the body to heal itself.

However, the practice of homeopathy provides a model that makes sense in light of modern medical economics. Clinically based research is accumulating that validates the "efficiency" as well as effectiveness of homeopathy. In addition, the nature of the homeopathic interview and the assumptions of self-healing in response to the remedy are only two of the many factors that contribute to the mutually satisfying nature of the physician-patient relationship in homeopathic practice.

References

1. Hahnemann, S: *Organon of the medical art*, Ed: W. Brewster O'Reilly, Redmond, WA, 1996, Birdcage Books.
2. Allen TF: *Encyclopedia of pure materia medica*, A record of the positive effects of drugs upon the healthy human organism, 12 vols, New Delhi, India, 1988, B Jain Publishers Pvt. (original 1874).
3. Kent JT: *Lectures on homeopathic materia medica*, New Delhi, India, 1986, B Jain Publishers Pvt.
4. van Zandvoort R: *The complete repertory*, Version 3.0, MacRepertory Computer Program, San Rafael, California, Kent Homeopathic Associates (computerized version).

Suggested Readings

Borland D: *Homeopathy in practice*, Beaconsfield, England, 1982, Beaconsfield.

Panos MB, Heimlich J: *Homeopathic medicine at home*, Los Angeles, 1980, JP Tarcher.

Schmidt P: *The homeopathic consultation: the art of interrogation*, Delhi, India, 1954, B Jain.

Ullman R, Reichenberg-Ullman J: *The patient's guide to homeopathic medicine*, Edmonds, WA, 1995, Picnic Point Press.

Vithoulkas G: *Science of homeopathy*, New York, 1980, Grove Press.

Weil A: *Health and healing*, Boston, 1983, Houghton Mifflin.

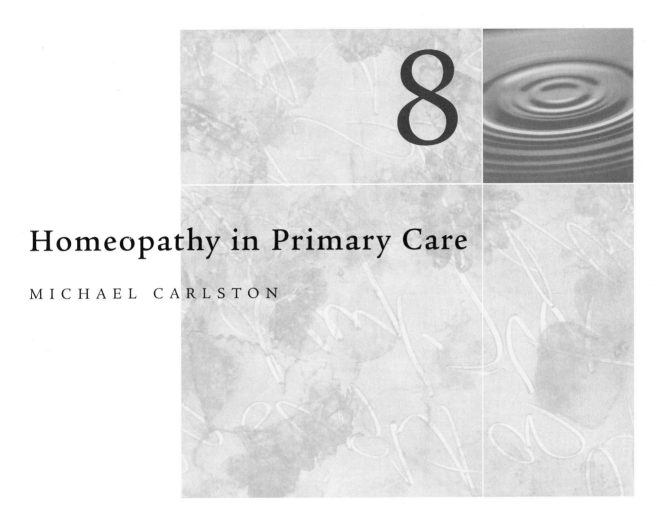

Homeopathy in Primary Care

MICHAEL CARLSTON

WHEN IS HOMEOPATHY LIKELY TO BE SUCCESSFUL?

Consideration of any form of healing must include some thought about conditions for which it is useful. As Hahnemann wrote in the opening line of the *Organon of Medicine*, "The physician's highest calling, his only calling, is to make sick people healthy—to heal, as it is termed."[1]

What is our responsibility if not to help our patients? What is homeopathy good for? When is its use appropriate and when not?

Although these are simple questions, simple questions are often the most difficult to answer and simultaneously the most instructive. Remember that the view of disease in homeopathy is quite different from that of conventional medicine. The very different understanding of disease and health necessitates complicated answers to these simple questions. Simply put, because homeopaths define disease quite differently from conventional physicians, comparing success by disease categories is problematic.

For two centuries the homeopathic refrain has been that we treat the patient, not the disease. The point of this statement is that all patients are unique; their conventionally labeled *disease* is only part of who they are. Disease labels do not fully describe the imbalance in a person's health. Further, each person diagnosed with a certain conventional disease is significantly different from others with the same disease. The diagnosis is an imprecise label for the totality of a patient's condition. Homeopathic treatment focuses on the unique pattern of each person's response. Common aspects of that response are not particularly helpful when choosing the homeopathic remedy.

As a very simple example, consider a patient with pneumonia. A cough is quite common, indeed rarely absent, in this disease and thus minimally helpful to the homeopath. Of the hundreds of homeopathic remedies recorded for use in coughs, only a handful of them are likely to be useful for a given patient—and for each patient, one remedy is the best. The absence of a cough, or a cough that has unusual characteristics (sound, instigating or ameliorating factors) can be quite helpful because of its uniqueness, its individuality. This rich complexity of factors requiring consideration increases dramatically when the patient suffers from chronic health complaints and subtle consideration of all elements of the patient's health become necessary.

Homeopaths rarely associate remedies with specific diagnoses. Instead we speak of the *sulphur patient* or the *phosphorus patient*, recognizing the pattern of the patient's reactions and temperament as primary. A sulphur patient can suffer many diseases, but the homeopathic remedy sulphur is expected to alleviate all of them. On the other side of the equation, in a room full of patients with diagnosis *x*, perhaps only one is a sulfur patient; the rest may need a different homeopathic remedy. No homeopath would expect every patient with a certain disease to respond to the same homeopathic remedy. In fact, homeopaths do not expect patients to improve unless the correct homeopathic medicine is selected from the massive list of possibilities.

Given these constraints, it is difficult to construct hierarchic lists of diseases graded by the degree of homeopathic effectiveness. Some homeopaths utterly reject the effort as futile and deceiving to those seeking to understand homeopathy. However, patients, and even many homeopaths, temper their ideology with pragmatism and recognize that certain conventionally defined diseases are more prone to response than others. A great number of the classical homeopathic texts of the past two centuries include lists of remedies recommended for consideration in patients with certain conventional diseases.[2-7] Always, however, is the essential precondition that the homeopath must select the correct homeopathic remedy for the individual patient.

Research Evidence of Effectiveness

One way to answer questions of effectiveness is by turning to published medical research. Unfortunately, the best homeopathic research to date has focused almost exclusively on placebo differentiation. Although there is still insufficient research to conclusively prove that homeopathic treatment is more than placebo, the amount of research devoted to demonstrating that homeopathy gives patients clinically meaningful improvement is at best a small drop in a very large bucket.

Perhaps the best experimental evidence is that supporting the use of homeopathy in allergic conditions, particularly allergic rhinitis (hay fever). One of the very first homeopathic trials published in a conventional medical journal investigated the use of a homeopathic medicine for hay fever symptoms.[8] The trial used a 30C dilution of mixed pollens and found a statistically significant improvement among patients in the treatment group by a variety of measures (see Chapter 6 for further discussion of these studies). The trial was one of a series conducted by Reilly and associates dealing with inhalant allergic disease. When they completed the third trial in the series and published their meta-analysis, the combined *p* value so strongly favored homeopathy ($p = .0004$) that the authors concluded, "Either answer suggested by the evidence to date—homeopathy works, or the clinical trial does not—is equally challenging to current medical science."[9] Although this conclusion is rather ambitious, and somewhat weakened by the latest trial in the series, other human and basic sciences studies and literature reviews support the contention that allergic rhinitis is the clinical arena with the strongest evidence for homeopathic effectiveness.[10-18]

Another form of allergic respiratory disease, asthma, was included in Reilly's series with similarly positive results. In spite of other favorable studies of homeopathic treatment of asthma, far too little published evidence of effectiveness exists to claim that the matter is settled.[19-21] However, it may be significant that asthma is the most common problem for which patients in America seek treatment from physician homeopaths.[22]

Ear infections (otitis media) are another respiratory disease leading patients to homeopathy and which has a modest amount of supporting research.[23-27] A number of interesting discussion points were raised by a trial conducted by de Klerk and published in the *British Medical Journal*.[23] This study highlights some of the difficulties in conducting homeopathic clinical trials. Two groups of children with recurrent upper respiratory illnesses (including acute otitis media [AOM]) received a classical homeopathic interview and lifestyle advice. One group received a homeopathic remedy, whereas the other took placebo. Both groups had a marked reduction in upper respiratory illnesses, but the homeopathic remedy group did not achieve a statistically significant superiority. In addition to the methodologic problems in the study (see Chapter 6), the significant improvement in members of the "control group," who received all components of homeopathic treatment except the medicinal globules, raises important questions and highlights our ignorance about the magnitude of effects caused by each component of a homeopathic intervention.

Additional clinical research suggests that homeopathy may be effective for rheumatologic conditions and menstrual disorders.[28-31] Some studies support, although others contradict, traditional homeopathic wisdom that homeopathy is useful for tension and migraine headaches.[32-38]

Clinical Reports of Efficacy

Homeopathy enjoys a very lengthy clinical tradition, and many cases have been recorded in precise detail. These case reports include sufficient detail to assess the response of the patients to their homeopathic treatment. Most case reports have only short-term follow-up and very few of them have independent verification. In the absence of further objective assessment, and given the previously mentioned concerns about disease categorization, the voice of clinical tradition deserves a critical hearing.

Traditionally, homeopaths have written that excessive tissue destruction, which occurs with end-stage disease, precludes a curative response to homeopathic treatment.[39,40] Cancer, heart disease, and arthritis, which have created marked joint deformities, are cited as examples in various texts. In spite of this belief, however, homeopaths commonly treat patients with these conditions, anticipating palliation rather than cure. Arthritis, for example is among the most common diagnoses of patients seeking professional homeopathic care in several studies.[22,41] Many homeopathic texts address the use of homeopathy in a variety of heart conditions, including congestive heart failure, arrhythmia, and angina.[42-44]

A relatively large number of articles in homeopathic and conventional medical journals address homeopathic treatment of cancer.[45-62] Many of these articles refer to the use of homeopathy as an adjunctive means to assist cancer patients with quality of life issues, such as adverse effects resulting from conventional cancer treatment.[63-65] Homeopaths tend to be extremely careful to avoid misleading patients about the abilities of homeopathy in serious diseases. As a result, the usual application of homeopathy for patients with cancer is as a complementary therapy.

Although somewhat tangential, there is a very interesting perspective on gastrointestinal cancer prevention arising from homeopathic theory. Morgan used homeopathic principles to explain the effectiveness of aspirin as a prophylactic for esophageal and colorectal cancer.[66] This action currently lacks a well-accepted conventional explanation,[67,68] as does quinine's effectiveness in malaria; in both instances, homeopathic theory offers a reasonable explanation.

Homeopaths and the homeopathic clinical literature indicate that homeopathy appears useful in conjunction with conventional treatments in many other disease conditions. Angina, carpal tunnel syndrome, elevated cholesterol, diabetes, hypertension, osteoporosis, acute pain, chronic pain, and rheumatoid arthritis are on this list. Many common medical problems are believed to respond quite well to homeopathic treatment alone. Some of these problems are anxiety disorders, back pain, chronic fatigue, immune dysfunction syndrome, digestive disorders, gastroesophageal reflux, sinusitis, and stress-related illnesses.

Patients appear to seek homeopathy for their health problems in a pattern very much in keeping with homeopathic opinion (Table 8-1). The diagnoses of patients seen by American physician homeopaths in Jennifer Jacobs' 1992 survey[22] closely parallel the preceding discussion.

For Whom Does Homeopathy Work Well?

Another way of considering homeopathy's effectiveness is to turn the question around into a more "homeopathic" form. Because homeopathy focuses on the individual rather than the disease category, instead of asking, "For what does homeopathy work

TABLE 8-1

Diagnoses of Patients Seen by Homeopathic Physicians

Diagnosis	Cases (%)
Asthma	4.9
Depression	3.5
Otitis media	3.5
Allergic rhinitis	3.4
Headache, migraine	3.2
Neurotic disorders	2.9
Allergy, nonspecific	2.8
Dermatitis, eczema	2.6
Arthritis, osteoarthritis	2.5
Hypertension	2.4

From Jacobs J, Chapman EH, Crothers D: *Arch Fam Med* 7(6):537, 1998.

well?" we can instead ask the question, "For whom does homeopathy work well?"

Homeopathy requires much of its patients. Homeopaths want to know all about patients' symptom patterns, lifestyle habits, and emotional makeup. As a result, patients who are self-aware can be easier to treat.

Even a self-aware patient must convey his or her understanding to the homeopath or the insight is lost. Some patients do not want to discuss the most important concerns in their lives, a choice that obviously impedes the homeopath's work. On the other side of the patient-physician relationship, a perceptive homeopath can communicate with a diverse range of patients (and is expected to perceive things about the patient that he or she has yet to perceive). Good communication between patient and practitioner is probably more important in homeopathic than in conventional medical practice.

Some patients interpret their experience through a blanket of preconceptions that can easily lead the homeopath astray. This is true of patients who are adamantly convinced that their problems stem from a particular source (often something they have read in a popular health book). Their opinions can be unshakable, even when many indications contradict their ready explanations. Such patients tend to ignore these messy contradictions. As a result, the patient presents a very neatly tied but false package of information. Patients who have experienced lengthy

poor-quality psychotherapy are often in this category. Inevitably, because homeopathic patients are usually asked to answer questions they had not considered in the past, they give a certain amount of incorrect information to the homeopath. The quantity of this misinformation is not usually sufficient to confuse an experienced homeopath.

As discussed earlier (see Chapter 7), treatments of all sorts can be suppressive. Although the suppressive treatment is most commonly a conventional medication, homeopathy or any other therapeutic method has the potential to obstruct the body's healing process. When obstruction occurs, the patient's pattern of symptoms becomes much more difficult for the homeopath to interpret; finding the correct homeopathic remedy is thus much more difficult. In addition, nonhomeopathic medications sometimes reduce or negate the effectiveness of the homeopathic remedy.

Traditionally defined adverse drug effects, such as dry mouth from using an antidepressant, can confuse homeopathic prescribing. The homeopath must determine which symptoms are true expressions of the body's healing process versus which are toxic effects from the prescription medication. Adverse effects induced by conventional treatment can necessitate specific homeopathic treatment as well, but that is a more complicated discussion and beyond the scope of this book.

BEYOND ILLNESS—DISEASE PREVENTION

Although homeopaths have traditionally claimed that homeopathy's health-improving effects prevent future disease, such as cancer, only limited evidence exists to substantiate these claims. De Klerk's study[23] is one of the few studies in which homeopathic treatment was evaluated over more than a few months. She found a significant reduction in rates of upper respiratory illness among her subjects. However, both the control and treatment groups improved, and the treatment group's superiority was just short of statistical significance.

Another study that perhaps links use of homeopathic or anthroposophical treatment with disease reduction was conducted in New Zealand.[69] Investigators surveyed a population (students attending Rudolph Steiner schools) whose philosophy encourages the use of anthroposophical and homeopathic treatments in place of conventional medication including antibiotics. After controlling for confounding factors, the children who received antibiotics in the first year of life were four times as likely to develop asthma than the other children.

These findings add support to the growing body of evidence for what has been called the *hygiene hypothesis*.[70] There has been a precipitous rise in childhood asthma throughout the wealthier countries in the world. This is true despite significant improvements in nearly all known asthma risk factors. The hygiene hypothesis attributes much of this deterioration in the health of our children to overzealous removal of infectious agents from our bodies and environments. Infections appear to help the maturation of the human immune system. Interference with that process, no matter how well intentioned, may lead to increased tendency to atopic diseases, including asthma. Treatments such as homeopathy, which offers alternatives to antibiotics, could thus play a significant part in reducing the risks of future disease.

Proof that the use of homeopathy (or avoidance of conventional medications) leads to healthier populations would be much more than a decorative feather in a homeopath's cap. If the belief that homeopathy leads to greater emotional balance and improved immune functioning is correct, a reduction in disease rates would inevitably follow homeopathic treatment. However, contentions like these should be examined carefully and systematically before claims are made. I have heard it said that homeopathic patients simply don't get cancer. I have seen otherwise. Certainly, we all share death's end point. More subtle investigations of disease rates are necessary to prove or disprove the important question of homeopathy's effect on disease prevention.

HEALTH RISKS ASSOCIATED WITH HOMEOPATHIC MEDICINE

Within the infant rind of this small flower, poison hath residence and medicine power.

WILLIAM SHAKESPEARE (from *Romeo and Juliet*)

Any substance that can heal can also cause harm. Every medicinal substance has adverse effects as well as beneficial. Human life cannot exist without the sun, but solar radiation causes cancer. Water is essential to life, but excessive amounts can kill. Love may be the sole exception, but that is for poets to decide. The use of homeopathy must entail some risk. What are those risks?

When Is a Poison Not Poisonous?

First, we will consider injury from the homeopathic treatment itself. Many homeopathic medicines are made from poisonous substances. The dilution process used by homeopathic pharmacists almost always negates this potential cause of harm.

Because of confusion about homeopathic pharmaceutic nomenclature, I used to receive many calls from poison control centers inquiring about pediatric patients who had swallowed entire bottles of *Belladonna* 30C. They recognized the name *Belladonna*, also known as *deadly nightshade*, because it is toxic. Although the name justified their concern, what they did not know was that homeopathically prepared *Belladonna* 30C has so little *Belladonna* remaining that it would take a mass greater than that of our galaxy to contain a toxic dose. Certainly the harm from swallowing such a mass would be the primary concern!

Think of the most toxic substance you know. Most of them are chemical toxins, which are poisonous in doses on the order of a millionth of a gram. Because this is an extremely small quantity, a patient would have to take many doses of a homeopathically prepared 6X-strength remedy made from that substance to suffer that level of exposure. Because 6C is customarily the most material dose used (i.e., 1 part in 1,000,000,000,000), and 12C (1 part in 1,000,000, 000,000,000,000,000) and 30C (1 part in 1,000, 000,000,000,000,000,000,000,000,000,000,000, 000,000,000,000,000,000,000,000) doses are common, conventional toxicity issues are nearly irrelevant.

In spite of the drastic dilution involved in the preparation of homeopathic remedies, *homeopathic* does not automatically mean *safe*. The smallest grain of plutonium could kill you and anyone who came into contact with your remains for many thousands of years. Avoiding homeopathic medicines made from toxic substances in potencies less than 12C is prudent, particularly during pregnancy.

Neglect of Appropriate Care

In addition to directly toxic effects from the homeopathic remedy, other potential causes of harm to homeopathic patients exist. One of these is any suffering the patient may experience from delaying more effective treatment. Although the homeopathic treatment itself may not cause harm, the patient's condition could deteriorate during the trial of homeopathy.

The evidence is fairly strong that this risk is not presently significant. Because few patients seek homeopathic care without first trying conventional medicine, the possibility of homeopathic treatment delaying conventional treatment is quite low. In addition, many homeopathic practitioners are trained in conventional medicine, and all others who complete formalized homeopathic training in the United States or United Kingdom are taught when to refer for conventional treatment. The recent Boston survey conducted by Lee and Kemper[71] (see Chapter 4) reminds us that, although the risk is small, it is not nonexistent—some homeopaths do not recognize when they need to refer patients for conventional treatment. Professional homeopaths without conventional medical training must know when referral is necessary to ensure the safety of their patients. The inadequate level of clinical supervision in homeopathic training, already identified as a problem by the homeopathic community, may aggravate the referral problem.[72] Diligent efforts in the educational arena are necessary, because the rising popularity of homeopathy seems likely to increase the number of patients seeking homeopathy before they have tried conventional medicine.

My own clinical experience gives me a further, potentially insoluble, cause for concern. Over the years, a significant number of new patients have come to see me for treatment of problems that had been misdiagnosed by other conventional physicians. Seeking relief, these patients come to my practice unrelieved by conventional treatment, when they actually had *not yet received* conventional treatment because they were misdiagnosed. Dissatisfaction with treatment, for whatever cause, leads patients to try other means to feel better. Although this problem begins with a misdiagnosis provided by conventional medicine, it comes to roost in the population of patients seeking homeopathic treatment.

Aggravations and Provings

Homeopaths use some words with meanings unique to homeopathy. Two terms important to this discussion of adverse effects of homeopathic treatment are *aggravations* and *provings*.

The term *aggravation* refers to the temporary worsening of symptoms that commonly occurs when a patient takes a homeopathic remedy for a chronic condition. The term is quite descriptive, and it is easy to imagine that homeopathic patients may have devised the name. An aggravation classically proceeds along specific lines with the "deeper" problem (i.e., the mental/emotional or severe physical pathology) flaring up within days after beginning the homeopathic treatment; lesser disorders become more intense as the more serious problems remit. Not only is the homeopathic aggravation a common experience, it is so well recognized that homeopaths and homeopathic patients are sometimes disappointed when it does not occur. The homeopathic aggravation is welcomed as a herald of better times to come.

Hahnemann named his clinical trials of homeopathic medicines *provings*. Provings were experiments to determine precisely what symptomatic responses were characteristic of certain homeopathic medicines. These characteristic symptoms then became the indications for using that homeopathic remedy to help patients recover. A patient who takes a homeopathic medicine for too long will develop symptoms attributable to that excessive dosage. Akin to a conventional overdose, this circumstance is also called a *proving*. There is controversy within the homeopathic community about whether these proving symptoms will always go away of their own accord. Although this matter is controversial precisely because it is so rarely seen, concern about the possibility is the reason many classical homeopaths are uncomfortable with the popularity of homeopathic self-care. This concern is heightened with the use of combination remedies because the greater the number of remedies a patient takes, the greater the likelihood of sensitivity to one of them. Adding to the concern is the false popular belief that homeopathy can *never* cause any harm, making it unlikely that patients will identify the cause of ill effects they experience.

The uncertainty and broad questions surrounding this issue of homeopathic adverse effects can be answered only by careful study. Several long-term patient observational surveys are currently under way. Hopefully more definitive information will come out of these surveys. Because of homeopathy's very long track record and reputation for safety, significant problems appear extremely unlikely; however, the matter remains unresolved.

HOMEOPATHY: FROM MEDICAL SPECIALTY TO "DO-IT-YOURSELF"

Two apparently diametrically opposed points of view about the use of homeopathy exist. Accordingly, opinions about the necessary training and experience are as contradictory. Pierre Schmidt, one of the most highly regarded French homeopaths of the twentieth century, reportedly said, "It takes five years of full time practice to become a competent worker in homeopathy, ten years to become a craftsman and twenty five years, if you have the aptitude, to become a master." Yet 80% of the use of homeopathy in the United States is now self-care. Few of the people self-medicating with homeopathy have even the most basic understanding of homeopathic principles. How do we reconcile this trend with Schmidt's opinion, and what does this perplexity teach us about appropriate professional use?

The deeper truth underlying this seeming contradiction is quite simple. Although it is easy to use a few homeopathic remedies to treat minor acute illnesses based upon a few symptomatic indications, the complex evaluation process required to successfully treat chronic conditions is an entirely different matter. When Dr. Schmidt spoke of the many years necessary to learn the basics of homeopathic practice, he was acknowledging the quantity of information that must be mastered and the subtlety of understanding needed to skillfully use that information to treat chronic conditions.

Any reasonably intelligent person can quickly learn to apply homeopathy in a limited way. Several years ago, the director of a homeopathic pharmaceutic company told me of meeting a conventional physician at a Club Med. This physician learned of my friend's work and then showed him his kit of five homeopathic remedies. Although he knew only a little about when to use these remedies and essentially nothing about any other homeopathic medicines, he routinely prescribed those five homeopathic remedies in his medical practice.

As the average conventional physician starts to include bits and pieces of complementary medicine into practice, homeopathy can be a piece of the puzzle. Although useful for others, this piecemeal approach is unlikely to be of much help to the group of patients currently seeking professional homeopathic treatment. Those patients are looking for help with chronic problems that conventional medicine has not relieved. Homeopathic band-aids will not help them. They will continue to seek out physicians who specialize in homeopathic care for much more intensive chronic—sometimes called *constitutional*—care.

Physicians who specialize in homeopathy are growing in number, but are still quite rare in the United States. Our number may generously be estimated at nearly 1000. Because homeopathic specialists typically spend more than an hour with each new patient and close to 30 minutes with every returning patient, relatively few Americans have access to a homeopathic specialist.

How Is Homeopathy Different for the Physician?

Although most discussions of complementary medicine address the differences in clinical interaction from the patient's point of view, the physician's side of the interaction is also different. This is particularly true when the therapy is homeopathy. These differences can have a significant impact on the physician's ability to achieve therapeutic success and enjoy his or her work.

The physician has to spend more time with each patient and take a much more careful history than is required when practicing conventional medicine. This degree of attention can be very demanding. Each practitioner must develop insight about the way that patients interact with his or her personality, and must also learn to recognize his or her pattern of interaction with various types of patients, because these behavioral patterns are important clues to remedy selection. An inevitable mathematic consequence of the time required for each patient and the limited number of hours in a day is that homeopathic physicians tend to have lower incomes than conventional physicians. This is true despite the fact that homeopaths often charge each patient more for their services. Other disadvantages for the physician include the years required to learn the practice and following this achievement, enduring the criticism of less open-minded members of the medical community.

If these negatives were the sum total of the physician experience of homeopathy, it would be difficult to imagine homeopathy surviving two years, let alone two centuries! However, the many aspects of homeopathic care that are rewarding for the physician overwhelm these few negatives.

Although some physicians do not like the depth of patient interaction necessitated by homeopathy, many others find it much more satisfying then the usual 8 to 10 minutes and out-the-door routine sadly common these days. Paying careful attention to each patient enriches the interaction for the physician *and* the patient. Each patient is unique, and that individuality makes every clinical interaction more interesting. No patient is just a snotty nose or a backache.

The degree of attention necessary in homeopathy also helps the physician learn about the process of disease and recovery. One simple example is the clinical management of AOM in children. Antibiotics have been the routine treatment for decades. As research evidence accumulates that antibiotics should play a more limited role, conventional management is slowly evolving. For even longer than conventional physicians have been using antibiotics for AOM, clinical records show that homeopaths have successfully managed these patients without antibiotics. Following my conventional training I was very uncomfortable learning to manage AOM without reverting to antibiotics. However, I quickly learned that my patients did well without antibiotics. In fact, my clinical experience is that they appear much less likely to develop subsequent episodes of AOM if I manage the case without antibiotics.

Along these lines, homeopathy has a lengthy tradition of reducing patient use of prescription medication. If this can be done successfully, as homeopaths maintain, limiting only the use of needless antibiotics could be very beneficial to our society at a time when we face a rising, and very frightening, tide of antibiotic resistance. Taken a step further, if a physician can successfully treat a patient without exposing him or her to potentially significant adverse drug reactions, is it ethical not to make the attempt?

One reason that homeopathy helps reduce the use of conventional medication is that it offers the physician a therapeutic choice. Although conventional medicine provides fantastic tools to help patients, especially those with end-stage disease, too often the adverse effects of those powerful tools outweigh the benefits for common minor problems experienced by many of our patients. A few years ago, when I was developing a course introducing complementary medicine to primary care physicians, I asked conventional colleagues what problems were most frustrating in clinical practice. Dismayingly, their list was nearly identical to the National Ambulatory Medical Care Survey list of the 10 most common conditions seen by U.S. primary care providers.

Antibiotic overuse is one of the most serious problems facing conventional medicine today, particularly in the pediatric population. Among parents and physicians, many conflicting views contribute to this overuse.[73-78] Similarly, adult patients and their physicians appear to have difficulty reaching an understanding about appropriate antibiotic use, in part because of poor communication and unrealistic or even contradictory expectations.[79-81] Physicians often justify inappropriate antibiotic prescriptions by reporting that they feel pressured by their patients' demands for antibiotic treatment.[82] For homeopathic patients, homeopathy is an acceptable or even sought-after alternative to antibiotics. Certainly no evidence exists at this time that choosing homeopathy as an alternative to inappropriately prescribed antibiotics is harmful to patients. The opposite appears far more likely.

The clinical experience of homeopathy is different from the clinical experience of conventional medicine. This is true for the physician and for the patient. Although it is true that homeopathy can place more demands on the practitioner, many clinicians so strongly prefer the homeopathic clinical relationship that the disadvantages become insignificant.

SUMMARY

A person who wishes to investigate homeopathy need go no further than the office of a homeopathic specialist to grasp the unique qualities of the therapy. Details of homeopathic theory and findings of modern scientific investigations of homeopathy help us understand homeopathy. However, the heart of homeopathy is most easily examined in the clinician's office. The clinical experience calls patient and physician back to an earlier age, when the healing relationship was built less upon technology and more upon human qualities.

The primacy of the clinical relationship is homeopathy's most essential, most appealing, and most frustrating characteristic. It is entirely in keeping with Hahnemann's advocacy of *healing the patient*, as the physician's sole responsibility. It is what attracts patients and physicians hungry for an alternative to modern medicine's worst techno-failings. Its soft subjectivity appalls scientists who are firm in their conviction that all gaps in our knowledge will be filled by finer instrumentation. In many ways, it represents the essential conflict between the *art* and *science* aspects of medicine.

References

1. Hahnemann S: *Organon of medicine*, ed 6, Los Angeles, 1982, JP Tarcher.
2. Agrawal YR: *Homeopathy in asthma*, Delhi, 1985, Vijay Publications.
3. Borland D: *Homeopathy in practice*, Beaconsfield, England, 1982, Beaconsfield.
4. Burnett JC: *On neuralgia: its causes and its remedies, with a chapter on angina pectoris*, New Delhi, 1990, B Jain.
5. Dewey WA: *Homeopathic therapeutics*, ed 3, New Dehli, 1975, B Jain.
6. Farrington EA: *Therapeutic pointers (to some common diseases)*, New Delhi, 1988, B Jain.
7. Hering C: *The homeopathic domestic physician*, ed 14 (American), New Delhi, 1984, B Jain.
8. Reilly DT, Taylor MA, McSharry C et al: Is homoeopathy a placebo response? Controlled trial of homoeopathic potency, with pollen in hayfever as model, *Lancet* 2(8512):881-886, 1986.
9. Reilly D, Taylor MA, Beattie NG et al: Is evidence for homoeopathy reproducible? *Lancet* 344(8937):1601-1606, 1994.
10. Weiser M, Gegenheimer LH, Klein P: A randomized equivalence trial comparing the efficacy and safety of Luffa comp.-Heel nasal spray with cromolyn sodium spray in the treatment of seasonal allergic rhinitis, *Forsch Komplementarmed* 6(3):142-148, 1999.
11. Ludtke R, Wiesenauer M: [A meta-analysis of homeopathic treatment of pollinosis with Galphimia glauca], *Wien Med Wochenschr* 147(14):323-327, 1997.
12. Poitevin B, Davenas E, Benveniste J et al: In vitro immunological degranulation of human basophils is modulated by lung histamine and Apis mellifica, *Br J Clin Pharmacol* 25(4):439-444, 1998.
13. Sudan BJ: Total abrogation of facial seborrhoeic dermatitis with extremely low-frequency (1-1.1 Hz) "imprinted" water is not allergen or hapten dependent:

a new visible model for homoeopathy, *Med Hypotheses* (6):477-479, 1997.
14. Linde K, Clausius N, Ramirez G et al: Are the clinical effects of homeopathy placebo effects? A meta-analysis of placebo-controlled trials, *Lancet* 350(9081):834-843, 1997 (published erratum appears in *Lancet* 1998 351[9097]:220,1998).
15. Linde K: [Are there proven therapies in homeopathy?], *Internist (Berl)* 40(12):1271-1274, 1999.
16. Kleijnen J, Knipschild P, ter Riet G et al: Clinical trials of homoeopathy, *BMJ* 302(6772):316-323, 1991 (published erratum appears in *BMJ* 302[6780]:818, 1991).
17. Taylor MA, Reilly D, Llewellyn-Jones RH et al: Randomised controlled trial of homeopathy versus placebo in perennial allergic rhinitis with overview of four trial series, *BMJ* 321:471-476, 2000.
18. Lancaster T, Vickers A: Commentary: larger trials are needed, *BMJ* 321:476, 2000.
19. Campbell JH, Taylor MA, Beattie N et al: Is homeopathy a placebo response? a controlled trial of homeopathic immunotherapy in atopic asthma, *Am Rev Respir Dis* 141:A24, 1990.
20. Lewith GT, Watkins AD: Unconventional therapies in asthma: an overview, *Allergy* 51(11):761-769, 1996.
21. Lane DJ, Lane TV: Alternative and complementary medicine for asthma (editorial), *Thorax* 46(11):787-797, 1991.
22. Jacobs J, Chapman EH, Crothers D: Patient characteristics and practice patterns of physicians using homeopathy, *Arch Fam Med* 7(6):537-540, 1998.
23. de Lange de Klerk ES, Blommers J, Kuik DJ et al: Effect of homoeopathic medicines on daily burden of symptoms in children with recurrent upper respiratory tract infections, *BMJ* 309(6965):1329-1332, 1994.
24. Friese KH, Kruse S, Moeller H: [Acute otitis media in children. comparison between conventional and homeopathic therapy], *HNO* 44(8):462-466, 1996.
25. Friese KH, Kruse S, Ludtke R et al: The homoeopathic treatment of otitis media in children—comparisons with conventional therapy, *Int J Clin Pharmacol Ther* 35(7):296-301, 1997.
26. Harrison H, Fixsen A, Vickers A et al: A randomized comparison of homoeopathic and standard care for the treatment of glue ear in children, *Complement Ther Med* 7(3):132-135, 1999.
27. Mudry A: [Controversies concerning acute otitis media], *Arch Pediatr* 6(12):1338-1344, 1999.
28. Gibson RG, Gibson SL, MacNeill AD et al: Homeopathic therapy in rheumatoid arthritis: evaluation by double-blind clinical therapeutic trial, *Br J Clin Pharmacol* 9:453-459, 1980.
29. Fisher P, Huskisson EC, Turner P et al: Homoeopathic treatment of fibrositis, *Lancet* 336(8720):954, 1990.
30. Seidl MM, Stewart DE: Alternative treatments for menopausal symptoms. systematic review of scientific

and lay literature, *Can Fam Physician* 44:1299-1308, 1998 (published erratum appears in *Can Fam Physician* 44:1598, 1998).

31. Kass-Annese B: Alternative therapies for menopause, *Clin Obstet Gynecol* 43(1):162-183, 2000.
32. Whitmarsh TE: When conventional treatment is not enough: a case of migraine without aura responding to homeopathy, *J Altern Complement Med* 3(2):159-162, 1997.
33. Whitmarsh T: Evidence in complementary and alternative therapies: lessons from clinical trials of homeopathy in headache (editorial), *J Altern Complement Med* 3(4):307-310, 1997.
34. Walach H, Haeusler W, Lowes T et al: Classical homeopathic treatment of chronic headaches, *Cephalalgia* 17(2):119-126, 1997.
35. Ernst E: Homeopathic prophylaxis of headaches and migraine? a systematic review, *J Pain Symptom Manage* 18(5):353-357, 1999.
36. Vernon H, McDermaid CS, Hagino C: Systematic review of randomized clinical trials of complementary/alternative therapies in the treatment of tension-type and cervicogenic headache, *Complement Ther Med* 7(3):142-155, 1999.
37. Straumsheim P, Borchgrevink C, Mowinckel P et al: Homeopathic treatment of migraine: a double blind, placebo controlled trial of 68 patients, *Br Homeopath J* 89(1):4-7, 2000.
38. Whitmarsh T: More lessons from migraine, *Br Homeopath J* 89(1):1-2, 2000.
39. Kent JT: *Lectures on homeopathic materia medica*, New Dehli, 1971, B Jain.
40. Roberts HA: *The principles and art of cure by homeopathy: a modern textbook*, Rustington, England, 1936, Health Science Press.
41. Goldstein MS, Glik D: Use of and satisfaction with homeopathy in a patient population, *Altern Ther Health Med* 4(2):60-65, 1998.
42. Swayne JM: Survey of the use of homeopathic medicine in the UK health system, *J R Coll Gen Pract* 39(329):503-506, 1989.
43. Clarke JH: *Diseases of the heart and arteries*, New Delhi, 1987, B Jain.
44. *Small remedies and interesting cases II: Proceedings of the 1990 Professional Case Conference*, Seattle, 1990, International Foundation for Homeopathy.
45. Flinn JE: Bromium in acute lymphatic leukemia, *J Am Inst Homeopath* 58(7):213-214, 1965.
46. Bond W: Pathological prescribing, *J Am Inst Homeopath* 59(11):327-329, 1996.
47. Trexler HL: Carcinoma of the breast also treated by homeopathy, *J Am Inst Homeopath* 59(5):165-167, 1966.
48. Belloni L: [The intraorbital tumor of Field Marshal Radetzky cured by homeopathic therapy], *Gesnerus* 42(1-2):35-46, 1985.

49. Bradley GW, Clover A: Apparent response of small cell lung cancer to an extract of mistletoe and homoeopathic treatment, *Thorax* 44(12):1047-1048, 1989.
50. Ehring F: [Regression of over 150 skin metastases of malignant melanoma with complex homeopathic therapy], *Hautarzt* 40(1):23-27, 1989.
51. Mellor D: Mistletoe in homoeopathic cancer treatment, *Prof Nurse* 4(12):605-607, 1989.
52. Report of the joint Commission of the Royal Academy of Medicine on the analysis of publications concerning the study of homeopathic preparations aimed at immunotherapeutic treatment of AIDS and cancer, *Bull Mem Acad R Med Belg* 147(3-5):190-191, 1992.
53. Hauser SP: Unproven methods in cancer treatment, *Curr Opin Oncol* 5(4):646-654, 1993.
54. van der Zouwe N, van Dam FS, Aaronson NK et al: [Alternative treatments in cancer; extent and background of utilization], *Ned Tijdschr Geneeskd* 138(6):300-306, 1994.
55. Crocetti E, Crotti N, Feltrin A et al: The use of complementary therapies by breast cancer patients attending conventional treatment, *Eur J Cancer* 34(3):324-328, 1998.
56. Grootenhuis MA, Last BF, de Graaf-Nijkerk JH et al: Use of alternative treatment in pediatric oncology, *Cancer Nurs* 21(4):282-288, 1998.
57. Cassileth BR: Complementary therapies: overview and state of the art, *Cancer Nurs* 22(1):85-90, 1999.
58. Kasmann-Kellner B, Graf N, Elflein E et al: [Follow-up of retinoblastoma during homeopathic therapy], *Klin Monatsbl Augenheilkd* 214(4):aA12-aA16, 1999.
59. Van Dam FS: [Increased use of alternative diets and other alternative treatments for cancer patients: Houtsmuller (diet) is in, Moerman (diet) is out], *Ned Tijdschr Geneeskd* 143(27):1421-1424, 1999.
60. Malik IA, Khan NA, Khan W: Use of unconventional methods of therapy by cancer patients in Pakistan, *Eur J Epidemiol* 16(2):155-160, 2000.
61. Montfort H: A new homeopathic approach to neoplastic diseases: from cell destruction to carcinogen-induced apoptosis, *Br Homeopath J* 89(2):78-83, 2000.
62. Thompson E, Kassab S: Homeopathy in cancer care, *Br Homeopath J* 89(2):61-62, 2000.
63. Thompson EA: Using homoeopathy to offer supportive cancer care, in a National Health Service outpatient setting, *Complement Ther Nurs Midwifer* 5(2):37-41, 1999.
64. Thompson E, Hicks F: Intrathecal baclofen and homeopathy for the treatment of painful muscle spasms associated with malignant spinal cord compression, *Palliat Med* 12(2):119-121, 1998.
65. Oberbaum M, Yaniv I, Ben-Gal Y et al: A randomized, controlled clinical trial of the homeopathic medication TRAUMEEL S in the treatment of chemotherapy-induced stomatitis in children undergoing stem cell transplantation. *Cancer* 92(3):684-690, 2001.

66. Morgan G: Aspirin chemoprevention of colorectal and oesophageal cancers: an overview of the literature and homeopathic explanation, *Eur J Cancer Prev* 5(6):439-443, 1996.

67. Vainio H, Morgan G: Mechanisms of aspirin chemoprevention of colorectal cancer, *Eur J Drug Metab Pharmacokinet* 24(4):289-292, 1999.

68. Sandler RS, Galanko JC, Murray SC et al: Aspirin and nonsteroidal anti-inflammatory agents and risk for colorectal adenomas, *Gastroenterology* 114(3):441-447, 1998.

69. Wickens K, Pearce N, Crane J et al: Antibiotic use in early childhood and the development of asthma, *Clin Exp Allergy* 29(6):766-771, 1999.

70. Strachan DP: Family size, infection and atopy: the first decade of the "hygiene hypothesis," *Thorax* 55(suppl 1):S2-S10, 2000.

71. Lee AC, Kemper KJ: Homeopathy and naturopathy: practice characteristics and pediatric care, *Arch Pediatr Adolesc Med* 154:75-80, 2000.

72. Kreisberg J: Trends in homeopathic education: a survey of homeopathic schools in North America 1998, *JAIH* 93:75-84, 2000.

73. Liu HH: Overuse of antimicrobial therapy for upper respiratory infections and acute bronchitis: who, why, and what can be done? [editorial], *Pharmacotherapy* 19(4):371-373, 1999.

74. Barden LS, Dowell SF, Schwartz B et al: Current attitudes regarding use of antimicrobial agents: results from physician's and parents' focus group discussions, *Clin Pediatr (Phila)* 37(11):665-671, 1998.

75. Palmer DA, Bauchner H: Parents' and physicians' views on antibiotics, *Pediatrics* 99(6):E6, 1997.

76. Pichichero ME: Understanding antibiotic overuse for respiratory tract infections in children [comment], *Pediatrics* 104(6):1384-1388, 1999.

77. Schwartz RH, Freij BJ, Ziai M et al: Antimicrobial prescribing for acute purulent rhinitis in children: a survey of pediatricians and family practitioners [see comments], *Pediatr Infect Dis J* 16(2):185-190, 1997.

78. Watson RL, Dowell SF, Javaraman M et al: Antimicrobial use for pediatric upper respiratory infections: reported practice, actual practice, and parent beliefs [see comments], *Pediatrics* 104(6):1251-1257, 1999.

79. Gonzales R, Steiner JF, Sarde MA: Antibiotic prescribing for adults with colds, upper respiratory tract infections, and bronchitis by ambulatory care physicians [see comments], *JAMA* 278(11):901-904, 1997.

80. Britten N, Ukoumunne O: The influence of patients' hopes of receiving a prescription on doctors' perceptions and the decision to prescribe: a questionnaire survey, *BMJ* 315(7121):1506-1510, 1997.

81. Greenhalgh T, Gill P: Pressure to prescribe [editorial; comment], *BMJ* 315(7121):1482-1483, 1997.

82. Macfarlane J, Holmes W, MacFarlane R et al: Influence of patients' expectations on antibiotic management of acute lower respiratory tract illness in general practice: questionnaire study, *BMJ* 315(7117):1211-1214, 1997.

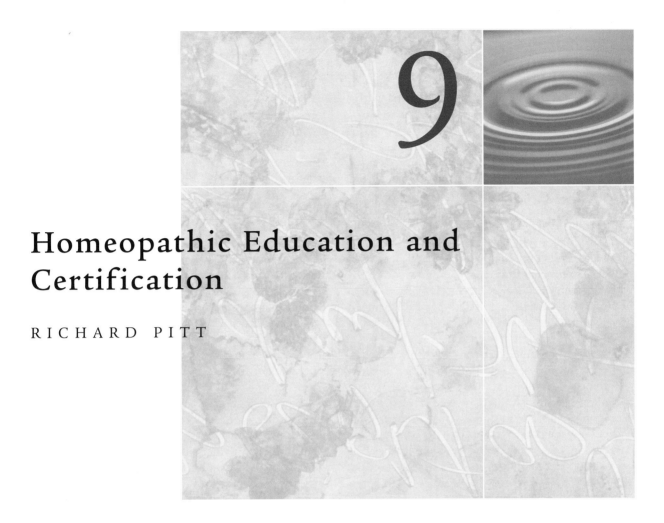

Homeopathic Education and Certification

R I C H A R D   P I T T

INTRODUCTION

Homeopathic education and certification have evolved significantly over the last 200 years. Homeopathy originally developed as part of the medical practice of physicians. Homeopathic physicians were required to have the same medical knowledge as any other physician, but applied homeopathic remedies based on homeopathic principles as opposed to allopathic medicines given for specific disease conditions. In the United States, as homeopathy became popular in the second half of the nineteenth century, homeopathy was taught in homeopathic medical schools. In most parts of Europe where homeopathy was practiced, a similar standard of training was established. As a distinct form of medical practice, homeopathy had its own licensing boards that defined standards for the profession. However, because homeopathy was not fully recognized in all states, common standards of practice were never fully established and regulated.

Medical licensure was not integrated into law in the United States until the second half of the nineteenth century, and even then standards varied considerably. It was only in the twentieth century that medical curricula and licensure became more uniform throughout the country.

As homeopathy became more popular, it was practiced not only by physicians but by many people who did not hold a medical license. This practice began with Samuel Hahnemann's second wife, Melanie. She continued to work in Paris after Hahnemann's death, although the authorities attempted to curtail her practice.[1] That homeopathy is practiced outside of medical licensure has since become one of the most contentious aspects of homeopathic history.

This controversy has grown in the last 20 years because many more nonmedical or lay homeopaths have trained and become practitioners. In the United States, there are probably more professional homeopaths (the term given to nonlicensed homeopaths) than licensed practitioners. This has occurred for a number of reasons. First, the growth of homeopathy within the ranks of physicians has been very slow. Although homeopathy was developed by a physician and was understood to be the practice of medicine by its adherents, it has struggled to be widely accepted. The dominant form of medical practice, known to homeopaths as *allopathy,* has come to define the practice of medicine. Homeopathy, whose philosophy and rationale challenges some fundamental tenets of modern science, has been unable to grow within the present framework of medicine. However, because homeopathy has always been defined as medicine, it has not created a separate legal identity outside of medical practice.

Therefore a nonphysician interested in practicing homeopathy must decide whether to become a physician to do so. A growing number have decided not to become physicians and have instead trained in private homeopathic institutions; they then practice without a medical license. This trend is compounded because no medical school in the United States has offered substantial training in homeopathy since the 1930s.

This predicament reveals fundamental questions. What is medicine, and how can it be defined, both legally and philosophically? Where does homeopathy, with its very different philosophy and methodology, fit into the conventional practice of medicine? How can people who want to practice homeopathy get the homeopathic and medical training necessary to become competent, recognized, and professional?

HOMEOPATHY, MEDICINE, AND THE LAW

Except for three states—Nevada, Connecticut, and Arizona—there are no licensing standards for homeopathic practice in the United States today. These states have homeopathic licensing boards, but none has been active in defining homeopathic standards and assessing professional levels of competency. As of 1999, to become certified through the Arizona licensing board, a licensed physician needs to complete just

40 hours of classical homeopathy training and 300 hours of some other form of alternative medicine, or only 90 hours of classical homeopathy. There is no actual examination process and no evaluation of homeopathic training. Arizona has established a professional designation for Homeopathic Medical Assistant, who can work under the direct supervision of a physician if 180 hours of homeopathic training has been completed. The other two states have not defined any homeopathic standards. Apart from the assistant category established in Arizona, these boards are open only to physicians.

In the United States, standards regarding the education and certification of homeopaths are largely established by various professional organizations working independently of regulatory bodies. People who want to practice homeopathy must decide whether they will gain a license as a medical doctor or another medical professional, or work as a homeopath without a license. Working with a license does not necessarily ensure any higher standard of homeopathic competency than working without one. Any health care license holds the practitioner to certain professional standards, which vary depending on the profession being licensed, and is also an assurance of certain formal education, but it does not ensure any particular competency in homeopathy.

In the United States, homeopathy is considered the practice of medicine, partly because the legal statutes determining medical practice of each state are extremely broad and partly because the Food and Drug Administration defines homeopathic remedies as drugs. In the California Business and Professions Code, Sections 2050-2079 pertain to medical practice. Section 2052 says the following:

Any person who practices or attempts to practice, or who advertises or holds himself or herself as practicing any system or mode of treating the sick or afflicted in this state, or who diagnoses, treats, operates for, or prescribes for any ailment, blemish, deformity, disease, disfigurement, disorder, injury, or other physical or mental condition of any person, without having at the time of doing so a valid, unrevoked or unsuspended certificate as provided in this chapter, or without being authorized to perform such act pursuant to a certificate obtained in accordance with some other provisions of law, is guilty of a misdemeanor.

Section 2068 states that nutritional advice can be given without being a medical doctor. In contrast to the definition of homeopathic remedies, herbs, vitamins, and other "natural" substances are defined as food supplements. Although homeopathic medicines are available over the counter, defining them as drugs influences the legal definition of homeopathic practice. However, the basis for giving a homeopathic remedy is generally very different from that associated with conventional drugs. As often stated by homeopaths, homeopathy treats the person, not the disease. The basis for choosing a particular remedy depends on individual characteristics of the whole person and not just the common symptoms of a given disease. Also, homeopathic remedies do not go through the same safety testing as conventional drugs, because their use was established prior to the FDA Act that "grandfathered" homeopathic medicines, recognizing their general acceptance as safe. Reassuring many, most homeopathic remedies are "potentized" to the point where the "energy" of the substance remains, but probably none of the physical substance from which the remedy is derived.

Homeopathic remedies therefore do not have the same potentially dangerous toxic side effects as conventional drugs; however, as with any substance that can have a powerful therapeutic effect, they can stimulate a strong response that, if not handled properly, can be dangerous in exceptional circumstances.

Defining homeopathy as medicine establishes contradictions that are not easy to resolve. In the nineteenth century, homeopathy and its philosophy struggled with an allopathic methodology that was underpinned by a traditional Newtonian perspective, an approach fundamental to all the physical sciences. Homeopathic philosophy did not fit into this model because of its radical position in believing in the concept of *energy* or *vital force,* and therefore it could never truly belong.

So if homeopathy is not medicine, as it has since come to be understood and defined legally, what is it, and how should its practice be defined? This question has not yet been resolved, and homeopathy finds itself still divided between two identities, one historical and the other philosophic.

HOMEOPATHY IN THE UNITED KINGDOM AND EUROPE

It is interesting to compare the situation in the United States with that of England. In 1946, when the National Health Service (NHS) was created in the United Kingdom, homeopathy was included among the methods of medical care available. Physicians who train in homeopathy can practice homeopathy within the NHS. These physicians pass an assessment process and are registered with the Faculty of Homeopathy. They are still accountable as physicians, but are allowed to practice homeopathy.

However, no legal medical statutes in England define who can or cannot practice homeopathy. The laws defining the practice of medicine in the United Kingdom are for doctors only. The concept of licensure for all professions is not applied. People can practice whatever they want under common law unless specific laws exist to the contrary. They cannot call themselves *doctor*s or prescribe allopathic medicines without a medical license, but they can practice homeopathy. Therefore the largest growth of homeopathic practitioners in the United Kingdom in the last 20 years has been in the number of professional (nonmedical) homeopaths. Professional organizations have been established to support the profession and define standards. New homeopathic schools work together to define curricula and are now are being accepted within the university system in England.

Early this century, as homeopathy declined in popularity in England as elsewhere, it was salvaged by nonmedical homeopaths. Most homeopathic medical doctors did not want anything to do with nonmedical homeopaths, but the most famous homeopathic doctor of his era, John Clarke, taught many nonmedical homeopaths and actively encouraged them to practice. This led to his estrangement within the homeopathic medical field, yet his influence ensured homeopathy's survival in the United Kingdom. The different legal situation in England, which didn't restrict the practice of homeopathy, aided the development of the nonmedical homeopath. Therefore the practice of homeopathy in England has always been divided between physicians and professional (lay) homeopaths, much as it is in Holland, Norway, Sweden, Australia, and New Zealand.

In Europe, only France and Austria have a situation similar to the United States, where, strictly speaking, homeopathy can be practiced only by physicians. In Germany, homeopathy can be practiced by physicians or by a separate category of practitioner called a *Heilpraktikur,* which is similar to a naturopathic physician in the United States or Canada.

MEDICALLY TRAINED VS NONMEDICALLY TRAINED HOMEOPATHS

In the United States, the main difficulty with homeopathy being practiced under a medical license is that the doctor's homeopathic competency is never assessed; the system defines only the physician's legal right to practice medicine. This is not necessarily the same thing as practicing homeopathy.

Some homeopathic physicians believe (from both a legal and professional point of view) that a person should be a physician to practice homeopathy. They believe that people who are not trained as physicians cannot be as competent as those who are; that they will not have the knowledge to treat more complex pathologic conditions and therefore will not do homeopathy justice. They believe also that homeopathy is medicine in the finest sense and that one has to be a physician to do it. Furthermore, they point out, it is not legal to practice without a license.

Professional homeopaths respond to this by stating that practicing homeopathy effectively does not require as much knowledge of medicine as does allopathic medicine. Homeopathy's unique philosophy and practice can be effectively applied with a relatively superficial (from an allopathic point of view) amount of medical knowledge. Most people seeing professional homeopaths already consult with a regular physician and often come with diagnosis in hand. The job of the homeopath is to take these people further than allopathic medicines have been able to take them. Professional homeopaths contend that a deep knowledge of homeopathy enhances their understanding of disease processes; therefore the most important thing is to be thoroughly trained in homeopathic principles.

A common point of view among professional homeopaths is that some physicians trained in homeopathy may tend to look at the patient from an allopathic perspective and apply homeopathic remedies from that point of view; such a practice, they believe, compromises the holistic viewpoint of homeopathic philosophy. This point was in fact emphatically stated many times by Samuel Hahnemann, the founder of homeopathy,[2] and has since been a major point of contention within homeopathic practice. Hahnemann had strong views regarding the damage caused by allopathic treatment, and was critical of any homeopath practicing homeopathy from an allopathic perspective. This perhaps necessarily extreme stance that Hahnemann took continues to affect homeopathy today, both within the profession and homeopathy's relationship to allopathy in general.

Therefore the debate as to how much medical knowledge is necessary to practice homeopathy is influenced by historical debates within homeopathy itself, and also reveals the different approaches within the umbrella of homeopathic prescribing. One approach emphasizes the importance of understanding the whole person and prescribing a remedy matching that subtle complexity (see Chapter 7). In this approach the medical diagnosis is unimportant. This approach can be contrasted with one that is more "medicalized," with remedies selected chiefly on the basis of allopathic diagnosis and pathologic changes. Although by no means mutually exclusive, these differing approaches reflect the different clinical directions within homeopathy and obviously demand markedly different conventional medical training for the homeopath.

For homeopathic physicians, one of the main challenges has been increasing awareness of homeopathy within conventional medicine. Until recently, not many conventional physicians knew what homeopathy was, and the attitude toward alternative medicine, including homeopathy, was generally negative. This lack of recognition and hostile attitude created a unique challenge for committed homeopathic physicians who looked for greater recognition of homeopathy but faced prejudice and antagonism within the profession. With the recent surge of interest in alternative medicine, this is now beginning to change; however, homeopathy is still not widely understood within mainstream medicine.

Although treated with greater tolerance in other countries, physicians who practice homeopathy abroad are also somewhat marginalized. One country in which homeopathy is well established within medical practice is India. There are over 100 homeopathic medical schools there, and graduates achieve the same status of physician as allopathic doctors. India is known for a greater mutual acceptance among medical professionals, and each modality is seen as a different aspect of medical practice. However, the standards of homeopathic knowledge do vary widely in India. Other countries in which homeopathy is more accepted within medical practice are Mexico, Argentina, Brazil, France, and England.

Given the complexities of legal definitions of homeopathic practice, the history of homeopathy's fight against allopathic dominance, and the matter of homeopathy being practiced by nonphysicians, it is quite a task to achieve consensus as to the standards of professional competency needed to define homeopathic practice. It is also a challenge to establish professional training programs, especially in the United States, when there is no licensure for the profession. This obstacle has the direct effect of limiting people's ability to make a living from homeopathic practice. It is also difficult to interest many physicians, who have already endured many years of study, to study for a few years more to attain adequate homeopathic skills.

Therefore, until homeopathy can establish its own standards and find a way to bridge the philosophic and political divisions it has faced for 200 years, it is hard to see how it will establish itself as a major healing system of health care.

THE PRACTICE OF HOMEOPATHY: PRESENT REALITIES

In the United States, homeopathy is practiced by people of all backgrounds, some licensed, some not. Apart from medical and osteopathic doctors who practice homeopathy, the main licenses under which homeopathy is practiced are acupuncture, chiropractic, physician's assistant, nurse practitioner, and naturopathy. Practitioners in these fields may practice homeopathy exclusively or in the context of their licensed profession. The state boards of each profession have scopes of practice that define what practitioners can do within their licensure. Some boards, especially acupuncture and chiropractic, have stated that homeopathy does not fall within their scope of practice. This means that in some states practitioners risk their license by practicing homeopathy.

Apart from a case in North Carolina, no medical doctor has been challenged for practicing homeopathy. The North Carolina Medical Board ordered George Guess, MD to desist from using homeopathy and to practice only conventional medicine, arguing that homeopathy was not within the scope of medical practice. Instead, he moved to Virginia. In part because of this case, a law was then passed in North Carolina making it unlawful to censure a physician solely for

practicing unconventional therapy. Since then, North Carolina reinstated Dr. Guess' full license to practice homeopathy or conventional medicine as he chose.

Some physicians who practice homeopathy do so exclusively. They do not practice allopathic medicine but use their medical license to practice homeopathy. Other physicians see homeopathy as an adjunct to their regular practice and incorporate it into their practice to varying degrees. Opinions as to whether homeopathy is a profession in its own right or an adjunct to conventional practice vary from practitioner to practitioner.

Some physicians see homeopathy as a specialty within medicine, and believe homeopathic physicians should be seen as specialists. This position gives a greater credibility to the profession than the view that homeopathy is merely an adjunct modality subsumed within conventional medicine. However, other people argue that even this view obscures the fundamental differences of philosophy between homeopathy and allopathy.

Some homeopaths therefore believe that some kind of legitimacy needs to be created for homeopathy distinct from allopathy and medicine at large. Most people who follow this line of thinking are professional homeopaths and do not have any other medical license. Professional homeopaths do not see homeopathy as a specialty of medicine, because they cannot practice medicine and do not have any legal recognition for what they do within the medical licensing system.

Whatever freedom professional homeopaths have to practice depends on the state and to some extent the town and county in which they practice. Because they practice in the gray area of the law, their situation is somewhat unpredictable; no legal precedent has been established regarding professional homeopathic practice. In California, the State of California threatened to take a professional, nonlicensed homeopath to court for practicing medicine without a license, but the practitioner did not pursue the case and ceased practicing. The only other legal incident involving a professional homeopath was in Connecticut, which, ironically, has a homeopathic medical board. A professional homeopath was reported to the Connecticut Department of Health, which instructed the Connecticut Homeopathic Medical Examining Board to come to a legal determination of whether the practitioner was practicing medicine without a license. The Department of Health had previously taken a very aggressive position against the practice of midwifery but eventually lost the case in the courts. Eventually, the case against the homeopath was dropped because the Department of Health could not prove that she was practicing medicine without a license. The lawyer representing the homeopath made the case that the Connecticut Homeopathic Medical Examining Board had no jurisdiction over the homeopath in question, because she was not licensed through the board.

Although all nonlicensed professional homeopaths face this risk in practicing homeopathy, most feel safe enough to practice. They cannot accept insurance, and many make it clear that they are not practicing medicine and do not diagnose disease. Some practitioners require that their patients have a regular physician and undergo relevant diagnostic procedures before coming for homeopathy. The challenge many homeopaths face is to make a living by practicing a discipline that is relatively unknown and not eligible for insurance benefits.

The interest of professional homeopaths lies in defining homeopathy under either a separate homeopathic medical license or certification, mandated by the state, or by establishing self-regulation for the profession without state licensure. The latter option appeals to some homeopaths who feel that conventional medicine claims an unwarranted monopolistic power to define what is good in healing practices. This population of homeopaths would also support the idea that licensure of any kind does not necessarily benefit the profession—that if homeopathy were to have its own medical license, the profession would be accountable to the dictates of the state, which could enforce standards that compromise homeopathic philosophy. State regulation could also impose limits of practice that are antagonistic to ideas of freedom of practice.

However, every profession needs to have standards. Without clearly defined and applied standards of practice, homeopathy cannot seriously be called a profession. But given the diversity of homeopathic practitioners in the United States and the historical and political realities, defining a single profession with one level of professional competency has not been achieved.

This situation is further complicated by the fact that many practitioners may practice what they *call* homeopathy, but what they practice is fundamentally different from the principles of classical homeopathy laid down by Samuel Hahnemann. Using low potencies only, combination remedies, or remedies given for "drainage" or for specific diseases, they classify their practice as homeopathy, although many homeopathic professionals would not. Calling the practice *homeopathy* just because homeopathically potentized remedies are used is not acceptable for many classical homeopaths and threatens to further confuse the problem of defining homeopathic practice.

HOMEOPATHIC CERTIFICATION ORGANIZATIONS

Five organizations are recognized as playing a role in defining and measuring standards of homeopathic competency in North America. Each has different levels of requirements for certification. The following is a description of each organization and its requirements.

The oldest organization of the five is the American Board of Homeotherapeutics (ABHT). This organization was formed in 1959 and certifies medical and osteopathic doctors only. There are presently 70 diplomates (D.Ht.) of this board. Historically, it was members of this organization that helped keep homeopathy alive earlier this century.

Another certifying body is the Homeopathic Association of Naturopathic Physicians (HANP). HANP represents naturopathic physicians who practice homeopathy. Naturopathy is licensed in 11 states, and homeopathy is included to varying degrees in the curriculum of naturopathic medical schools. Some naturopaths practice little or no homeopathy, whereas others practice it exclusively. In 1989, the HANP began to certify naturopaths practicing homeopathy and now has 66 certified homeopaths (DHANP).

The North American Society of Homeopaths (NASH) is a certification and professional organization established to define professional standards and represent professional homeopaths who do not practice under any other licensure. Professional homeopaths, who used to be called *lay* homeopaths, have been active in gaining legitimacy for their own standards of competency, irrespective of the legal ambiguity in which they practice. This organization was modeled after a British organization called the Society of Homeopaths. Although its membership is exclusively professional homeopaths without medical licenses, the Society of Homeopaths is the largest professional organization in the United Kingdom. In the United Kingdom, everyone is free to practice homeopathy and other nonmedical forms of healing. There are no licensing laws that limit its practice. Standards are regulated within the profession; as long as a professional homeopath does not pretend to be a medical doctor, there are no restrictions on the ability to practice.

Many professional homeopaths in the United States believe they should have the same right to practice as in the United Kingdom, and they do not think that defining homeopathy under medical statutes is an appropriate way to control the practice of homeopathy. It is a good example of how different political climates determine the legitimacy of homeopathy's practice, without regard to actual homeopathic standards.

Professional homeopaths have felt the need to define their own standards and to support their fellow practitioners in the United States and Canada. Because the NASH is modeled its English counterpart, it functions as both a certification and professional membership organization. The HANP also serves both functions. The other boards function exclusively as certification boards. As of July 2001, NASH had 148 certified members (RSHOM). In May 2000, NASH enacted a change in its policy by allowing both licensed and nonlicensed practitioners to join, thus offering membership to all practicing homeopaths.

The Council for Homeopathic Certification (CHC), established in 1991 to set up a standard of professional competency for all practicing homeopaths, is represented by homeopaths from all professions in which homeopathy is practiced. Recognizing the great variety of practitioners in North America, the CHC saw that establishing one standard that could be accepted by all homeopaths would be an important step in unifying the profession. It recognized that many people practicing homeopathy under licenses of other professions, such as acupuncturists, chiropractors, and nurse practitioners, have had no representation or avenue for professional evaluation. The CHC also represents a large number of professional nonlicensed homeopaths. As of December 2000, it had 218 certified homeopaths (CCH) as members.

The homeopaths certified by the CHC come from the following professions and backgrounds—doctors, naturopaths, physician assistants, nurse practitioners, chiropractors, acupuncturists, British-trained homeopaths from the Society of Homeopaths, Indian-trained physicians, professional nonlicensed homeopaths, and others. The board of the CHC includes representatives of all the professions that are certified through the CHC. This breadth was established to ensure equal representation within the homeopathic profession. In May 2000, NASH and the CHC agreed to use exactly the same certification process. This agreement allows applicants to undergo a single process to be certified through the CHC and registered and certified through NASH. Because NASH is a professional membership association and the CHC is solely a certifying agency, this arrangement clarifies and complements the function of each organization.

Another organization is the National Board of Homeopathic Examiners (NBHE). Like the CHC, this organization was originally formed to establish a national standard for the profession. Since then, NBHE has mainly represented chiropractors and its board has been dominated by chiropractors. Although this group formerly certified all homeopaths, it now certifies only homeopaths who practice under some form of health care licensure. Many of those certified have gone through educational programs connected to NBHE. This has raised some questions regarding conflict of interest. As of 2000, NBHE had approximately 160 certified homeopaths (DNBHE), 80 of whom practice in Florida.

One of the continuing difficulties involved in establishing closer relationships among the certifying organizations is the issue of medical standards. This issue has been a source of disagreement among the various communities in the United States and Europe. The problem is compounded by the legal definition of homeopathic practice in the United States. Also, because each organization has its own agenda to support its own community, it has been difficult to establish a closer working relationship.

One other issue among the various organizations is the level of homeopathic competency each seeks to measure. The process of defining a suitable professional standard for practice is open to much debate. How much knowledge should a person have to be deemed competent? How much experience and training should a homeopath have? How much medical knowledge? Given the diversity of homeopathic practice, these issues are not subject to easy agreement; thus the various organizations have different levels of educational requirements and standards of evaluation.

CERTIFICATION STANDARDS

The following is a list of certification requirements for the various certifying organizations.

1. Prerequisite hours of training: All the organizations require a certain number of hours of training in classical homeopathy. More specific information about this training appears later in this chapter.

   ABHT: 150 hours (from an approved school or course)

   HANP: 350 hours (from an HANP-approved school)

   NASH: 500 hours (from established training programs or a combination of training programs and seminars; up to 250 hours can come from approved correspondence training, with 1 hour of credit given for every 4 hours of training)

   CHC: 500 hours of training (subject to the same qualifications as for NASH)

   NBHE: 300 hours of training

2. Prerequisite level of practical experience and/or clinical training: Each organization requires a different level of experience. Because they are establishing levels of professional competency and there are few internship programs, actual practical experience is required. Individuals can be in practice prior to being certified because no legal license is being issued.

   ABHT: Homeopathic practice for 3 years

   HANP: Homeopathic practice for 1 year and 100 hours of preceptorship

   NASH: Homeopathic practice for 1 to 2 years or a combination of formal clinical supervision and clinical practice

   CHC: The same as NASH

   NBHE: None required

3. Medical training prerequisites:

   ABHT: Proof of medical license, open only to MDs and DOs

   HANP: Proof of naturopathic license, open to NDs only

   NASH: Proof of cardiopulmonary resuscitation certificate and college-level anatomy and physiology certificate; a pathology program is also required if the anatomy and physiology is completed through an approved correspondence program

   CHC: Same as NASH

   NBHE: Proof of health care license

4. Case submission requirements: This criterion is to provide evidence of clinical experience and competency.

   ABHT: 10 chronic cases are to be submitted, five with 1 year of follow-up analysis and five with 3 years of follow-up analysis

   HANP: 5 chronic cases with 1 year of follow-up analysis

   NASH: 5 chronic cases with 6 months of follow-up analysis (until 1999 NASH also required two video cases with 6 months of follow-up analysis)

   CHC: 5 chronic cases with 6 months of follow-up analysis

   NBHE: Must take a live case before examiners during the oral examination

5. Curriculum vitae requirements: Each organization requires certain information on its applicants:

   ABHT: References from two current members

   HANP: References from two current members

   NASH: Details of training and experience in homeopathy and other fields, details of current practice, and three professional references

   CHC: Details of training and experience in homeopathy and other fields, details of current practice, and three professional references

   NBHE: Details of training and experience in homeopathy and other fields, details of current practice, and 1 professional reference

6. Examination process:

   ABHT: A 3-hour examination, mostly multiple-choice questions on homeopathic philosophy, case management, repertory, and materia medica

   HANP: The same examination process as the ABHT

   NASH: Since 1997, same as the CHC examination

CHC: A 7-hour examination involving a multiple-choice section on homeopathic philosophy, materia medica and medical sciences, and an essay section on homeopathic case analysis. Applicants must pass each section in sequence before attempting the next

NBHE: A 6-hour examination, mainly multiple-choice questions

7. Oral examination process:

ABHT: A 2-hour review of submitted cases, a review of live cases, and other practice management issues

HANP: A review of submitted cases and practice management issues

NASH: Same as the CHC examination

CHC: A 1-hour phone interview to review practice management issues, professional practice concerns, and the applicant's general biographic information

NBHE: Required to take a live case in front of two examiners, analyze relevant issues, and recommend appropriate remedy

8. Continuing education requirements:

ABHT: Every 3 years, those certified must satisfy all of the following: complete 30 continuing medical education credits (e.g., seminars), submit one article to the *Journal of the American Institute of Homeopathy,* perform a preceptorship for at least one student, and give a lecture or presentation

HANP: Every year, 12 hours of training from seminars, or 12 hours teaching or supervising students, submitting articles, or writing examination questions

NASH: Every year, 14 hours of training need to be completed, or 14 hours teaching, submitting articles to journals, doing a homeopathic proving or other research, or writing examination questions

CHC: The same requirements as NASH

NBHE: Every year, 12 hours of training are required from an approved program, and also one of the following: submitting an article, writing 20 questions, teaching in an approved school, or submitting a case study

HOMEOPATHIC EDUCATION

Because homeopathy does not have a distinct license in the United States, from legal and economic points of view it cannot be defined as a separate profession. Therefore the structural resources and economic incentives to establish full-time professional training programs leading to a career and sustaining wage do not exist.

A person who wants to study homeopathy in the United States has certain choices. First, he or she must decide whether to be licensed in a particular profession. Because there is no license in homeopathy, a license as some sort of health professional can be an umbrella for practicing homeopathy. The choice of licensure depends on many factors. People commonly choose one of the following: medical or osteopathic doctor, physician's assistant, nurse practitioner, acupuncturist, or chiropractor. There are advantages and disadvantages to each choice. However, once a person has obtained a license, he or she must still learn homeopathy, which is equally or more difficult to study and practice.

An already licensed person who wants to study homeopathy has a variety of choices. The most common form of professional homeopathic study are 3- to 4-year part-time programs that allow students to continue to work in existing jobs. Most students coming to these programs have jobs and families and need the flexibility to study at home. These programs normally meet once a month on a weekend, or for 3 days, with the rest of study being done at home. The homework requirements for successful completion of these programs are considerable. Graduates may or may not be granted a specific certification on completion. Most of these programs give only a certificate of completion and recommend that graduates gain certification through one of the five certifying organizations.

This model of training is based on schools established over the last 20 years in England and the rest of Europe. However, in Europe, because homeopathy and homeopathic education have become more established, there are now full-time programs. Grants are now available in England, because some programs are linked to the university system.

If homeopathy was a legally licensed or certified profession in the United States, homeopathic schools would develop full-time programs, obtain funding and student loans, and be able to attract larger numbers of students. Many homeopaths dream of the idea of homeopathic medical schools, but this possibility is stifled by the political and legal situation. However, even in regard to this vision, there are arguments over how much medical knowledge would be taught in proportion to the amount of homeopathic knowledge. One of the observations that homeopaths have made of other professions, such as naturopathy, acupuncture, and especially osteopathy, is that in their attempt to become more acceptable to the mainstream medical model they have emphasized conventional medical knowledge at the expense of their own therapeutic model. This makes some homeopaths wary of making homeopathy more "medical."

This last point is fundamental in understanding homeopathy's relationship with allopathic medicine. Hahnemann railed against the homeopaths he saw as compromising homeopathic principles and copying allopathic methods. This polarization, perhaps necessary in Hahnemann's day to establish the distinct identity of homeopathic methodology, created an antagonistic and competitive relationship between homeopathy and allopathy. It also created antagonism among homeopaths.

The weakest part of most homeopathic education, both in the United States and abroad, is in clinical training and evaluation. Graduates leave a program with varying degrees of homeopathic knowledge but have not had the opportunity to practice under supervision and gain the evaluation necessary to define professional competency. This means that graduates entering practice must learn as they go. This limitation is being rectified as more schools are implementing clinical work into their programs. However, it is fair to say that most schools do not have the resources to give students the kind of individual mentorship necessary for entering professional practice.

Homeopathic Training Programs

There are approximately 10 professional part-time programs in the United States and another 5 in Canada. Some of these programs accept only licensed practitioners. Most, however, accept people with or without a medical license. Criteria for joining the program are usually 2 years of college, age of 21 years or older, and a willingness and ability to study. Some schools include human sciences training if not already completed, but most ask students to get anatomy and physiology from local colleges and may offer a correspondence pathology program.

Homeopathic Training in Naturopathy Schools

Naturopathic programs are the only licensed programs in which homeopathy is included substantially in the curriculum. Three accredited schools in the United States—in Washington, Oregon, and Arizona—train naturopaths. A naturopathic school in Connecticut is seeking accreditation, and a Canadian naturopathic school is also seeking accreditation in the United States.

Homeopathy is included in the curriculum of all these schools, but to varying degrees. Homeopathy is only one modality of many in which a licensed naturopath can practice. Most of the schools offer homeopathy as an elective for those who want to study it more deeply. However, it is debatable whether any of these programs alone are enough to give the level of homeopathic training, including clinical work, necessary for professional competency. Most naturopaths who want to study homeopathy also do extra seminars to complete their training. The naturopathic school in Seattle offers up to 200 hours of lectures, 50 to 100 hours of supervised case analysis, and up to 180 hours of homeopathic clinics. The naturopathic school in Oregon offers 144 hours of homeopathy with an elective of another 144 hours. Students can then do up to 200 hours of homeopathic clinics.

Although practiced throughout the United States, naturopathic medicine is licensed in only 11 of them—Alaska, Arizona, Connecticut, Hawaii, Maine, Montana, New Hampshire, Oregon, Utah, Vermont, and Washington. It is also licensed in Puerto Rico and registered in the District of Columbia. There are lobbying and popular movements pushing for naturopathic licensure in California, Colorado, and Minnesota.

Naturopathy's struggle is similar to homeopathy's; many people who practice naturopathic methods are not licensed and do not believe they have to be licensed naturopathic physicians to do their work. This controversy has affected the drive toward licensure in various states. The concern has been whether naturopathic licensure would create an exclusivity of practice for naturopaths. Recently a naturopathic bill was introduced in North Carolina that distinctly creates an exclusive right to practice all modalities listed within the naturopathic bill, which includes homeopathy. The bill has not currently become law. In California, another naturopathic bill has been written that states that no monopoly would be created of any modality mentioned in the bill. The movement toward the licensure of naturopathy throughout the United States has faced determined opposition from other naturopaths who oppose this whole process and, as they see it, the monopolization of naturopathic techniques to one school of thinking.

Some naturopaths who learn naturopathy apart from a licensing program do so through correspondence training programs. One of the criticisms from licensed naturopaths is that these programs are ineffective and superficial. There are obvious limits to most types of correspondence programs, an issue faced by homeopathy as well.

Correspondence Training and Apprenticeship

Quite a few people in the United States and Canada train through homeopathic correspondence programs, often because there are no on-site homeopathic programs available in many parts of the country. As with many on-site programs, the quality of correspondence programs varies considerably. The major criticism of these programs is that correspondence learning is not sufficient. An evaluation of skills gained through an ongoing, personal relationship with teachers is a more rigorous approach to homeopathic education. The lack of a major clinical component is also a significant problem, as it is with all schools.

Traditionally, one way in which homeopaths learned was through apprenticeship. Spending time with experienced homeopaths and observing their practice has always been an important experience for developing homeopaths. This tradition goes all the way back to Samuel Hahnemann, the founder of homeopathy. However, today this is rarely a major form of learning for aspiring homeopaths.

Homeopathic Training in Medical Schools

Various forms of alternative medicine are now being included into conventional medical training. A 1995

study by Michael Carlston, MD, the first national survey of alternative medical education in the United States, revealed the extent of this inclusion. At the time of the study, one third of medical schools were teaching something about alternative medicine. An additional 5% of medical schools planned to begin instruction, and another 7% were considering alternative medicine instruction. Nearly 10% of American medical schools were offering some instruction about homeopathy. One third of the schools planning to expand their alternative medicine instruction intended to include homeopathy as a part of that expansion.[3]

Other surveys have since demonstrated more than a doubling in the number of U.S. medical schools offering instruction in complementary and alternative medicine, confirming the expansionist trends evidenced in Carlston's survey.[4,5] The evidence suggests that the homeopathic presence in conventional medical schools has expanded even more rapidly than CAM overall. A 1997-1998 AMA survey found that 71 medical schools (56.8%) taught medical students about homeopathy. Sixteen of those (12.8% of all U.S. medical schools) included instruction about homeopathy within required coursework.[6]

Homeopathic Seminars and Lectures

The final way of studying homeopathy in North America is through various seminars or accumulating hours through a combination of programs. Although many such programs are designed to be postgraduate or continuing education seminars, students can learn their homeopathy this way in combination with self-study. In the past, when even fewer training programs were available, many homeopaths had very little in the way of educational choice. Even some of the most respected homeopaths of this generation had to learn homeopathy in this piecemeal approach. Seminars are offered in many different ways. Weekend seminars with particular teachers, 1-year postgraduate programs in the form of 3 to 5 weekends of instruction, summer school programs through the National Center of Homeopathy, and intensive 1-week workshops are available. All contribute toward the education of the homeopath, yet none can be described as a school that should or could take responsibility for the evaluation and development of a student's learning.

The Future of Education

Although homeopathic education has come a long way in the last few years, it is in need of further development. Full-time schools cannot be created at the moment because homeopathy does not have the kind of legitimacy and popularity to create demand for such programs. For students to commit time and money to the study of homeopathy, they need some form of assurance that a living can be made once they are qualified. Unfortunately this is not the case at the moment.

There are four main options for further establishing homeopathic education:

1. Include homeopathy as a fundamental part of medical curriculum for doctors and nurses. Homeopathy would therefore grow within the medical practice of physicians, nurses, and others.
2. Create a medical license for homeopathy and have separate homeopathic medical schools similar to those established by naturopathy.
3. Create an alternative form of legitimacy, such as certification or registration, under the laws of each state, and create schools to teach to the appropriate level.
4. Establish a political climate in which homeopathy, among other alternatives, can be practiced freely without restriction and state regulation.

Arguments for and against each of these options exist.

The major risk of the first option is that homeopathy would be subsumed within an allopathic model of thinking and its philosophic integrity compromised, similar to the process that has afflicted other professions that took this path. On a positive side, the integration of homeopathy within conventional medical practice would allow homeopathy to gain acceptance among medical professionals and with the general public.

The biggest obstacles to the second option are political and financial. Creating a separate licensure is extremely expensive and complex. Homeopathy needs significantly more practitioners and a greater degree of unity than is presently the case.

The third and fourth options bring up challenges similar to the second, but on a lesser scale. Some people fear that an alternative form of certification would diminish homeopathy to the level of a profession such as massage, and that homeopathy would thereby give up its struggle as a viable medical alternative to allopathic medicine. This option could separate the medical and nonmedical parts of the homeopathic community. For most practitioners without a medical license, one of these options would provide an appropriate form of legitimacy, because it defines homeopathy as separate from existing medical licensure. It would not preclude medical doctors from practicing homeopathy and working within the scope of medical practice, but it would establish a parallel legitimacy, with a practitioner's scope of practice being defined according to the level of homeopathic and medical training he or she has received.

THE DEBATE ON LICENSURE FOR HOMEOPATHY

Given the political reality of medical licensure in the United States and the definition of homeopathy as the practice of medicine, homeopathic education will not change dramatically until homeopathy can be established legally through legislation. However, that is not likely in the near future in most states. Homeopathy does not have the resources, the professional unity, or the popularity within mainstream society to achieve this.

However, each state has its own political dynamic, and various options are available. In April 2000, a law called the Complementary and Alternative Health Care Freedom of Access Bill was passed in Minnesota. Its focus is to address the legal barriers that limit consumer access to complementary and alternative forms of health care. The bill affects licensed physicians who wish to offer alternative therapies, and also unlicensed practitioners in fields that do not have licensure (e.g., naturopathy, homeopathy, massage, and body work). The bill does not enforce standards of practice upon these professions but establishes the right of people to choose these therapies and to practice them as long as no harm is done. A practitioner has to submit certain documentation to a client as to the nature of his or her practice and get written informed consent, but that is basically all that is required. This bill is radical because it circumvents existing medical licensure. It is focused on the freedom of access; its only concern being that people can choose whomever they want to see as long as no harm is done.

This bill may bring into question the traditional route that various professions have taken to establish legitimacy.[7] Acupuncture and chiropractic became legal through licensure. Licensure establishes the right to practice a therapy by establishing state and federal sanction of standards of practice and professionalism. Practitioners with a particular license have to practice within certain established guidelines, and are accountable to the profession and, to some extent, to the state sanctioning bodies that monitor the profession. However, licensure establishes the exclusive right to practice that therapy. No one else can practice it. The exclusivity of licensure is criticized in many circles. In the nineteenth century, state licensing laws for medicine were often revoked because of the monopoly it created.[8] Nearly five centuries ago, Henry VIII's pronouncement establishing the right of all of his citizens to responsibly attempt to provide health care to each other was instigated by the perception that the orthodox physicians were taking financial advantage of patients through their monopolistic power. A common criticism of licensure is that rather than protect the public against unscrupulous and unqualified practitioners, it actually serves to protect the economic and political power of the profession licensed. This accusation has been leveled at the medical profession, among others.

This exclusive right and power leads many in alternative medical professions to fear that their profession will become subsumed under general medical practice, with the right to practice alternative therapies limited to medical doctors. The exclusivity clause has also been criticized from a constitutional point of view, especially from a more libertarian standpoint.[9]

Also, instead of protecting the public from unsafe practice, it can be argued that professional licensure instead subverts real accountability for damage done to patients. A professional monopoly allows one group to protect its own and persecute outsiders. Licensure can allow the medical profession to dictate what is good and not good for our health, establishing dependency on the medical profession and the economic and political systems that support it. This culture of dependency was stated in a seminal work by Ivan Illitch,[10] in which he stated that iatrogenic (drug- or medicine-induced) disease has three strands—physical, social, and cultural. His main point is that the political consequences of institutional power and authority create a dependency on the authority of the expert, a process that has serious personal and collective ramifications.

HOMEOPATHY AND MEDICINE: THE DEVELOPMENT OF THE HOMEOPATH

Putting the philosophic and political arguments about licensure aside, the question still arises as to whether a homeopath should be governed by the same restrictions and responsibilities as a medical doctor. Does what we do as homeopaths involve the same kind of risk as what most physicians do? Many homeopaths would answer *no*. Although a person coming to see a homeopath may have a serious problem that many need immediate medical intervention, is that the reality of everyday practice for most homeopaths?

In one study,[11] 79.8% of homeopathic patients had previously seen a conventional doctor for their problems, 91% had received nonhomeopathic treatment, 91% saw another health provider first, and 80% were using some form of self-help. Most people seeing a homeopath have seen other medical providers first and are coming to the homeopath for an additional form of treatment. This means that the homeopathic role is not primarily diagnostic and disease centered, but is "complementary" to the role of the physician. Therefore, given the levels of skills required, it can be said that the homeopath needs to know enough medicine to understand normal and pathologic processes within the body, but does not need the same knowledge as a physician unless he or she functions in a primary care medical capacity.

Also, because homeopaths do not give drugs with a specific toxic effect, but rather a homeopathic remedy that stimulates the body's own healing capacity, it can be argued that the risks involved in homeopathic practice are generally less than for a physician. This is not to say that homeopathic remedies are harmless and involve no risk (because any therapy that can do good has the potential to do harm), but that the risks are of less consequence.

Therefore most professional homeopaths would like to see homeopathy legitimized, either by using a freedom of access model such as in Minnesota or by being certified in each state. These solutions allow the profession to maintain primary responsibility for its standards of practice and do not create an exclusive right to practice. This system would mirror how homeopathy is practiced in England. The homeopathic profession therefore needs to develop its own standards and establish organizations that can support the necessary professional structures.

In Europe this is being done through two organizations—The European Council for Classical Homeopathy and the International Council for Classical Homeopathy. These councils have prepared a document that outlines the amount of homeopathic and medical knowledge necessary for homeopathic practice; this document can serve as a template for homeopathic schools and professional and certifying bodies. In the United Kingdom, there are now professional nonmedical homeopaths working within the National Health System. In Europe, each country has its own standards and professional organizations. Some have a more formal relationship with government than others. However, with the greater centralization created by the European Union, it is likely that homeopathic levels of education and practice will become more standardized in the next few years. In the United States and Canada, there have been recent attempts to follow the European model and create a broad document that can help define standards of practice and education for the whole profession. These attempts have been initiated by the Council for Homeopathic Education (an organization created to accredit homeopathic educational programs) and supported by the CHC, NASH, and ABHT, among others. Homeopathy in the United States and Canada is generally some years behind Europe, but in the last few years the explosion of interest in homeopathy and other alternative systems of healing is propelling the profession to define its standards of practice more clearly.[12,13]

FUTURE CONFLICTS AND CHALLENGES

The greatest challenge to homeopathy today is to produce skilled practitioners. Dedicated study for many years is required to consistently provide good homeopathic care. History has shown that physicians do not necessarily become better homeopaths than nonmedical homeopaths. It is important to maintain standards of homeopathic practice and create schools that can offer a high level of training.

A threat to homeopathy is the dilution of standards of practice to make homeopathy more acceptable to the general culture and mainstream medicine. This struggle is similar to the struggle of 100 years

ago. Some homeopathic principles are not easy to reconcile with prevailing views of health and disease. The holistic view of homeopathy, with its emphasis on treating the whole person and its critique of the suppressive effects of many modern medical drugs, still does not fit into conventional thinking. Some believe that homeopathy will not thrive until a philosophic shift occurs in medical and scientific thinking, a shift that is consistent with homeopathic and holistic thinking.

Another challenge, from the more conservative medical circles, is the "debunking" of homeopathy. As more people seek treatment from various practitioners of alternative medicine, the economic consequences of this trend will draw more attention to alternative practices. This will include homeopathy, which already has had a tumultuous relationship with allopathic medicine.[7] In the last few years, various legal actions have been filed against individual homeopaths and homeopathic pharmacies, and research that purports to show the ineffectiveness or danger of homeopathy has been published. One recent study, published in the *Archives of Pediatrics and Adolescent Medicine*,[14] asked questions of 38 homeopaths, including a question regarding a hypothetical medical scenario of high fever in a newborn child and another regarding advice given about vaccination.

The study was designed to assess the medical knowledge of licensed and nonlicensed homeopaths and also their opinions on the subject of vaccination, a controversial subject within many fields of alternative medicine. The study revealed that a high number of nonlicensed homeopaths did not make the right decision regarding the treatment of fever and also gave "negative" opinions regarding the issue of childhood vaccination. Although there may be some use to the first question, the second reveals the underlying agenda of the study, which is to expose the "questionable" practices of professional homeopaths and basically cast homeopathy in an unfavorable light. This is only one of many studies in which the agenda of the researchers was not impartial, but rather to undermine homeopathy.

Other studies that seemed to validate homeopathic methodology have been severely criticized by mainstream medical thinkers,[15] even when they conform to conventional double-blind methodology. Such critics often reveal their own prejudices, thinly disguised as objective science. Many homeopaths believe that homeopathy will be truly accepted only when advances in pure science are able to prove the validity of the concept of *energy* or *vital force* and the effect of homeopathic potencies. Others believe that homeopathy will always remain a marginalized system of practice because it demands too much of the practitioner and client.

The practice of homeopathy illustrates a broader struggle in defining who has the right and the skill to heal. Good health is not a right determined by law or medical knowledge, but by a combination of many factors, perhaps the most important of which is encouraging people to take a greater responsibility for their own health and well-being.

Fundamental to homeopathic philosophy is the principle of self-cure. Also fundamental is the idea that health is not merely an absence of symptoms but a dynamic state of physical and mental equilibrium in which an individual is able to establish and maintain health without dependence on drugs, doctors, or therapy. Health is a process toward freedom, not greater dependence, and homeopaths say this is what distinguishes homeopathic thinking from that of allopathic medicine and the limits of a materialistic "Newtonian" model.

SUMMARY

Given the challenge it faces, it is imperative that homeopathy define itself politically and legally to carve its appropriate identity in our society—an identity consistent with the principles and practice of this 200-year-old system of healing.

To do this, the profession must produce competent practitioners. We need schools that can offer a budding homeopath the level of education necessary for professional practice. The difficulty in creating the needed level of education is the lack of an appropriate legal definition for homeopathy. The profession must establish the unity necessary to define itself and work toward legitimacy as it creates competent practitioners. This will require that certification and professional organizations work more closely together on standards of practice and education so the profession can be strong enough to define itself. It will require the various organizations to do the legal work, state by state, to determine appropriate forms of legitimacy. It will also require the medical and nonmedical parts of the homeopathic community to come together and create a united front to give the necessary strength to the profession. This will help not only unite the homeopathic profession, but also redefine medicine and healing and establish the role of homeopathy in the future.

References

1. Handley R: *A homeopathic love story: the story of Samuel and Melanie Hahnemann,* Berkeley, Calif., 1990, North Atlantic Books.
2. Hahnemann S: *Organon of the medical art,* O'Reilley WB, editor, Decker SR, translator, Palo Alto, Calif., 2000, Birdcage Books.
3. Carlston M, Stuart MR, Jones W: Alternative medicine education in US medical schools and family practice residency programs, *Fam Med* 29:559-562, 1997.
4. Association of American Medical Colleges: *Curriculum directory 1997-1998,* Washington, DC, 1997, Association of American Medical Colleges.
5. Wetzel M, Eisenberg DM, Kaptchuk TJ: Courses involving complementary and alternative medicine at US medical school, *JAMA* 280:784-787, 1998.
6. Barzansky B, Jonas HS, Etzel SI: Educational programs in US medical schools, 1997-1998. *JAMA* 280(9):803-808, 827-835, 1998.
7. Shoon CG, Smith IL, editors: *The licensure and certification mission—legal, social and political foundations,* New York, 2000, Professional Examination Service (published by Forbes Custom Publishing).
8. Coulter H: *Divided legacy: the conflict between homeopathy and the American Medical Association,* vol 3, Berkeley, Calif., 1982, North Atlantic Books.
9. Young D: *The rule of experts—occupational licensing in America,* Washington, DC, 1987, Cato Institute.
10. Illitch I: *Medical nemesis, the expropriation of health,* New York, 1975, Pantheon.
11. Goldstein M, Glik D: Use of and satisfaction with homeopathy in a patient population, *Altern Ther Health Med* 4:60-65, 1998.
12. Eisenberg D, Kessler RC, Foster C et al: Unconventional medicine in the United States, *N Engl J Med* 328:246-252, 1993.
13. Eisenberg DM, Davis RB, Ettner SL et al: Trends in alternative medicine use in the United States, 1990-1997: results of a follow-up national survey, *JAMA* 280:1569-1575, 1998.
14. Lee AC, Kemper KJ: Homeopathy and naturopathy: practice characteristics and pediatric care, *Arch Pediatr Adolesc Med* 154(1):75-80, 2000.
15. Davenas E, Beauvais J, Arnara M et al: Human basophil degranulation triggered by very dilute antiserum against IgE, *Nature* 333(6176):816-818, 1988.

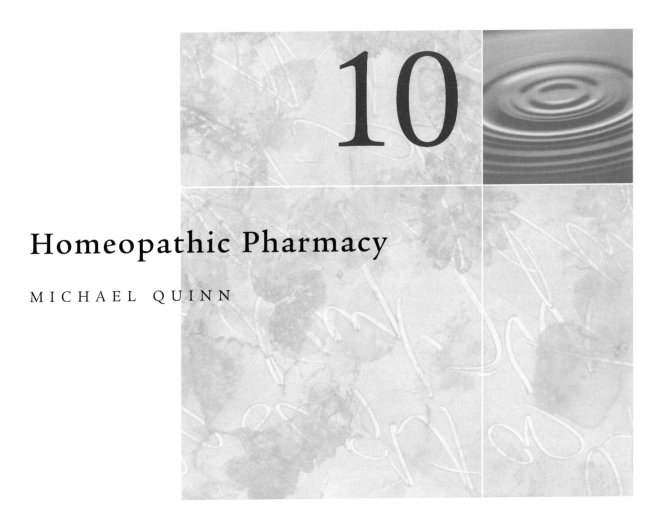

10

Homeopathic Pharmacy

MICHAEL QUINN

If every substance is capable of causing symptoms when the dose is high enough, and if a poison is a substance that causes symptoms, then every substance is a poison. Therefore every drug is a poison. Therefore the practice of medicine, or medicinal therapy, is primarily the selection of the correct poison for each patient, and secondarily a question of dosage. ∾

INTRODUCTION

Homeopathic pharmacy, like homeopathy itself, was the creation of Dr. Samuel Hahnemann. Hahnemann's first empiric discovery was the Law of

Similars, which he first described in 1795.[1] This law states that to cure a patient of a particular set of symptoms, the correct prescription is a medicine that will cause the exact same set of symptoms in a healthy person. In the beginning, homeopathic pharmacy was indistinguishable from traditional pharmacy. Hahnemann practiced homeopathy for several years using conventional doses of medicines before he developed the unique methods used in homeopathic pharmacy.[2] Because Hahnemann was administering medications that were capable of causing the very symptoms his patients suffered, it was necessary to deviate from the contemporary practice of giving large doses. Hahnemann's next line of research was to discover how small a dose he could give while maintaining clinical activity. In contrast, in allopathic medicine, the question of dosage is more often how large a dose can be given without reaching the point where the drug causes more problems than the disease. Hahnemann succeeded in developing a system that allowed him to dilute the drug to such a low level that it had no toxicity and yet retained its ability to relieve symptoms.

By 1799, Hahnemann had developed his unique method of making homeopathic medicines,[2] methods that have been both a blessing and a curse upon homeopathy to this day. The methods of homeopathic pharmacy are a blessing because they allow us to prepare medicines of great efficacy and low toxicity; they are a curse because the practice of drastically diluting medicines appears so irrational that most observers have concluded a priori that the methods of homeopathic pharmacy result only in placebo doses. Homeopathic medicines appear to be placebo doses because of the great dilutions employed in their preparation. However, the experience of homeopathic physicians around the world for 200 years suggests that they are not placebos.

Great caution should be exercised before declaring any superficially unexplainable or implausible phenomenon a fraud or placebo. Declaring that something doesn't work because it is not understood is naïve and unscientific. Homeopathic physicians and pharmacists, whose common experience is that homeopathic medicines do work, spend little time wondering what the mechanism of action of homeopathic remedies is. Like their busy clinical brethren in allopathic medicine, homeopathic physicians and pharmacists spend most of their time prescribing and dispensing the very best medicine for their patients.

More than 2000 substances from the mineral, vegetable, and animal kingdoms have been used as homeopathic medicines. The definition of what is or is not a homeopathic medicine relies more upon the way in which it is prescribed than the way in which it is prepared. In fact, a new medicine must first be demonstrated useful when homeopathically prescribed before it is accepted for inclusion in the Homeopathic Pharmacopoeia of the United States (HPUS),[3] the Food and Drug Administration's (FDA) recognized compendium for the production of homeopathic medicines in the United States. In other countries, such as Germany, the regulation of homeopathic medicines is oriented more to how they are prepared rather than how they are prescribed.

The fundamental processes employed in homeopathic pharmacy today are identical to those that

Hahnemann developed. Although they have evolved in the last 200 years, the goals of these processes are remarkably consistent with the goals of the procedures that Hahnemann described. In general, these procedures may be described as follows:

Step 1: Prepare a relatively concentrated solution of the chemical, animal, or plant extract.

Step 2: Dilute the concentrated solution in water or a water-ethanol mixture.

Step 3: Vigorously pound the vial holding the solution against a firm but resilient surface; this pounding is referred to as succussion.

Further steps are simply the alternating repetition of Steps 2 and 3.

To prepare a homeopathic medicine from table salt (sodium chloride), these steps are accomplished in the following manner:

Step 1: Prepare a 10% weight/volume solution of sodium chloride in water (i.e., dissolve 0.5 g of NaCl in water sufficient to yield 5 ml).

Step 2: Prepare a 1:10 dilution of the solution prepared in Step 1.

Step 3: Vigorously pound the solution prepared in Step 2 ten times against a firm but resilient surface, such as a book or hard rubber pad on a counter.

Now label the solution prepared in Step 3 *Natrum muriaticum* (Latin for "sodium chloride") 1C.

Homeopathic Terminology

Term	Definition
AAHP	American Association of Homeopathic Pharmacists
AHPA	American Homeopathic Pharmaceutical Association
Attenuation	Process of preparing homeopathic remedies
Continuous fluxion	Continuous-flowing-water method
Dilution	Decreasing concentration of raw material
Dynamization	Process of preparing homeopathic remedies

(Continued)

FDA	Food and Drug Administration
Fluxion	Flowing-water method of potentization
Hahnemannian	New-vial-each-step preparation method
HPUS	Homeopathic Pharmacopeia of the United States
Korsakovian	Single-vial preparation method
Maceration	Soaking of raw material in alcohol
Mother tincture	Source alcoholic liquid
OTC	Over-the-counter
Potentization	Process of preparing homeopathic remedies
Succussion	Forceful pounding of vial against resilient material such as book or rubber pad
Tincture	Alcoholic liquid
Centessimal	One to one hundred (1:100)
Decimal	One to ten (1:10)
Quinquageni-millesimal	One to fifty thousand (1:50,000)
LM	Quinquagenimillesimal dilution process
Q	Quinquagenimillesimal dilution process
X	Decimal dilution process
C	Centesimal dilution process
K	Korsakovian dilution process
CH	Centesimal Hahnemannian dilution process
CK	Centesimal Korsakovian dilution process
D	Decimal dilution process
M	1000C
1M	1000C
10M	10,000C
XM	10,000C
50M	50,000C
LM	50,000C (technically correct, but confusing usage)
CM	100,000C
MM	1,000,000C

The solution prepared in Step 3 is called *1C: C* because it represents a 1:100 dilution of the sodium chloride and is therefore a *centessimal*, or *C*, dilution, and *1* because it is the first vial so prepared. To prepare the 2C from the 1C, repeat Steps 2 and 3 with the following change. In Step 2, prepare a 1:100 dilution rather than a 1:10 dilution, because Step 1 is eliminated. Then succuss this vial ten times and label the vial *Natrum muriaticum* 2C.

All subsequent vials are prepared from the previous vial (i.e., the 3C is prepared from the 2C, the 4C is prepared from the 3C, and so on). Each preparation cycle consists of two steps, a 1:100 dilution followed by succussion of the new vial. The concentration of sodium chloride in the 2C vial is thus one part in 10,000, and the concentration of sodium chloride in the 3C vial one part in 1 million. This process is often referred to as *potentization*, or *attenuation*, of the raw material, and the resulting medicines are referred to as *potencies*, or *attenuations*. Thus the 3C vial could be referred to as the 3C potency of *Natrum muriaticum* or the 3C attenuation of sodium chloride.

The process described above is the core process of homeopathic pharmacy. This process should be used in every homeopathic pharmacy in the world and has been used as described for 200 years. Every other process used in homeopathic pharmacy either prepares materials for this core process or uses the solutions prepared by this core process. This process may be continued without end. Homeopathic physicians in the United States regularly use homeopathic medicines that have been carried to 10,000 cycles of dilution and succussion. Paradoxically, most homeopathic physicians agree that homeopathic medicines become clinically stronger with increasing cycles of dilution and succussion (i.e., a medicine so prepared gives greater relief in more severe illnesses than one prepared with only a few cycles of dilution and succussion).

Homeopathic physicians and pharmacists acknowledge that the chemical concentration of the original substance in such a preparation is so dilute as to be physiologically inactive after only a few cycles of dilution and succussion, and that the concentration will reach zero after 12 such cycles. After 12 cycles of 1:100 dilution, the theoretic concentration of the original substance is $(1 \times 10^{-2})^{12}$ (or 1×10^{-24}), a dilution sufficient to remove every molecule of the starting substance according to the limit suggested by Avogadro's Number (6.02×10^{23}), the number of atoms in 12 g of carbon. However, because it is the common, everyday experience of thousands of homeopathic physicians and pharmacists that homeopathic medicines do in fact work after more than twelve cycles of dilution and succussion, most of them believe that the activity of homeopathic medicines is attributable to some as yet unrecognized phenomenon that occurs in the solvent. Does water have the ability to store information? Well, do sand and rust have the ability to store information? Sand and rust do indeed store vast amounts of information as silicon chips and the iron oxide coating on computer hard disks. If information can be stored in sand and rust, it is premature to assume that information cannot be stored in water. Some physicists now believe that water can store information, specifically information contained in stable crystalline structures.[4,5]

The entire process of making a homeopathic medicine consists of the following steps:

1. Selection of a raw material
2. Trituration of raw material (if not soluble in water or alcohol) by grinding with mortar and pestle
3. Preparation of liquid potencies by dilution and succussion
4. Medication of blank pellets with liquid potencies
5. Drying of medicated pellets
6. Packaging of medicated pellets in vials for use

Homeopathic pharmacists obtain raw materials as described in the *HPUS*. Homeopathic manufacturing laboratories purchase the exact materials needed to make homeopathic medicines out of metals, salts, elements, and compounds of the *materia medica*. For example, very-high-purity gold leaf is used to prepare homeopathic gold, or *Aurum metallicum*, the Latin name for metallic gold. (Because Latin names of homeopathic remedies were used in Hahnemann's *Materia Medica Pura*[6] in 1811 and have been in continuous and unchanged use internationally for 191 years, they are generally used for most homeopathic medicines. As in the case of species names for plants and animals, the use of Latin names has proven advantageous.)

Botanical and animal sources are collected from clean healthy specimens free of infestation with parasites, and prepared according to the traditional methods described in the *HPUS*. Most plants are prepared for use as homeopathic medicines by first making a hydroalcoholic extract. The correct part of the plant is collected at the right time of the growing season, according to traditional homeopathic practice and as described in the *HPUS*. The plant material is cleaned of any dust, dirt, or insects; finely chopped; and thoroughly mixed. A small sample of the mixed plant material is weighed and dried in an oven to calculate its water content. Once the dry weight of the plant material is known, alcohol and/or water is added to the wet mixed plant material to produce a 10% dry plant weight/volume preparation (Table 10-1). This preparation is shaken daily and stored for 1 to 2 weeks before filtering and collecting the filtrate. This filtrate is referred to as the *mother tincture*. A tincture is a substance that contains ethanol, and this one is called the *mother tincture* because all of the other dilutions come from this original source.

All chemical substances readily soluble in water are prepared exactly as previously described for sodium chloride. For all substances readily soluble in water/ethanol mixtures, the process is exactly as described, but a water/ethanol mixture is substituted for water. For substances that are not soluble in water or water/ethanol mixtures, Hahnemann developed another process that converts insoluble substances into a form amenable to the core process. To make a homeopathic medicine out of an insoluble substance such as gold, the material is triturated. Trituration is a prolonged grinding of the material mixed with lactose, using a mortar and pestle. Gold is triturated by placing 1 g of highly pure gold leaf and 99 g of lactose into a clean mortar and grinding with the pestle for 1 hour. Because the gold has been "diluted" by a factor of 100, the material prepared by this trituration is labeled *Aurum metallicum* 1C. To prepare gold 2C, 1 g of the 1C is added to 99 g of lactose in a clean mortar and pestle and triturated for 1 hour. This material is collected and labeled *Aurum metallicum* 2C. One g of the gold 2C and 99 g of lactose are added to a clean

Homeopathic Pharmacy

Any substance can be made into a homeopathic remedy.

Question: Is the substance readily soluble in water or ethanol?

YES (e.g., salt, pulsatilla)	NO (e.g., gold, silica)
Prepare the mother tincture = 1X potency Prepare a 10% (w/v) solution (e.g., 10 g NaCl) in a total of 100 ml water, or use 200 g of a plant containing 50% water (and therefore 100 g water and 100 g plant substances) in the fresh state in 1000 ml water and ethanol 10 g NaCl/100 ml = 10% (w/v) 100 g dry plant/1000 ml = 10% (w/v) Plants should soak in the water/alcohol for 7-14 days and are then filtered to obtain the mother tincture	Triturate in mortar and pestle for 1 hour at each step

Start with	Mix into and grind into	New Potency
1 g raw material	99 g lactose→	1C
1 g of 1C	99 g lactose→	2C
1 g of 2C	99 g lactose→	3C

Add I g of the 3C to 100 ml water to make the 4C and continue as under C potencies

Steps Needed to Make X and C Potencies from the Mother Tincture

X potencies			C potencies			
Dilution Ratio	# of Suc-cussions	New Potency	Dilution Ratio	# of Suc-cussions	New Potency	Grams of ingredient/1g of finished product
1:10	10	2X =	1:10	10	1C	0.010000000000 10 mg
1:10	10	3X				0.001000000000 1 mg
1:10	10	4X =	1:100	10	2C	0.000100000000 100 µg
1:10	10	5X				0.000010000000 10 µg
1:10	10	6X =	1:100	10	3C	0.000001000000 1 µg
1:10	10	7X				0.000000100000 100 ng
1:10	10	8X =	1:100	10	4C	0.000000010000 10 ng
1:10	10	9X				0.000000001000 1 ng
1:10	10	10X =	1:100	10	5C	0.000000000100 100 pg
1:10	10	11X				0.000000000010 10 pg
1:10	10	12X =	1:100	10	6C	0.000000000001 1 pg

Preparation of LM Potencies (Quinquagenimillesimal or Q Potencies)

Start With	Add To	Of	Number of Succussions	Yields
0.062 g of 3C	500 drops	18% ethanol	0	Solution A
1 drop of Soln A	100 drops	95% ethanol	100	LM 1 liquid
LM 1 liquid	#10 pellets	(soak and then dry)	0	LM 1 pellets
1 LM 1 pellet	1 drop	water	0	Solution B
1 drop of Soln B	100 drops	95% ethanol	100	LM 2 liquid
LM 2 liquid	#10 pellets	(soak and then dry)	0	LM 2 pellets
1 LM 2 pellet	1 drop	water	0	Solution C
1 drop of Soln B	100 drops	95% ethanol	100	LM 3 liquid
LM 3 liquid	#10 pellets	(soak and then dry)	0	LM 3 pellets

mortar and pestle and triturated for 1 hour. This material is then collected and labeled *Aurum metallicum* 3C. At this point the "dry" dilutions of gold can be converted into liquid dilutions, which can then enter the core process of liquid dilution and succession. This conversion is made by adding 1 g of the *Aurum metallicum* 3C powder to a sufficient quantity of water/ethanol to total 100 ml. After the 3C powder dissolves, the solution is succussed ten times and labeled *Aurum metallicum* 4C. The 5C is prepared exactly as described in the core process.*

Trituration by hand is a laborious process that can be accomplished more efficiently and safely with various mechanical means. One such device is called a *ball mill*. A ball mill is similar in design to a rock polisher or rock tumbler. It consists of a cylindrical porcelain jar with a tight lid. The material to be triturated is placed into a jar along with 99 times as much lactose and the extremely hard "balls" that will grind the material (small cylinders are now used because they grind more effectively than balls). The closed jar is placed on two horizontal rollers. When the motor is turned on the rollers turn, forcing the cylindrical jar to rotate also. The porcelain or carborundum rollers roll over the material and lactose constantly for hours, reducing the material to a very fine powder. Ball mills are extensively used in science and industry to grind materials wherever exceptionally fine powders are needed. The use of a ball mill for trituration produces better results than hand trituration and is also much cleaner for the workplace and safer for the pharmacist or technician. Homeopathic materials are triturated for many hours to produce the final 3C triturate that is used to prepare liquid potencies.

Centessimal medicines are prepared as described above, diluting the raw material at a ratio of 1:100, followed by succussion at each step. One variation in the core process that is widely used is to substitute a 1:10 dilution ratio for the 1:100 ratio. Medicines prepared with a 1:10 dilution are succussed 10 times at each step, just as centessimal medicines are succussed. Medicines prepared with a 1:10 dilution ratio are labeled with a 1X, 2X, 3X, etc., or (as more commonly used in Europe) with a 1D, 2D, 3D, etc., and are known as *decimal medicines*.

Another variation, which is used to prepare LM, 50 millessimal, Q, or quinquagenimillesimal medicines, adds a 1:500 dilution step to the 1:100 dilution step of the centessimal process to achieve a dilution ratio of 1:50,000 at each step. The 1:50,000 dilutions are then succussed 100 times at each step rather than the 10 times used for centessimal and decimal medicines. LM medicines are used much less often than centessimal or decimal medicines, but their use has increased significantly in the last 15 years. These methods are summarized and compared in Table 10-1.

Centessimal and decimal medicines may be prepared in either Hahnemannian or Korsakovian methods. The Hahnemannian method uses one vial for each step, whereas the Korsakovian method uses only one vial no matter how many steps are carried out. To make a Hahnemannian 12C, twelve vials will be used. In the preparation of a Korsakovian 12C only one vial will be used. In the Korsakovian method, the dilution is carried out by emptying the vial of 99% of its contents, refilling it, succussing it, and so on. In general, the Hahnemannian method is used for the first 12 to 200 steps, and the Korsakovian method is used thereafter. The addition of the letter *H* or the letter *K* to the label indicates which method has been used to prepare that medicine.

The *HPUS* recognizes 16 classes, Class A to Class P, in the method of preparation of the raw material for entry into the core process of centessimal or decimal dilution and succussion.[3] Each medicine is monographed in the *HPUS* so that all the particular and pertinent details of its preparation are described. The official names of homeopathic medicines are defined in the *HPUS* as well.

The repetitive nature of the decimal and centessimal preparation processes allows them to be easily performed by machines designed for that purpose. In his elegantly illustrated article, Winston[7] describes the various types of automated systems used over the years. Because the mechanism of action of homeopathic remedies remains uncertain, it seems prudent to use mechanical processes that simulate as closely as possible the manual processes that have been used successfully for 200 years.

In the laboratory in which I work, the production equipment was designed by engineers who measured my arm from elbow to closed hand in order to build a mechanical arm of the same length. They measured

---

*To be true to Hahnemann's instructions for preparing triturations, the 99 g of lactose is added in three additions of 33 g, each followed by 20 minutes of mixing and grinding after each of the three additions. His method ensures a more uniform and complete mixing of the raw material into the lactose.

how far up and down I moved the vial while vigorously succussing it, and how fast I moved. These data were used to produce the drive system that pounds the mechanical arm against a firm rubber pad from a height of 5 inches, 20 times in 2 seconds. The force of the succussion is equivalent to dropping, by gravity alone, your closed fist against a table from a height of 15 inches. The blow is powerful enough that you would never put your finger between the vial and the rubber pad! To prevent cross-contamination, each production machine is in a separate room that is supplied by highly pure, HEPA-filtered air (i.e., air that has passed through high-efficiency particulate air filters).

Homeopathic medicines are prepared for use by patients as hydroalcoholic liquids or in dry forms. The dry forms are commonly either lactose powder or sucrose/lactose pellets that have been medicated with the hydroalcoholic liquid solution of the desired homeopathic remedy. For example, to prepare the pellet form of a homeopathic medicine in the 30C strength, the 30C alcoholic solution of at least 88% alcohol is added to a quantity of sugar pellets in a 1% volume/weight ratio. For example 10 ml of 30C solution added to 1000 g of sugar pellets medicates the pellets to the 30C strength. This is a sufficient quantity of alcoholic solution to moisten the entire quantity of pellets. The medicating solution needs to be at least 88% alcohol to prevent the dissolution of the sugar pellets. The mass of pellets is then shaken so that the medicating solution is evenly distributed. The solution is allowed to soak into the pellets for at least 5 minutes, and the pellets are then dried. However, a small quantity of the hydroalcoholic solution remains trapped inside the sugar pellets. The dried pellets are then packaged and labeled as the 30C strength.

FOOD AND DRUG ADMINISTRATION REGULATIONS

Homeopathic medicines have been used in the United States continuously since 1835.[8] The Food and Drug Administration of the United States was created by the Food, Drug, and Cosmetic Act of 1906. Homeopathic medicines were not specifically mentioned in the 1906 Act. The *HPUS* was added to the list of official compendia for the manufacture of drugs in the United States in the revisions to the Food, Drug, and Cosmetic Act enacted in 1938.[9] In the 1980s, the FDA met with representatives of the homeopathic pharmaceutical industry and with homeopathic physicians to establish an updated regulatory position regarding homeopathic medicines. In 1988, the FDA published a set of guidelines defining the conditions under which homeopathic medicines can be produced and sold in the United States.[10] This document reaffirms in the modern era the legality of the manufacture and sale of homeopathic medicines in the United States. It also reaffirms the primacy of the *HPUS* in determining what is a homeopathic medicine and defining the methods of preparation of homeopathic medicines in the United States.

The toxicity of homeopathic medicines is dependent on the specific toxicity of their source materials, the potency or level of dilution of the preparation, and the size of the dose administered. A quick comparison of the toxicity of common over-the-counter (OTC) medications with one of the most toxic homeopathic products listed in the *HPUS* demonstrates the inherent safety of homeopathic medicines. Arsenic is used as a homeopathic medicine to treat the various symptoms found in patients exposed to toxic amounts of arsenic when those symptoms arise in the course of disease, but not necessarily during an acute arsenical intoxication. The *HPUS* states that the lowest potency (the closest concentration to the raw material) of metallic arsenic that can be sold OTC is 8X, or its equivalent, 4C. As shown in Table 10-1, the concentration of metallic arsenic in the 8X or 4C product is 10 ng (nanograms) per gram of drug product. This is equal to 10 parts per billion (ppb), which is less than the 50 ppb allowed in drinking water. Table 10-2 lists comparative values for commercially available bottles of aspirin, acetaminophen (Tylenol), and homeopathic metallic arsenic in the most concentrated OTC dosage allowed by the *HPUS*. No homeopathic pharmaceutical firm is actually selling homeopathic metallic arsenic at this concentration. From Table 10-2, it is clear that homeopathic medicines are far safer than these common OTC drugs. Clinical statistics bear this out. In 1995, there were 2 million contacts with Poison Control Centers in the United States. There were 1 million emergency room visits for treatment of poisoning, of which 79,000 were for poisoning from analgesic, antipyretic, and antirheumatic medications.[11] A MedLine search

TABLE 10-2

Comparative Values for Aspirin, Acetaminophen, and Homeopathic Metallic Arsenic

	Aspirin	Acetaminophen	Homeopathic Arsenic
Common dose	325 mg	325 mg	10 ng per g of 8X (theoretical maximum)
Quantity of doses per container	100 tabs	100 tabs	100 g
Quantity of drug per container	32.5 g	32.5 g	1 µg (1/1,000,000 g)
Number of doses needed to produce severe toxicity in a 10-kg child (1-year-old) (200 mg/kg for aspirin or acetaminophen, and 1 mg/kg for homeopathic arsenic)	5 tablets	5 tablets	10,000 g
Number of toxic doses per container for 10-kg child	20	20	0.00001 (1/10,000)
Ratio of toxicity compared to homeopathic arsenic 8X	200,000 times more toxic	200,000 times more toxic	

in June 2000 uncovered no reports of poisoning from a homeopathic medicine in the United States from 1995 to 2000.

The FDA and the homeopathic pharmaceutical industry have worked closely together because of their mutual concern for the proper and safe manufacture and use of homeopathic medicines. One concern that the FDA and the HPUS committee share is that some drug manufacturers of nonhomeopathic products might try to use the HPUS to circumvent the extraordinarily expensive new drug approval channels of the FDA. The HPUS has adopted guidelines for review and acceptance of new medicines submitted to it to ensure that any new medicines are indeed homeopathic medicines and not conventional medications seeking to avoid the proper channels for new drug approvals. The Compliance Policy Guideline published by the FDA in 1988 specifically states that "agency compliance personnel should particularly consider whether the homeopathic drug is being offered for use or promoted significantly beyond recognized or customary practice of homeopathy."[10]

The *HPUS* defines the homeopathic strengths at which each homeopathic medicine may be sold in both prescription and nonprescription channels. The sale of a homeopathic medicine in nonprescription channels is generally allowed only when the chemical concentration of the medicine is so low that it poses a very low risk—even if a small child were to consume the entire contents of the package. The scrupulous concern for the welfare of the general public exhibited by the homeopathic pharmaceutical industry, homeopathic physicians and pharmacists, and the *HPUS* committee, as well as the intrinsically safe nature of homeopathic medicines, have yielded an extraordinary safety record for homeopathic medicines in the past 165 years.

References

1. Hahnemann S: Essay on a new principle for ascertaining the curative powers of drugs, and some examinations of the previous principles, *Hufeland's Journal* 11:391-439, 456-561, 1795.

2. Haehl R: *Samuel Hahnemann: his life and work*, New Delhi, 1985, B Jain (originally published in 1922).

3. Homeopathic Pharmacopoeia Convention of the United States: Criteria for eligibility of drugs for inclusion in the HPUS, *Homeopathic pharmacopoeia of the United States*, Washington DC, 1996, Homeopathic Pharmacopoeia Convention of the United States.

4. Lo Shui-Yin: Anomalous state of ice, *Modern Physics Letters B* 10(19):909-919, 1996.

5. Lo Shui-Yin: Physical properties of water with I_E structures, *Modern Physics Letters B* 10(19):921-930, 1996.

6. Hahnemann S: *Materiamedica pura*, New Delhi, 1995, B Jain (originally published in 1811).

7. Winston J. *A brief history of potentization machines*, Br J Hom 78(2):59-68, 1989.

8. Coulter HL: *Divided legacy: the conflict between homeopathy and the American Medical Association, Science and Ethics in American Medicine 1800-1910*, Berkeley, Calif., 1982, North Atlantic Books.

9. Middleton R: Regulation of the homeopathic industry, *CJHP* 5(12):8, 1993.

10. Food and Drug Administration: Compliance Policy Guideline 7132.15 (5/13/88), *Conditions under which homeopathic drugs may be marketed*, Washington, DC, 1988, Food and Drug Administration.

11. McCaig LF, Burt CW: Poisoning-related visits to emergency departments in the United States, 1993-1996. *J Toxicol Clin Toxicol* 37(7):817-826, 1999.

Suggested Readings

Kayne S: *Homeopathic pharmacy—an introduction & handbook*, Edinburgh, 1997, Churchill Livingstone.

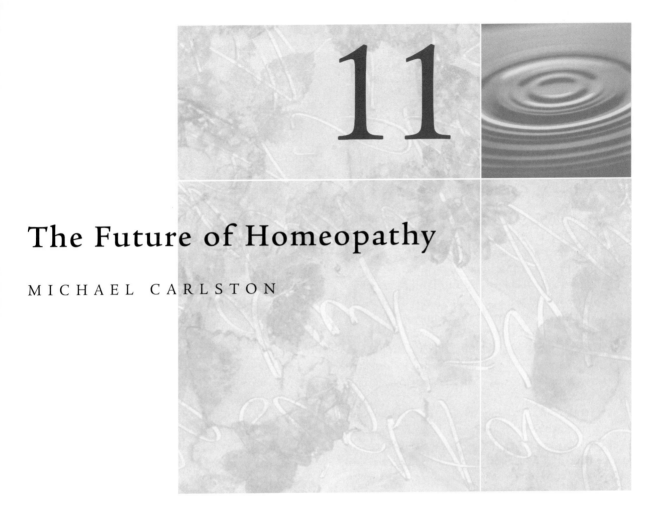

The Future of Homeopathy

MICHAEL CARLSTON

Most physicians believe that the theories of homeopathy are so contrary to conventionally accepted scientific principles that they simply must be false. Some research suggests otherwise. If favorable results continue to accrue in clinical homeopathic research, attention will focus on basic science investigations to help us understand how homeopathy works. If basic science research eventually provides sound explanations for the clinical effects of homeopathy, the implications will be remarkable. This scenario, however, is a collection of *ifs*—not an inevitability. Furthermore, establishing such a formidable base of evidence will require a great deal of time. Although more likely than even a few years ago, this still-distant possibility and its repercussions will not be discussed further in this chapter.

What is the ideal role of homeopathy in health care? The consensus answer of conventional physi-

cians has long been a simple, "None." Many in the homeopathic community have argued that conventional medicine is inherently damaging to patients' well-being and should be abandoned. As is usually the case when otherwise rational people assume such extreme and mutually exclusive positions, a middle ground is likely to emerge. Where is this middle ground?

SELF-CARE

Homeopathy's identity as a viable self-care choice was established long ago. On the American frontier in the nineteenth century, conventional physicians were a rarity. Homeopathy was one of the few medical treatments available to a mother forced to provide health care to her family. Conventional medicine of the day was an unwelcome expense and relatively ineffective, or even harmful, by today's standards.

The rapid growth of homeopathy today is largely a result of the influence of the self-care market. Although patients have many health care choices, homeopathy is attractive, because to many it represents a gentler option. Homeopathy seems to be more harmonious with the view shared by many that conventional physicians are too eager to use needlessly strong medicines. This population prefers gentler options such as homeopathy.

The sociologist Paul Ray recently defined a group he called *cultural creatives*.[1,2] This segment of the population is characterized by their values, including environmentalism, feminism, concern about global issues, and the importance of spiritual matters. They are affluent, well educated, and like to explore new cultural experiences. They center their lifestyle choices on health and ecological advocacy. Cultural creatives are a large and expanding segment of the American population (44 million in 1997, per Ray's estimate).[2] In a 1999 survey, 71% of this group reported buying homeopathic remedies.[3]

Patients who treat themselves and their families with homeopathy do so almost exclusively for minor problems. Because the effectiveness of most conventional therapies for minor problems is limited and prone to causing adverse effects, homeopathy may be a better choice. Even if homeopathy is of no benefit, clinical trials and lengthy clinical experience show that it is much less likely to cause adverse effects than over-the-counter products and conventional medicines. Self-care has been an important niche for homeopathy and might be a good role for homeopathy in the future.

WELLNESS/HEALTH PROMOTION AND DISEASE PREVENTION

Homeopathic philosophy defines illness more broadly than conventional medicine. Homeopathic treatment attempts to alleviate many minor dysfunctions that are believed precursors to more serious disease. If homeopathy successfully treats such precursors, homeopathic treatment can both promote health and prevent disease; however, this has not been proven.

The most pervasive belief of homeopathic practitioners and patients is in the importance of minimizing the use of medications. Avoiding adverse effects caused by conventional medicine is, by definition, health-promoting. We know that homeopathic patients do not utterly reject conventional medicine. With a fair degree of certainty, we also know that they almost always choose professional homeopathic care after conventional medicine has failed. It is reasonable to assume that overall, the use of homeopathy currently has a positive effect on health, if only by preventing the adverse effects of needless conventional medication. For example, tracking my prescribing patterns of children with acute otitis media, community prescribing patterns, and research data about antibiotic response, I have been preventing well over 100 needless antibiotic prescriptions a year for this condition. Responsible homeopathic care significantly reduces adverse effects of medication.

Does avoiding the overuse of prescription medication improve community health? One study in New Zealand suggests it does.[4] Investigators studied children attending Waldorf Schools because the students' families generally preferred homeopathic and anthroposophical medicines to conventional medicines, including antibiotics. The investigators compared students who had received antibiotics with those who had not. Controlling for other risk factors, they found that children who received antibiotics in the first year of life were four times more likely to develop asthma than the other children. Children who received antibiotics only after their first birthday were 1.6 times as likely to develop asthma as antibiotic-free children. This single study is inadequate to draw broad conclusions, but other studies suggest the same interpretation.[5-8] To raise an even more controversial topic, another recent study suggests that immunizations may make children more likely to later develop asthma.[9] Medical research is acquiring evidence that shows that getting sick can be good for us. The homeopathic philosophy of minimizing treatment instead of needlessly interfering with the process seems to be congruent with this new understanding. Similarly, the principle of using like to cure like, acting directly along the lines of the body's own response, makes sense and may facilitate the immune system's process of learning.

Although these are the homeopathic ideals, we must recognize that reality can be more complicated. Homeopathic adherents can be tempted by subtle indications and sometimes use homeopathic remedies when no treatment is necessary. I have seen patients take a remedy after slightly bumping a toe and then another a short time later because they sat in an air conditioner draft. Clearly no intervention was needed for either experience. People who use homeopathic remedies in this way simply trade one form of overmedication for another. Because of homeopathy's lower rate of side effects, homeopathic overtreatment may be preferable to allopathic overtreatment, but this misuse subverts some of the benefits of homeopathy.

Does suppression (hampering the body's expression of symptoms and its fight to regain equilibrium) cause harm? Homeopaths believe so. My clinical experience convinces me that it can. Adverse effects from suppressive treatment are subtler or less common than my homeopathic training indicated, but they are evident. Homeopathy is not blameless. Improper use of homeopathy can suppress and injure patients. If homeopathy can stimulate healing, there is no theoretic reason that it could not cause harm.

COST EFFECTIVENESS

There are preliminary data from England and France regarding cost effectiveness of homeopathic treatment. Fisher surveyed patients at the London Homeopathic Hospital and compared the cost of their treatment with that associated with the standard local treatments.[10] He found that homeopathic care significantly reduced expenditures over a 1-year follow-up. General information from the French national health service indicates similar savings.[11]

Homeopathic care saves money by reducing patient expenses for medication. Jacobs and associates found that physician homeopaths used conventional medicine 60% less often than conventional physicians.[12] Swayne documented a similar trend in the United Kingdom.[13] The 100 or so needless antibiotic prescriptions for otitis media that I *do not prescribe* each year may save the patients' families approximately $2000 in medication costs.

Jacobs's survey also documented other practice patterns with the potential to cut costs. Physician homeopaths ordered laboratory tests less than half as often as conventional physicians. Even more dramatic was the difference in the use of other diagnostic services; conventional physician use is nearly five times higher than that of homeopathic physicians.

If patient outcomes are similar, homeopathy should reduce health care costs solely on the basis of reducing use of conventional health care system resources—prescription medications, laboratory and other diagnostic testing. If, as believed by homeopathic practitioners and patients, use of health care services drops following homeopathic treatment, health care costs would further decline.

The number of *ifs* in the preceding paragraph is a good indication of our uncertainty about this issue. The few findings we have are open to alternative interpretations. Because most patients seek professional homeopathic treatment after already trying conventional medical care, conventional physicians may have already completed diagnostic evaluations by the time patients first visit a homeopathic physician. In fact, it may be possible that homeopaths order additional tests, thereby actually increasing diagnostic expenses. Homeopathic remedy selection is almost entirely uninfluenced by conventional laboratory diagnostics, so it is easy to assume that homeopathic care would reduce diagnostic costs. Despite this assumption, we have no firm evidence that a homeopath seeing the same patient at the same stage of diagnostic evaluation would order any more or less testing than a conventional physician.

Another caveat arises when we consider visit costs. Homeopathic physicians on average charge more for each visit than conventional primary care physicians. This is probably a result of the much longer duration of homeopathic visits. This increase tempers our cost-saving optimism. If homeopathic treatment causes patients to use fewer medical services overall, homeopathy could still prove more cost effective in spite of the higher per-visit charge.

There are no published data on the incomes of homeopathic practitioners. However, my informal surveys suggest that the income of an average physician homeopath is roughly half to two thirds that of a primary care physician practicing in the same locale. Although a conventional physician may see three times as many patients and receive only twice the income, is it accurate to say this physician is more cost effective if he or she also orders more tests and prescribes more-expensive medication? At this point it is not possible to draw any conclusions. We can neither advocate nor abandon homeopathy on the basis of cost considerations.

AN EXPANDING ROLE FOR HOMEOPATHY

Just as many cultural creatives choose homeopathy for self-care, they also embrace professional homeopathy for their medical care when the need arises. The stress of serious illness does not transform them into hypocrites. As this group ages and its enthusiasm for all forms of complementary medicine continues to spread to other segments of the population, there will be a rising demand for complementary medicine services, including homeopathy, among hospitalized patients.

Perhaps the area of greatest concern is the interaction of complementary medicines with conventional treatments. Whereas evidence accumulates that some herbs alter human metabolism and thus the action of some prescription medications, there is no evidence that homeopathic medicines do so. Interactions are important when the medications are most necessary and the patients are the sickest. If we continue to gather evidence of homeopathy's effectiveness and the absence of harmful reactions with conventional medications, homeopathy could move to the forefront of the movement of complementary and alternative medicine therapies into hospitals.

It would be misleading to consider cultural creatives as the only group driving the popularity of homeopathy. Ray identifies another group he calls *traditionalists*, or *heartlanders*. This group, which represents 29% of the American population, sustained homeopathy over many decades. Although the growth of homeopathy in the past 15 years has been remarkable, all indications are that it will continue to grow at a significant pace in the coming years.

EDUCATION

Homeopathy has much to offer physicians-in-training. The homeopathic interview teaches respectful and concentrated attention to the patient's problems. The thoroughness of the classical homeopathic interview demands that the practitioner work carefully. This careful process helps lead the physician or other health care practitioner to the correct conventional diagnosis and homeopathic remedy.

All health care providers must learn from our patients if we are to help them. There are far too many unknowns to allow us to stop learning after completing professional training. Homeopathy continues to teach practitioners by forcing us to think a little differently and observe the results of our interventions. By challenging our assumptions, homeopathy helps us learn the best ways to help our patients and challenges our tendency to use a particular treatment just because it is the status quo.

Patients also learn from homeopathy. Gaining a tool to use for minor illnesses when conventional treatments have little to offer can be helpful. Learning about health and self-care techniques is useful. Perhaps most important is the self-empowerment patients experience as they begin to take responsibility for their health in even a limited way. Instead of continuing as passive consumers, they become active participants and often implement other healthful lifestyle habits.

WHAT CAN HOMEOPATHY OFFER?

As a profession, homeopaths often express alternative views about other health practices—from Hahnemann's contrarian advocacy of exercise to questions about long-term effects of antibiotics raised by today's homeopaths. The homeopathic community is not the only group to question orthodox standards, but the consistency with which it has done so has created a dissident identity for homeopathy. This dissident tradition has raised the hackles of conventional physicians for generations.

Criticism can create a beneficial dialog. Even if the orthodox position eventually proves correct, the process of critical examination forces us to apply careful scientific methods and consider alternative explanations. Homeopathy and other forms of alternative medicine ask questions that continually require conventional medicine to define itself and to confirm that correct choices are made. Historically, sometimes these alternative opinions have been proven correct. How many physicians today advocate bloodletting for pneumonia? Against a storm of controversy, homeopaths argued that conventional practice was not only ineffective, but harmful to the weakened patient. There have been many other examples of orthodoxy being proved wrong through the decades; the most recent example is always the most controversial, because it lacks the objectivity that comes only with the passage of time.

In recent decades, conventional medicine's focus has become increasingly technologic. Scientific advances have dramatically changed our lives and in many ways improved our health. The promises of technology are exciting. However, the realities of the adverse repercussions of our advanced technology are disappointing to many.

In an exuberant rush to embrace technology, physicians increasingly rely on it to diagnose and treat our patients. Unfortunately, this reliance appears to have blunted our clinical acumen. Many believe that medicine has become depersonalized as a result and that we must find a better balance between heart and mind. Much to our detriment, the art of listening to the patient has withered, damaging the relationship between patients and physicians. Homeopathy can help us sharpen the clinical skills neglected in recent decades.

Homeopathic values emphasize that the patient's inner being is of paramount importance. Traditionally, this means the patient's mental and emotional functioning are considered more subtle indications of well-being than physical symptoms. Health does not end with the body, and most homeopaths do not believe that disease starts there either. Beginning with Hahnemann, many of the most important homeopaths in history loudly proclaimed the paramount importance of a person's spiritual well-being. Disease and health originate from that most essential core of a human being. Hahnemann wrote:

When man falls ill it is at first only this self-sustaining spirit-like vital force (vital principle) everywhere present in the organism which is untuned by the dynamic influence of the hostile disease agent. It is only this vital force thus untuned which brings about in the organism the disagreeable sensations and abnormal functions that we call disease.[14]

Few conventional physicians disregard the importance of their patients' thoughts and feelings. Medical research continues to demonstrate the impact of emotions on physical illnesses. Similarly, many conventional physicians consider spiritual wellness an important aspect of their patients' health. However, Hahnemann went a step further by formally incorporating this perspective into homeopathy's founding document, thereby institutionalizing the belief.

In addition to the desire to minimize the use of medication, so fundamental to homeopathy, other aspects of homeopathic philosophy offer potential benefit to modern patients and physicians. One such belief is in the importance of the long-term view. Homeopaths believe that homeopathic treatment for chronic conditions takes a long time. Patients are told to expect to feel worse in the first few weeks of treatment but to look for lasting improvement over months. There are many repercussions of an attitude shift that accepts or even extols short-term suffering as a means to achieve long-term relief. Although developing patience is beneficial for many of life's circumstances, it is a great challenge to many patients in this impatient time. Observing the healing process and seeking to work in concert with that clinically visible process, physicians can also learn patience.

In the final analysis, the term *complementary medicine* describes homeopathy quite succinctly. Homeopathy is a counterbalance to orthodox medicine. It brings different qualities to the healing partnership and the health care delivery system. Homeopathy's strengths are conventional medicine's weaknesses, and vice versa. Although the marked difference between conventional medicine and homeopathy can lead to easy rejection of homeopathy, it may just as easily be the very reason homeopathy is so valuable.

References

1. Ray PH, Anderson SR, Anderson R. *The cultural creatives: how 50 million people are changing the world.* New York, 2001, Three Rivers Press.
2. Ray PH. The emerging culture. *American Demographics,* February 1997. Available at www.demographics.com. Accessed April 10, 1998.
3. Food Marketing Institute: *Shopping for health, 1999: the growing self-care movement,* Washington, DC, 1999, Food Marketing Institute.
4. Wickens K, Pearce N, Crane J et al: Antibiotic use in early childhood and the development of asthma, *Clin Exp Allergy* 29(6):766-771, 1999.
5. Droste JH, Wieringa MH, Weyler JJ et al: Does the use of antibiotics in early childhood increase the risk of asthma and allergic disease? *Clin Exp Allergy* 30(11): 1547-1553, 2000.
6. Gemmell CG: Antibiotics and neutrophil function—potential immunomodulating activities, *J Antimicrob Chemother* 31(suppl B):23-33, 1993.
7. von Hertzen LC: Puzzling associations between childhood infections and the later occurrence of asthma and atopy, *Ann Med* 32(6):397-400, 2000.

8. Strachan DP: Family size, infection and atopy: the first decade of the "hygiene hypothesis," *Thorax* 55 (Suppl 1):S2-S10, 2000.

9. Kemp T, Pearce N, Fitzharris P et al: Is infant immunization a risk factor for childhood asthma or allergy? *Epidemiology* 8(6):678-680, 1997.

10. Fisher P: Cost effectiveness of homeopathy, presented at Homeopathic Research Network's Fourth Scientific Symposium, Homeopathic Research Network, Washington, DC, 1998.

11. Boiron T, President and CEO of Boiron USA: Personal communication, November 15, 1998.

12. Jacobs J, Chapman EH, Crothers D: Patient characteristics and practice patterns of physicians using homeopathy, *Arch Fam Med* 7(6):537-540, 1998.

13. Swayne J: The cost and effectiveness of homeopathy, *Br Homeopath J* 81:148-150, 1992.

14. Hahnemann S: *Organon of medicine*, ed 6, Los Angeles, 1982, JP Tarcher.

Suggested Readings

Garrett L: *The coming plague: newly emerging diseases in a world out of balance*, New York, 1994, Penguin Books.

Ray PH, Anderson SR, Anderson R: *The cultural creatives: how 50 million people are changing the world*, New York, 2001, Three Rivers Press.

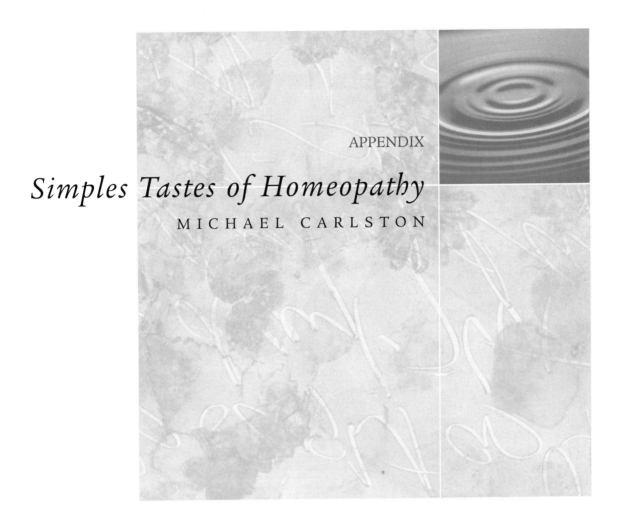

APPENDIX

Simples Tastes of Homeopathy

MICHAEL CARLSTON

Hahnemann used the motto *Aude sapere* ("Dare to taste and understand") in his advocacy of homeopathy. Following Hahnemann's admonition, this appendix provides specific information the reader can use to experience a small dose of homeopathy. The following examples are simplistic and do not reflect the full complexity of classical homeopathic medicine, particularly as it should be applied in chronic conditions. In each instance many other possible remedy selections exist. However, as "tastes" they might whet the reader's appetite for a fuller consideration of clinical homeopathy in more complicated circumstances. Other texts (a good recent example being the series of case conferences published by the International Foundation of Homeopathy in Seattle) provide detailed examples and discussions of the use of classical homeopathy in clinical practice.

In addition, please be advised that these suggestions are not intended to take the place of professional medical care. My assumption is that the reader is a health care professional seeking information to test homeopathy on himself or herself, patients, or family members.

DOSAGE GUIDELINES

Aphthae—Canker Sores

In acute episodes, particularly when the origin is infectious (e.g., herpes stomatitis), **Mercurius vivus** can be useful. These patients usually drool quite a lot, have bad breath, and feel worse during the night.

Croup

There are three homeopathic remedies most commonly used to treat croup. When fear is a defining characteristic, *Aconitum napellus* given hourly is the first choice. If it is not helping after two doses, either *Spongia tosta* or *Hepar sulphuris calcareum* is likely to help. *Hepar* is the better choice if the child is chilly and quite irritable.

Ear Infections—Otitis Media

The sicker the patient, the more rapid the response. A child with a high fever and crying with ear pain should be significantly improved in less than 1.5 hours. Give the medicine (as indicated by pain) from every hour, when the picture is as intense as described above, to once a day, when the child is nearly well and spontaneously complains of momentary ear pain only occasionally. It is quite important to avoid giving the remedy when the patient is symptom free, because given without regard for the patient's clinical improvement, the remedy will cause the patient to become sick again. If no improvement is elicited after two doses of the medicine, change the prescription.

Although the most certain way to end the recurrent cycle of acute otitis media is with the child's chronic medicine, finding that medicine requires a good deal of training. Unlike other chronic complaints, curing the patient of the tendency toward recurrence is often accomplished by the successful homeopathic treatment of a single episode of acute otitis media.

Belladonna. Symptoms are sudden in onset with high fever and much pain, flushed cheeks, and cold feet with hot body during the fever. Problems tend to be on the right side. Patient is bothered by noises and light.

Chamomilla. Very irritable. Capricious mood. Patient wants to be carried around (but nothing satisfies). Often needed when the ear infection occurs during teething.

Hepar sulph. Very chilly and irritable. Ear worse with any touch or cool air. Often associated with sore throats. Ear infection often associated with hard, dry cough (e.g., croup).

Mercurius vivus. Ear infection with very bad breath, sore throats, and drooling. Often worse at night. Can be associated with oral aphthae (e.g., herpes stomatitis).

Pulsatilla. The patient is clingy but sweet. Patient desires attention but demonstrates little (or no) irritability. Ear infection occurs at the end of a cold with thick nasal discharge. Little thirst (otitis probably due in part to dehydration). As slow in onset as the *Belladonna* type is fast. Manifests on the right side. Symptoms of upper respiratory infection include cough that might make the patient retch. Feels better with open air.

Silica. Difficult to prescribe, because the patient and the clinical picture are mild and typically unexpressive. Slowly developing ear infection. Patients are often chilly but have a sweaty head and/or feet. Prominent, swollen glands.

Acute Emotional Distress

Aconitum napellus is indicated for patients in a state of **hysterical fear.** Often useful following a traffic accident or disaster (e.g., earthquake) when the patient is convinced death is imminent. (Also often needed in croup when the child wakes in a similar state of panic.)

Arsenicum album. Fearful like aconite but associated with extreme restlessness. Often needed with food poisoning. Worse from midnight to 2 AM. Very chilly.

Gelsemium is a common homeopathic prescription for **stage fright.** Its characteristic symptoms are familiar to most people—weakness (especially felt in the knees or abdomen) with trembling. This fear state usually comes about in anticipation rather than in response to a frightening event. *Gelsemium* is also often used in acute influenza, because the pattern of symptoms is quite similar—weakness and trembling.

Ignatia amara can be very useful for patients who have recently suffered a significant personal loss. Common symptoms include weeping easily (often the tears will appear at unexpected times), tightness in the throat (globus hystericus), sighing, and myoclonic jerks when falling asleep.

Gastroenteritis

Although homeopathic medicine does not obviate the need for proper rehydration feeding practices, research confirms the experience of two centuries that remedies can assist this process.

Arsenicum album is undoubtedly one of the most common remedies for this variety of problems particularly when food poisoning is the cause. The patient is chilly, restless, and has profuse watery, acrid diarrhea. Nausea can be quite pronounced with ineffectual retching. The patient can be quite weak and is often fearful. Although the pains are burning, warmth (drinks or environmental heat) often makes the patient feel better. They tend to be worse during the night (midnight to 2 AM).

Carbo vegetabilis is for conditions characterized by abdominal distention and eructations with rumbling in the abdomen and nausea. It is as if something is rotting in the digestive tract. Food poisoning often creates a *Carbo vegetabilis* state. Although chilly, patients strongly desire open air and loosening of their clothing.

Phosphorus is very similar to *Arsenicum.* These patients experience profuse watery diarrhea, which can be acrid or even bloody at times. Symptoms come on or are greatly aggravated right after eating. A classic *Phosphorus* symptom is that of digestive upset triggered after drinks warm up in the stomach. An unusual but memorable characteristic (like *Veratrum album*) is simultaneous vomiting and diarrhea. These patients crave cold drinks and salty foods. Like *Arsenicum,* fear is common, particularly when alone, but *Phosphorus* patients are easily reassured and quite pleasant company.

Phosphoricum acidum is much like *Phosphorus,* but these patients are considerably more debilitated and feel weak immediately after an episode of diarrhea. They crave moist fruits.

Podophyllum's hallmark is painless yellow diarrhea at 4 AM. The illness most often comes on after eating fruit in hot weather. Eating often triggers a loose stool.

Mercurius vivus diarrhea is very acrid, creating a good deal of irritation and discomfort, occasionally including rectal spasms. Bad breath is common, and these patients are worse during the night, including profuse night sweats. These patients tend to be very thirsty for cold drinks.

Nux vomica is indicated for stomach pain and indigestion brought on by excess—overwork or overindulgence. These patients are chilly, irritable, and sensitive to noises, lights, and odors. They find their abdominal pains difficult to relieve because of ineffectual retching and rectal urging. They desire spicy foods, cold drinks, and alcohol. Food poisoning can be causative factor.

Sulphur, perhaps the most common homeopathic remedy, inevitably has a role to play in digestive complaints. An irritable, perhaps fearful patient with acrid, excoriating diarrhea that drives him or her out of bed at 5 AM is classic symptom picture. These patients feel hot and dislike warm foods or environments.

Sepia's principal digestive indications are nausea and sensitivity to odors. Homeopaths often use *Sepia* for nausea during pregnancy, in addition to gastroenteritis when the characteristics match.

Veratrum album patients are similar to *Phosphorus* patients but lack their fears. They have copious painless watery diarrhea, sometimes at precisely the same unfortunate moment that they vomit. The vomiting can be painful. They have an unquenchable thirst for cold drinks, which aggravate the vomiting. Patients experience extreme restlessness, particularly reflected in their mental state.

Headaches

Belladonna patients have headaches, often pounding, on the right side with flushed, hot face. Patients are very sensitive to noises and light.

Bryonia alba should be considered when motion markedly intensifies the headache and firm pressure relieves the headache.

Nux vomica is indicated when the headache comes on following a time of overwork or overindulgence (alcohol or food). Often the patient needing this remedy for a headache will suffer from concurrent gastrointestinal distress of some sort.

Injuries

Homeopathic remedies are expected to alleviate discomfort and accelerate healing. As with all other conditions, the remedies are taken as indicated by the severity of the injury (e.g., broken leg: q15min; muscle strain: tid).

For injuries with bruising, think *Arnica montana.* The classic indication for *Arnica* is such sensitivity that the bed feels too hard. For good or ill, *Arnica* is often given routinely for injuries without consideration of more specific features. If it does not help, further consideration regarding the precise quality of the symptoms is necessary.

Bryonia alba is used for sprains or injuries aggravated by motion. The patient wants to hold the area quite still. Symptoms are improved by pressure. Patient is often irritable when spoken to. The patient might bring the image of a hibernating bear to the mind of the physician.

Rhus toxicodendron is indicated for sprains or other injuries that feel better with motion. Symptoms are worse when beginning to move, but are better with continued motion (like a rusty hinge). Also, patients feel better from warmth. (Do not ignore the conventional use of cold to treat acute injuries. Although these patients might feel better immediately with warm applications, like everyone else, cold is still better to treat acute injuries.) These patients are often remarkably restless.

Ruta graveolens can be useful for sprains and stiffness of tendons and injuries to the periosteum. These patients feel bruised and lame in limbs and joints. These patients feel worse in cold and wet conditions and when beginning to move. Like ***Rhus tox,*** they feel better from continued motion, although heat does not make them feel so much better as it does for ***Rhus tox*** patients.

Menstrual Cramps

Although dysmenorrhea is a chronic condition and rightfully the province of a professional homeopathic consultation and constitutional prescription, many patients can gain short-term relief simply with the use of ***Magnesia phosphorica.*** The principal relevant indications for this remedy are cramping pains that respond well to pressure and heat.

Motion Sickness

When the primary symptom is dizziness, treat with ***Cocculus;*** when the primary symptom is nausea, use ***Tabaccum.***

Teething

Sleepless nights caused by teething may be the most common and powerful inducement for parents of young children to try homeopathy. Although the popular over-the-counter homeopathic combinations for teething have earned a following, selecting the precisely indicated remedy should generate the most optimal response.

Chamomilla is the homeopathic teeth remedy *par excellence.* The indications are the same regardless of the diagnosis for which it is used (see also Ear Infections). The child is restless, changeable, and quite irritable. He or she wants to be carried but then wants to get back down, only to demand to get picked up again. When you give the favorite toy for which the child has been crying, he or she throws it across the room. This is ***Chamomilla.*** The child often experiences diarrhea that appears like chopped spinach (a sign of gastrointestinal distress).

Calcarea phosphorica can be useful for teething when the child is not so irritable as ***Chamomilla.*** These children spit up a great deal, and the vomitus is often sour smelling.

Urinary Retention in Newborns

Aconitum napellus. Crush 2 pills between two spoons and administer once by sprinkling into the newborn's mouth. ***Aconite***'s apparent success in these cases suggests that fright induced by the birthing process could be the cause of the urinary retention. This is not too surprising, given the nature of the event.

THINGS TO KNOW

Administration

Because the sense of taste can interfere with the action of homeopathic medicine, patients should not taste food or toothpaste when they take the homeopathic remedy, nor should they smell strong odors in the room. The patient should not touch the remedy. Using the bottlecap or a clean metal spoon is customary. Some manufacturers have designed their bottles specifically to allow easy administration of any desired number of pellets. The patient should allow the remedy to dissolve under the tongue and then wait a minimum of 15 minutes before eating or drinking anything other than water. The remedies must be stored carefully, away from heat (over 110° F) and sunlight. As with any medicinal substance, keeping homeopathic remedies out of the reach of inquisitive children is always a good idea.

Dosages

Potency issues are complicated and controversial. The simplest course is probably to use 12C, 30C, or 30X potencies to limit the frequency of repetition and to eliminate any possibility of adverse effects from the crude source material. A few guiding principles will assist you:

1. Always administer homeopathic remedies with an eye on the patient. Adjust potency and dosage regimen accordingly. The frequency of doses is determined by the severity of the illness or injury and the patient's response.
2. Potency is based upon the following factors:
   a) Availability: The correct remedy will work regardless of potency, although the frequency of administration may need alteration.
   b) Prescription certainty/remedy fit: A remedy that is an excellent fit will create a healing response in the patient in an extremely dilute/potentized dosage. A mediocre fit requires a more physiologic dose.
   c) Physicality: Many homeopaths believe that mental and emotional problems (e.g., anxiety or depressive states) require higher potencies (e.g., 1M, 200C) to be effective.

3. Dosage regimen
   a) As a *very* crude measure (for a problem of average severity), use one of the following doses: 30C three times/day; 12C (30X) four times/day; or 6C (12X) four to five times/day.
   b) Wean treatment as symptoms abate.
   c) Two to five pills is an adequate dosage for anyone, infant or adult.

Response

The speed of the patient's response to treatment is proportional to the speed and intensity of the illness. Aphthous sores that developed during illness go away over days (the pain should dissipate in hours), whereas a teething child will be better, either sleeping or in a significantly improved mood, in 5 to 30 minutes.

Suggested Readings

Cummings S, Ullman D: *Everybody's guides to homeopathic medicine,* Los Angeles, 1997, Tarcher.

Hering C: *The homeopathic domestic physician,* ed 14(Am), New Delhi, 1984: Jain Publishing (reprint)(original 1835).

Leckridge B: *Homeopathy in primary care,* Edinburgh, 1997, Churchill Livingstone.

Jonas W, Jacobs J: *Healing with homeopathy,* New York, 1996, Warner Books.

Ullman R Reichenberg-Ullman: *The patient's guide to homeopahtic medicine,* Edmonds, Wash., 1995, Picnic Point Press.

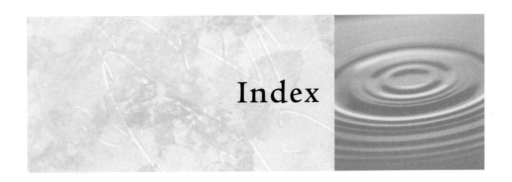

Index

Page numbers followed by f indicate figures; t, tables; b, boxes.